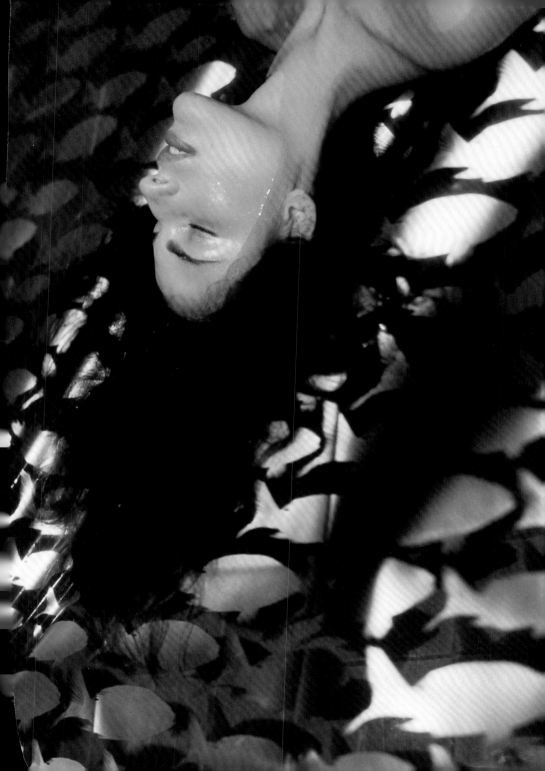

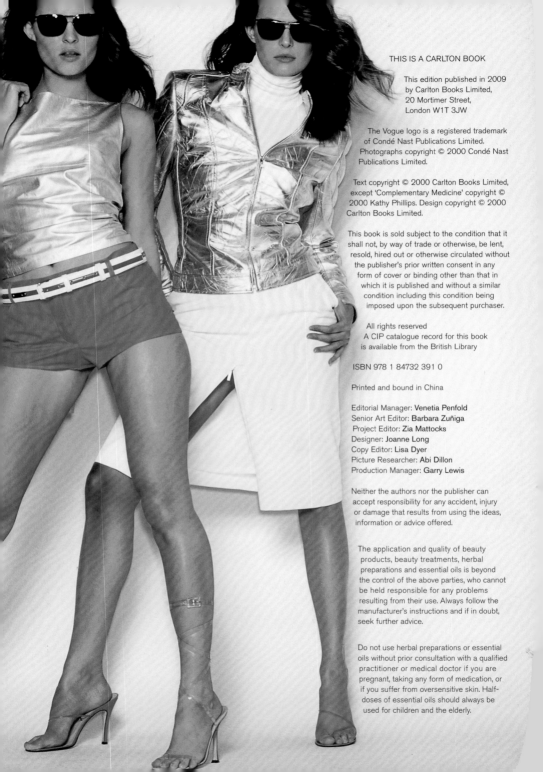

THIS IS A CARLTON BOOK

This edition published in 2009
by Carlton Books Limited,
20 Mortimer Street,
London W1T 3JW

ISBN 978 1 84732 391 0

Printed and bound in China

Editorial Manager: Venetia Penfold
Senior Art Editor: Barbara Zuñiga
Project Editor: Zia Mattocks
Designer: Joanne Long
Copy Editor: Lisa Dyer
Picture Researcher: Abi Dillon
Production Manager: Garry Lewis

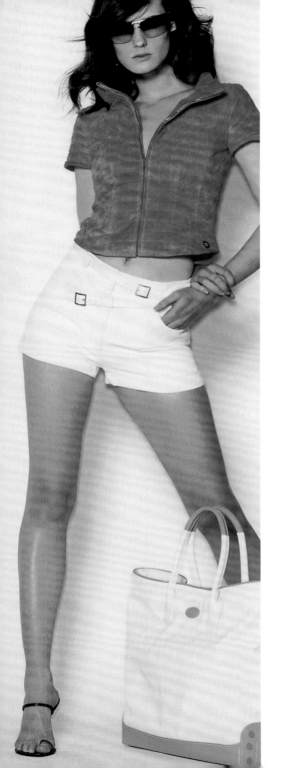

°VOGUE
beauty

bronwyn cosgrave

juliet cohen

rachel marlowe

kathy phillips

lizzie radford

CARLTON
BOOKS

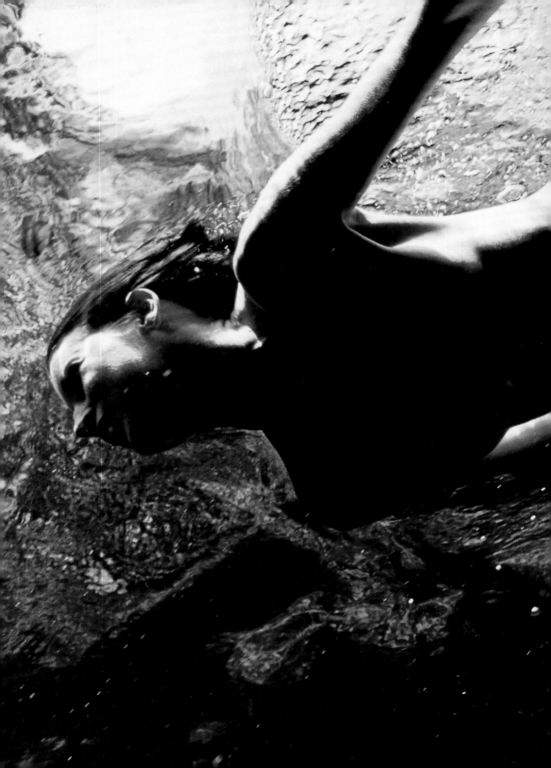

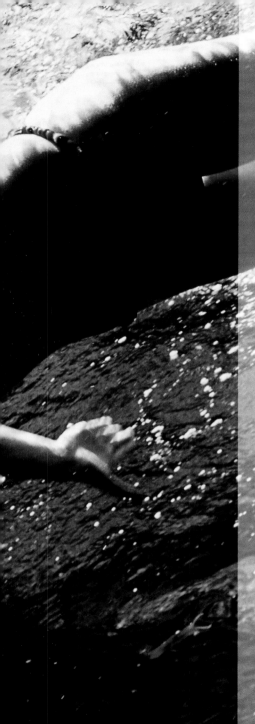

contents

Foreword   6
Kathy Phillips

What is Beauty?   8
Lizzie Radford

Beauty & Fashion   16
Lizzie Radford

1 The Body   38
Bronwyn Cosgrave

2 Skincare   88
Rachel Marlowe

3 Hair   166
Lizzie Radford

4 Make-up   212
Juliet Cohen

5 Scent   276
Lizzie Radford

6 Complementary Medicine   324
Kathy Phillips
with additional research Vikki Berg

Directory   388
Index   398
Acknowledgements   400

foreword

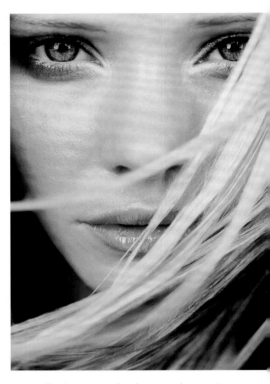

How you look matters. Not in a petty, superficial way, but because how you look reflects how you feel, and how you feel affects how you perform in all areas of your life. Strike it lucky in the gene pool and you can be good-looking, but with effort and intelligence you can be beautiful from the inside out. The *Vogue* woman is a mirror of her time, and *Vogue Beauty* reflects and celebrates the changing moods, attitudes and aspirations of society at the highest level. *Vogue Beauty* is a compilation of the latest research, information and professional opinion on the way we want to be beautiful now and how to achieve it. Its credo is style, quality and specialization.

Being beautiful is hard work. The high-maintenance woman, as she's been christened, is someone who has slotted all she needs to do into her daily routine and eliminated the junk. It's in with regular exercise, relaxation and good breathing, and out with unnecessary stress, as well as a whole list of unsuitable food and drink. In with an intelligent skincare routine and

out with heavy, caked-on make-up in favour of iridescent foundations and cunning concealers that take seconds to apply. In with pampering and indulgences that are mood-enhancing, and out with time-consuming treatments that are ineffective.

Beauty today is a body that is healthy, strong and energetic, skin that is radiant, hair that shines and bounces, good teeth, bright eyes and manicured hands and feet. But it is also about giving in to extravagances – mood-lifting treats that have a profound effect on everyone around you. For instance, scientists have proved that women who spray themselves with scent twice a day have improved moods and less anxiety and fatigue.

In *Vogue Beauty*, Lizzie Radford puts the perfume world into perspective, showing how your choice of scent accents your individuality and leaves a lingering presence; Rachel Marlowe steers you through the minefield that is skincare today and also attacks the burning issues of cosmetic surgery. Should today's woman go under the knife, opt for enhancement via toxins which freeze the muscles, galvanic currents which exercise them, lasers which eradicate lines, or choose collagen which plumps up the face? Bronwyn Cosgrave discusses the body positive, self-image, diet and exercise, and offers a holistic attitude as the path to perfection. My own particular contribution to this book is the chapter focusing on complementary medicine, because I believe that alternative therapies and cultures are showing us new frontiers to better health and greater longevity. Conventional medicine has not proved to have been effective in many areas of health. Preventative medicine offers a whole new arena of potential for women who want to feel, look and be their best selves. Lizzie Radford also cuts into the world of hair and dissects what makes a good-hair day. This chapter is all about the best crops and the subtlest colours — everything you need to know before you let your hair down. Of course, the book would not be complete without its creative intuition. For those who simply want to know all the very latest ways of applying make-up, Juliet Cohen has insider information from the cosmetics counter and from international make-up artists so that she can suggest with confidence which products and techniques you really cannot live without.

WHAT IS BEAUTY?

A modern beauty cannot be defined by her anatomically perfect proportions. In fact, she cannot be defined at all. Nor can she be stereotyped, pigeonholed or labelled any longer. This is the reason why today's ideas about beauty are new and different from ever before. Just as we all know beauty when we see it — we love it and want a piece of it — it just disappears into thin air when we try to define it. Beauty holds within it an allure, a charm, as well as considerable power, but it can also be elusive, frustrating and easily dissipated. The quaint old-fashioned notion of beauty as a gift from the gods, or a happy accident of birth, a combination of perfect measurements and fairy-tale colouring, is exactly that: quaint and archaic. It belongs to an era when beauty was a blessing endowed upon only a lucky few, and which faded once the first flush of youth had passed.

Modern beauty is a world away. Today it is about gloss, polish, vitality and style. It is a rich and varied picture — full of every exotic ethnicity, every skin colour, hair type and age. In fact, if we struggle to label today's version of beauty, we could say it is about individuality. If you flick through the pages of *Vogue*, you will see that there is no longer just one look to strive for, one icon to emulate or one fashion to follow. Beauty is as diverse, individual and idiosyncratic as the women we see around us. What matters now, and where the talent of the modern beauty lies, is to learn how to make the right choices, to make the most of your looks and to find time for yourself while you are at it.

This seismic change in attitude that enabled the world of beauty to become more accessible, obtainable and democratic has technology to thank. In this postmodern era, beauty has an international ground-breaking industry behind it. Where once women were indulged by cosmetic companies, only to be ticked off by dermatologists, now the genuine results and facts about products are available for us to see for ourselves. Today, the research and development departments of major cosmetic companies are the places to be. This is where exact sheets of human skin are grown in

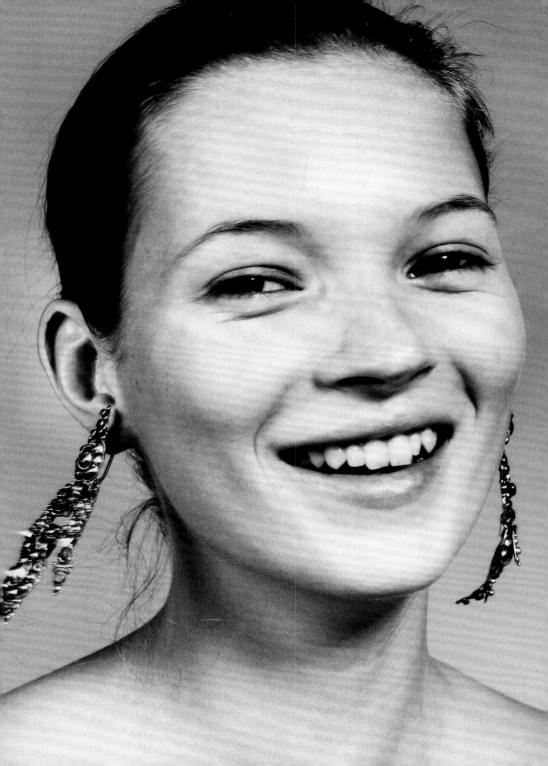

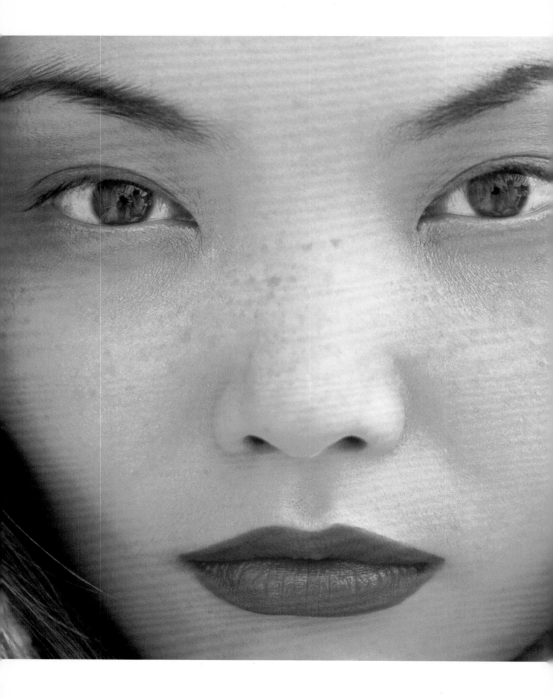

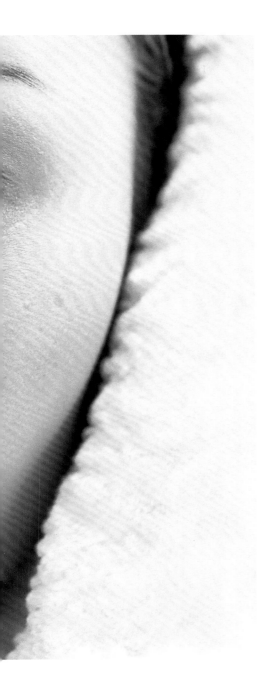

labs, where skin creams are designed that affect our mood and where fragrance molecules are created that can actually whiten the skin through inhalation (I promise, it's really true).

In fact, in the beauty industry today, almost anything is possible. Real progress has been made in antiageing, and it is not just in skincare – there is antiageing haircare and bodycare, too. We can prevent environmental skin ageing, which is 80 per cent of all skin ageing. We can remove body hair, birthmarks and scars permanently and safely, tan year round without sun damage, change the shape of our bodies, the colour of our eyes, our teeth and hair – all while appearing entirely natural. In fact, there is almost nothing that a woman, in search of her own style of beauty, cannot do to enhance her image.

According to make-up maestro Vincent Longo, the future of beauty has never looked so good. 'We have freedom of style now. There are so many different looks that women can tap into, as well as classic looks from the 1940s, 1950s and 1960s that they can revisit and modernize. The technology is amazing. Powders and foundations used to be difficult to blend and only the professionals knew how to use them, but now the quality of make-up is so good that you can apply it with your fingers and still look great. There are so many timeless beauty looks – the red lip, the pale lip or lip stains, the "no-make-up look", the "heavy make-up look", and so many different beauty icons – Jackie O, Mia Farrow, Audrey Hepburn, Diana, Cher, Gwyneth and so on. But it doesn't really matter which you choose. Modern beauty is really about enhancing your own features and looking pretty and approachable.'

But what are the new beauty rules now? If female individuality is celebrated on the catwalks of London, New York, Milan and Paris, and in the pages of glossy magazines, how are we to choose what to do, how to do it and to know if we are doing it correctly? The short and simple answer has to be that if it makes you feel good, then it must be right. The reason why the pursuit of beauty must feel right, and why fun and pleasure are vital to getting a look together, is that beauty really does come from within. If you are not having fun any more, then you are not doing it right. That may sound strange, with cosmetic tech-nology now such an advanced industry and those age-old barriers to beauty largely broken down, but no matter how perfect the make-up or how awe-inspir-ingly toned the body, if you are not achieving pleasure and enjoying yourself, then you are not getting the full benefit of what beauty can do for you.

Beauty should be about pleasure, not pain. It should be about fulfilling your potential, expressing your individuality and taking time for yourself. As scien-tists have found, when we enjoy our lives, our self-esteem improves, which in turn enhances our immunity and resistance to disease. French cosmetic giants Christian Dior, Chanel and L'Oréal teamed with the Centre Nationale de Recherche (CNRS) at Lyon University to research into the positive effects that pleasure gained from using beauty products has on health. The thesis was based on the idea that just as we all experience negative stress, so we can also experi-ence positive stress, which results from such experiences as being in love, eating wonderful food and, apparently, from using beauty products. We are not talking about the efficacy of

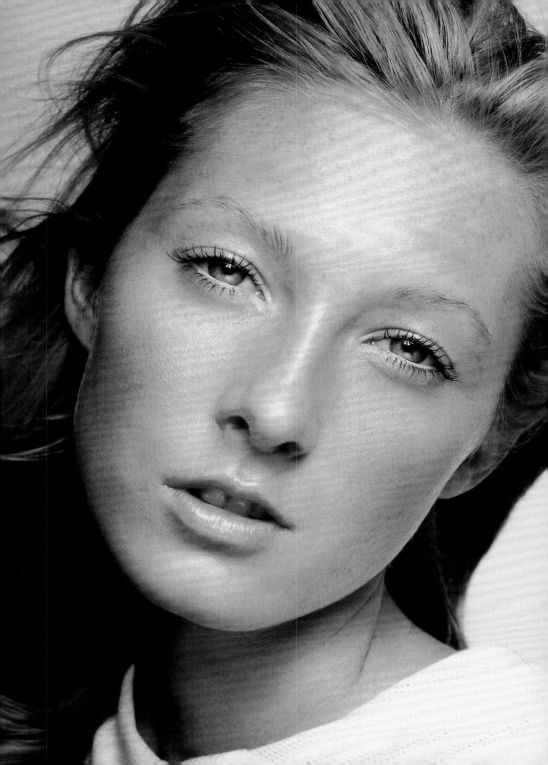

the products — whether they diminish wrinkles, plump up features or banish cellulite. We are talking about the wonderful fun of buying something deliciously naughty, running home with it and ripping open the shiny cellophane to reveal, for example, a box of the most beautiful, sweet-scented, glistening bath salts. Imagine: you turn on the bath, sprinkle the salts on top of the swirling water and watch as your daily bath turns into a flight from reality. Perhaps you are in a bougainvillea-clad Oriental spa, a steamy, scented Moroccan hammam or a big marble bathroom in a Parisian hotel — whatever; you get the message. You are transported to somewhere relaxing, your heart rate slows down, stress levels drop, you feel like a nicer person and — would you believe it? — you are starting to look more beautiful already.

Session hairstylist Guido Palau is one of the gurus of modern beauty. A hairdresser who works with designers and models to push back the boundaries, he experiments with what is regarded as acceptable and he always brings out the rare beauty in every woman he touches. 'There are now so many different types of beauty that we never had before. For example, models as different as Kate Moss and Karen Elson could only have happened now, when the rules about what's pretty or beautiful have liberated women. Generally, women today are more confident about beauty and are not being dictated to in the way that they were in the 1970s and 1980s.

'That's not to say that they are always satisfied with how they look, but they are more clever about beauty now and are more discerning about what's on offer. A beautiful woman today is a woman who is at ease with herself, not a woman who looks tortured by her beauty routine — too squeezed, too manicured or too artificial. In the 1980s looking great was a status symbol. It showed that you had the time and money to spend on yourself. But today the trend is towards getting the basics right and making it look very simple and natural. A woman may choose to have every beauty treatment, but she sure doesn't want to look like she has. Now she wants shiny, glossy hair, beautifully coloured and in the best condition possible, but she wants to tie it up herself and keep the look chic and simple.'

Dominique Szabo agrees. The senior vice president of global lifestyles and trends at Estée Lauder in New York, Szabo was the innovator behind Guerlain's Meteorites and Terracotta ranges and is an acknowledged visionary in her field. 'Modern beauty now is about finding balance. And having a good quality of life. The idea of classic beauty is fading; it is too perfect and women are tired of fantasy. They want what is real, clean and natural. You can see it instantly when you meet a woman. If she is at peace with herself, if she is real, healthy and balanced, then it just shines through and she is really beautiful. But it's the role that beauty will play in helping women to find their balance that is very interesting right now. Already we are seeing the birth of "intelligent" beauty products that are capable of either relaxing or energizing us, depending on what we need at the time we use them. And then there is this surge of interest in yoga, Pilates and t'ai chi – forms of exercise that build up strength and stamina, but also keep us centred and peaceful. Modern skincare, make-up and suntan technology is so sophisticated now that it is working on a deeper level to improve our looks. We are using antioxidants in skincare to improve the health of the skin, skincare benefits in make-up, and anti-skin-cancer technology in suntan products. These may make us beautiful on the outside but they are working on the inside, too.'

It was Estée Lauder who said in the 1960s, 'You wouldn't wear the same dress out in the evening as you would to play tennis. So why should you wear the same perfume?' She was right, and way ahead of her time. Today women's lives are so varied and our roles so diverse that it is difficult to imagine one style, let alone one make-up look, hairstyle or scent, fitting in with everything we have to do and every role we play. Women can become corporate executives in their twenties, first-time mothers in their forties and are constantly breaking the boundaries in their professions. Learning to dress the part and look and feel great is becoming a skill in itself. But we are lucky. We have the freedom to choose our own style; we have technology at our fingertips; and we know that in indulging ourselves we are really improving our health and well-being. I think that sounds like a very promising start.

BEAUTY & FASHION

Fashion is cyclical. Like economics and the weather, it is in perpetual motion, hitting new highs and lows almost daily. The relationship between beauty and fashion is intrinsic. It always has been. When Cecil Beaton, Horst P Horst and Irving Penn began photographing beautiful young models for the pages of *Vogue* in the 1950s, they knew instinctively that the look of elegance, refinement and chic they were after was not going to come from the clothes alone. The models were chosen for their elegant lines; they were not painfully thin, nor were they overtly sexual. Hair was always discreet and never daring enough to upstage the clothes. Make-up was artfully painted: the lips and nails rich and glossy, the complexion pale and powdered and the eyes carefully defined. Imagine those models in the same clothes, but with the hair and make-up of another era — perhaps with flat, matt panstick, Biba blackberry lips and huge painted eyelashes, or even extreme 1980s punk make-up. Would it have worked? Of course not. Hair, make-up and the line, curvature and attitude of the body are extensions of the designer's message.

Photographers, stylists, session hairdressers, make-up artists and models know this. Twice a year, year in and year out, the new fashion collections pound down the runways of New York, London, Paris and Milan. The clothes change, the mood alters and so does the hair and make-up. By now, we have probably seen it all, though perhaps not in every combination. The hair has been big, bold, flat, flicked, frizzed, curled and crimped. It has been short, even shorter and extra long with synthetic hair extensions. Make-up has swung from minimal to maximal; one season the girls look slutty with mussed-up mascara, the next they are paragons of suburban chic, with pussycat bows and the hair and make-up of 1950s Avon ladies. But without the free reign of the catwalk or magazine shoots, designers would never be able to let their creativity rip, raise a few eyebrows and, ultimately, influence how we want to look.

Where fashion leads the way, we follow — like it or not. The choice of clothes, shoes and make-up available is decided by shop buyers, who in turn are influenced

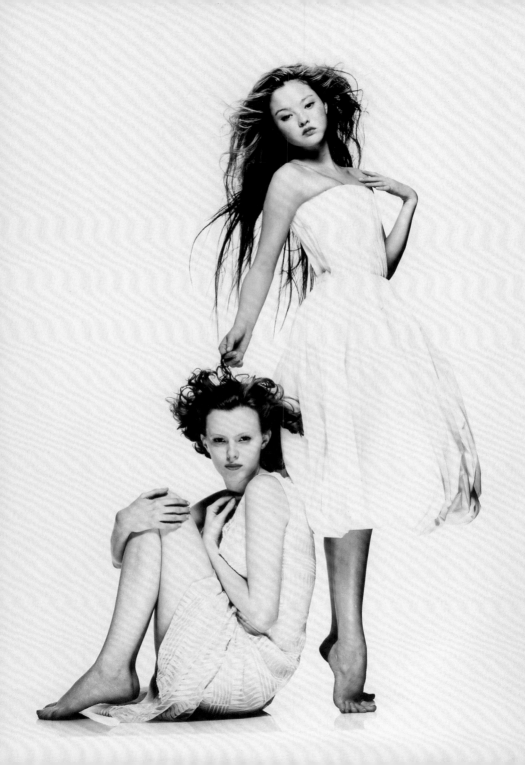

by international trends. But even when we think we are neatly side-stepping the fashion issues, and are instead dressing for work, religious occasions or camping holidays, we are making instinctive and subtle beauty choices. There are very few beauty rules today, but there are some, and they are all about beauty's relationship to clothes and fashion. For example, you would be pushing your luck to turn up for the evening in a John Galliano creation, wearing the same ponytail and fresh face that you had worn on the tennis court. Beauty may put the seal on the designers' vision, but we are still allowed room for our own creativity. No matter how strict the dictates, we all know how to buck a trend and adapt a look to suit our own face, figure and pocket, or at least we should. Following fashion to the letter may be fun, but it is only for the fearless. What is in one moment may be out the next; what is up will be down; what is black will be white; and what you may kill for one season, you would not be seen dead in the next. If you can anticipate the trends and know how to handle the curve balls, you will be better able to take control of a look and develop your own sense of style. But that only comes with perspective, so read on.

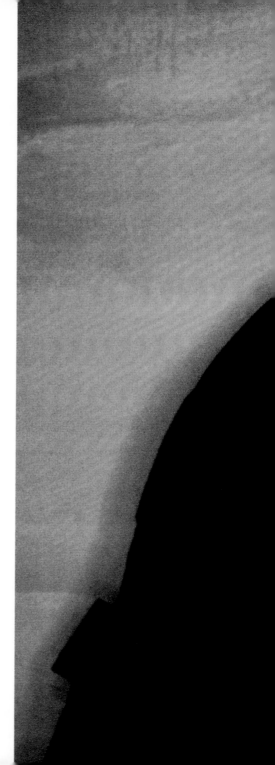

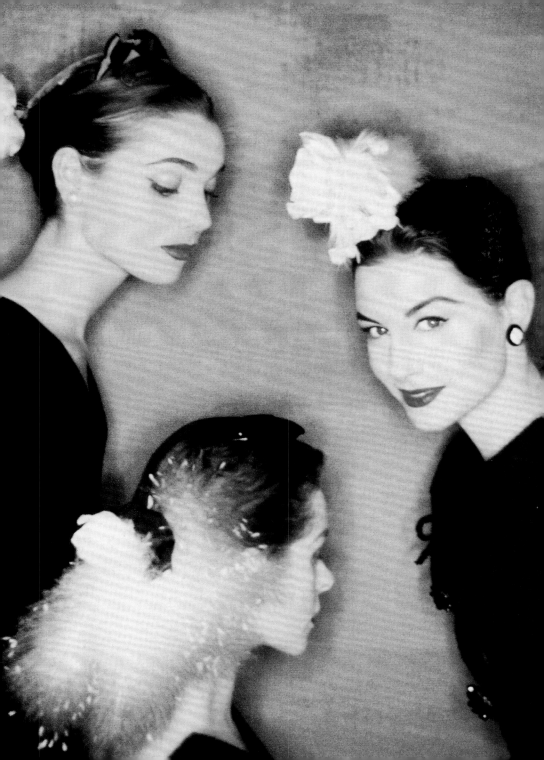

the 1950s

After years of wartime austerity, women craved to assert their femininity once again, so glamour and elegance became the trademarks of the decade. Immediately after the Second World War, fashion was still in the grip of a financial downslide. In Britain, unnecessary luxury was seen as unpatriotic and wasteful, and fabric was in short supply. During the war years, women worked in factories and on the land and left their children while they went out to work, but in the 1950s the roles reversed again. In the USA more than 50 per cent of female university students dropped out to marry and have children. The decade was destined to be one of propriety, traditional values and womanliness.

Christian Dior challenged all that. His New Look flagrantly emphasized a woman's best assets — her bust, waist and hips — with his lavish use of fabric, visible curves and restrained sexuality. He used longer, wider, fuller skirts, nipped-in waists and shapely jackets to create the new feminine line. Underwear was another important change to the silhouette. The bust, cleavage and waist were sculpted and displayed as the new erogenous zones. The new corsets were a triumph of artifice, as figures were 'perfected'. Marilyn Monroe, Jane Russell and Diana Dors all epitomized the look. The idea of 'perfecting' women was a major ethos behind the beauties of the day; this was not a live-and-let-live, let-it-all-hang-out decade. There were rules and you had to follow them. Anita Colby was a 1950s stylemaker who groomed aspiring young actresses into Hollywood stars. She sums up the attitude of the day in her 'four-week beauty and charm course': 'Measure yourself against the most popular girl in the school, or in the elevator operator's eyes … if your first impression is one of bulk, awkwardness, bad grooming, you may never make a second impression on the man you want in your life.' But she was not alone. Beauty was seen as a powerful tool to entrap or keep a man, and a woman had to know how to use it. Make-up was seen as 'corrective'. Often two shades of foundation were worn to create contours that would give the impression of the 'perfect' oval face shape. Likewise, lips were painted or drawn to conceal faults; tricks were used to paint the corners of the mouth upwards to make a woman look as if she was permanently smiling or to paint inside the lip edge to 'keep a dainty mouth'. And it was vitally important to 'know your type'. Each woman fitted neatly into a category: the cool blonde, the warm blonde, the cool brunette, the warm brunette, the cool redhead and the warm redhead. Make-up colours were available to 'correct' and 'perfect' each type. False eyelashes emphasized the feminine look and black liquid eyeliner, dark shadow and black, block mascara were staples. The flip side of the coin was the Audrey Hepburn look. Elegant and beautiful though she was, Audrey Hepburn was not playing for major sex stakes. She represented the gamine, youthful woman seen during the war. She was free-spirited, outspoken and did not have to play by the rules — beauty or otherwise.

Hair was roller-set, backcombed and sprayed. In fact, hairspray was the only widely available hair product. Girls

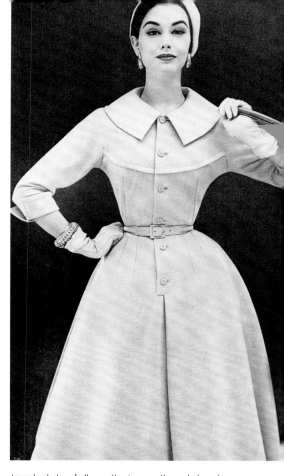

tended to follow their mothers' leads when it came to beauty regimes — going to the same hairdresser and wearing the same scent. But things were changing. On a visit to Rome in the early part of the decade, Audrey Withers, the then editor of British *Vogue*, was astounded to see Italian women wearing bare, brown legs and thong sandals — a look that is still popular today. The mood was set for the future.

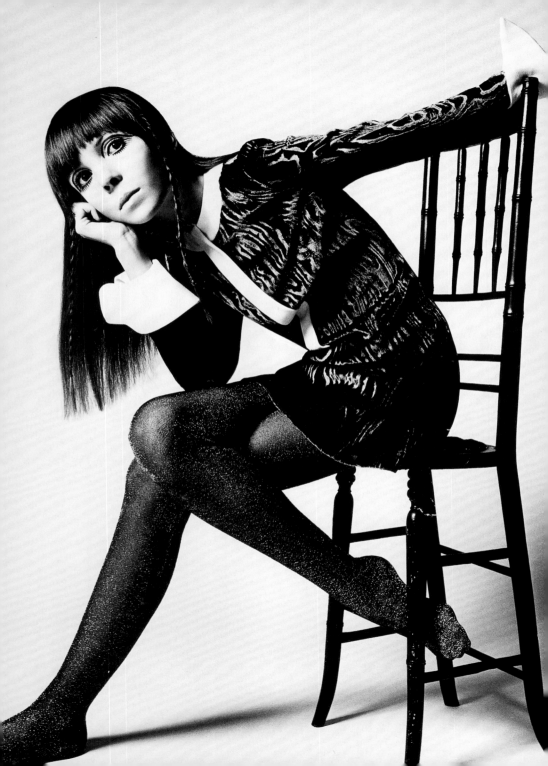

the 1960s

Liberation and defiance, in every sense, were the hallmarks of the 1960s. For the first time, fashion became democratic and young women were buying fun and fashionable clothes from both chain stores and incense-filled designer boutiques. Women craved whatever was decreed fashionable. Despite the apparent liberation from social and sexual norms, this was not a decade about individuality. Women were not being encouraged to break free and find themselves, but instead were moving from the traditional female role into a clearly defined psychedelic *belle époque*. The shock of the new was what counted most and clothes were worn as a badge of identity, a sign that you were modern, mobile and had arrived. You no longer had to use your mother's dressmaker to run up a new dress, or even seek her approval (no doubt she would not have approved). Quality and durability were no longer important when it came to clothes; novelty was paramount. Consumerism had taken hold. The reason why youth culture, fashion and music exploded during these years is that the post-war baby boom had come of age. Many of them were working and had a desire fuelled by income.

The sexual revolution had the greatest impact on women. For the first time in history, women could control their fertility, and so plan their futures and careers. No longer did they want to wear the structured clothes of the 1950s; instead they wanted freedom of movement, ease and shock value. As a result, underwear changed radically, and with it the shape of the female body. Girdles, corsets, stockings and suspenders were out. In came no-bra bras, tights and pretty little panties, which were often dotted with rosebuds and flowers because they would be visible when wearing a miniskirt.

Hair is often the most blatant social and political barometer, and it certainly was in the 1960s. According to John Frieda, who, alongside Trevor Sorbie and Vidal Sassoon, was changing the face of hairdressing at the time, 'When society loosened up, so did hair. Suddenly that rigid, "set" hair of the 1950s became much freer and women started to grow their hair long, wear it loose and natural. This was also the era of the "cut and blow-dry" and, of course, the Sassoon bob — an easy, no-fuss look that women could manage at home.' Wigs also came into their own, allowing women to change their look instantly, from gamine to space girl to romantic. Women may not have looked sophisti-

cated, but they were new, different and in control of their look.

Brigitte Bardot and Twiggy were the real beauty icons of the decade. Of course, their looks were poles apart: Bardot was overtly sexual and pouty, while Twiggy was almost childlike and naïve. Almost every woman tried to choose an element from one of them and run with the trend. Make-up was the final, vital, finishing touch to getting the look just right. No more borrowing mother's block mascara; young women now had their own trendy products and used them extravagantly. Eyes became the major focus of the face. Cosmetic companies like Max Factor developed new ranges of false eyelashes, liquid eyeliner, cake eyeliner, waterproof mascara and eyeshadow sticks — all for the first time. British make-up artist Barbara Daly remembers the look as being 'highly decorated': 'We painted a black socket line on the eyes, painted eyelashes on and wore a lot of blue and white eyeshadow.' Lipstick was also taken to the limit. Girls wore either white, pale pink, dark plum or bright orange. Pretty? Maybe. Sexy? Perhaps. Extreme? Definitely.

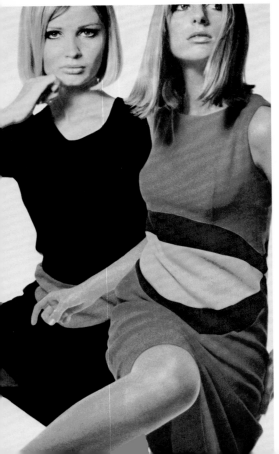

the 1970s

After a decade of optimism, and a feeling of community among the world's youth, the 1960s reached a stalemate. By the late 1960s and early 1970s worldwide economic and political misery was setting in. British sterling had been devalued in 1967 and cutbacks were biting hard; both Martin Luther King Jr and Robert Kennedy had been recently assassinated, the war raged in Vietnam and students were protesting in the streets of Paris. There was an international oil crisis and Italy was in the grip of her own terrorists, the Red Brigade. All this turmoil led the disillusioned youth to seek an 'alternative' society. Social conventions really broke down this time. Drugs, free love and sex were big news. Self-expression and inner freedom became a kind of Holy Grail. People wanted to feel close to nature again. They wanted peace and they wanted freedom from rules and social convention. Stylewise, the 1970s will always be known as the decade of the hippie. Even though not everyone espoused the hippie ideals, the look filtered down and influenced everyone's wardrobe

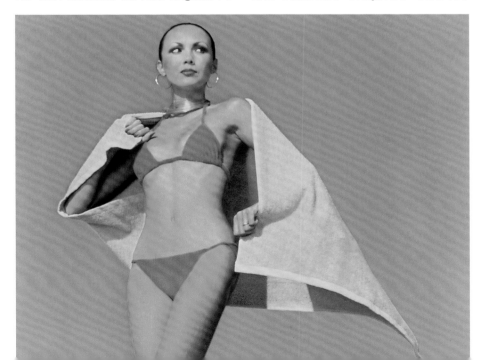

and beauty routine (or non-routine, as the case may have been). Hair grew longer, for men and women, men grew beards again for the first time since the Victorians and even female body hair became, almost, acceptable. As formality began to slide, clothes became more relaxed. Anything handmade or home-grown was adopted by the hippies, who loved embroidery, knitting, tie-dyeing and items that were nostalgic or mystical. The young were constantly searching and, unwittingly, redefining beauty.

As the decade wore on, an important anti-fashion trend was emerging, epitomized by Ralph Lauren, Laura Ashley and the world's apparently insatiable passion for denim. By the late 1970s denim was ubiquitous: men and women, young and old wore it; children and teen-agers wore it; and it came in every guise, from jeans to jackets, dresses, skirts and shirts, bags and hats. Just as fashion was rejected and the catwalk ceased to have relevance to most women, so beauty changed. Women did not want artifice any more; they wanted natural. Health food and vegetarianism became mainstream, and beauty products containing natural ingredients were everywhere. Avocado, lemon, yogurt, strawberry, green apple and wild musk were being used in shampoos, creams and fragrances for the first time. The first American scent to break the hold the French had on perfumery was Revlon's Charlie, launched in 1973. The ultra-modern scent seemed to epitomize a newfound freedom for women in the boardroom and the bedroom.

Clinique, the first offspring of the traditional Estée Lauder brand, was launched. Its approach was entirely new. Women no longer cared so much about superficial make-up, but were passionate about the skin underneath and Clinique's unique three-step skin-care and hypoallergenic products were the answer they craved. Calvin Klein arrived on the scene and declared, 'If you're really interested in clothes, then your body should be in shape.' Hair became wash 'n' wear. Women did not want to look as if they had nothing better to do than spend the morning at the hairdresser. They wanted clean, sexy, easy hair, like Farrah Fawcett, whose flicked-out style radiated good vibes. Health, super-sexiness and super-confidence were what it was all about.

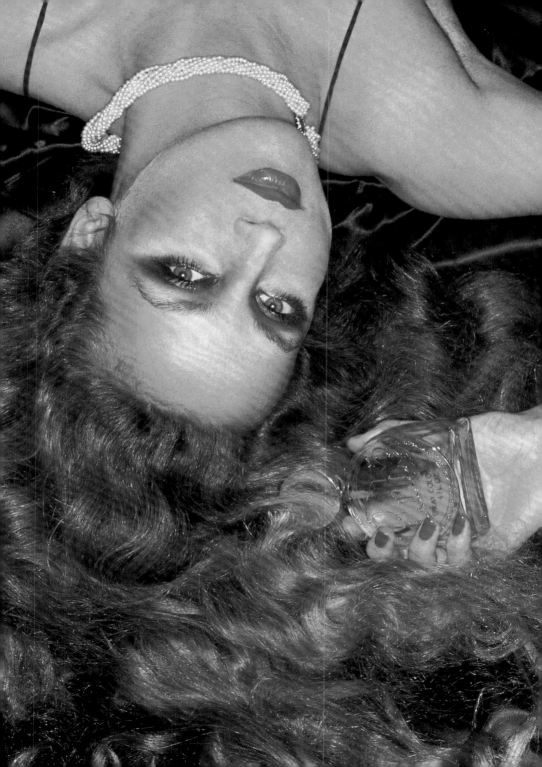

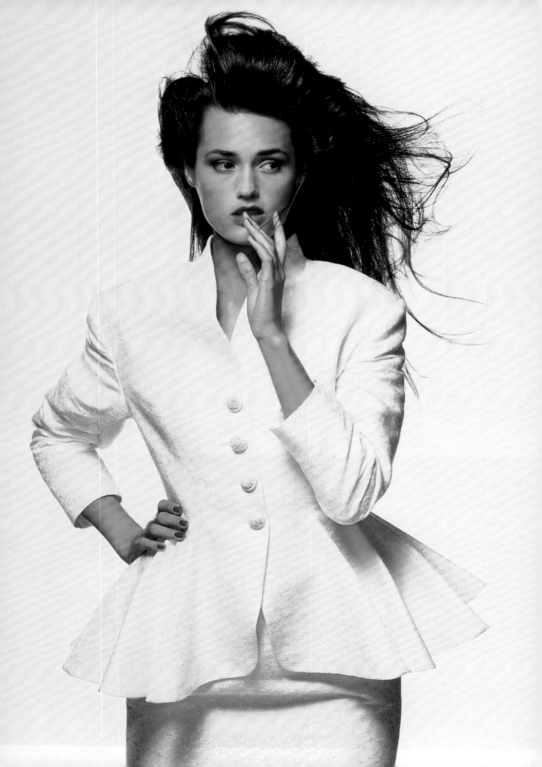

the 1980s

The 1980s is a decade that we have finally come to terms with, perhaps because those years of power dressing, big hair, matt make-up and legwarmers are now far enough in the past. The 1980s generation, Thatcher and Reagan's children, became known as the 'me' generation and the lust for money, power and all its accoutrements were well documented in films like *Wall Street* and books such as Tom Wolfe's *Bonfire of the Vanities*. Women were now really beginning to make headway in their careers and, in turn, were making money and wanted to show it. The house of Chanel had a massive revival. The Chanel suit, complete with shoulder pads and large gold buttons, quilted handbag and two-tone pumps, became the quintessential fashion statement – a look that filtered down from catwalk to sidewalk. The reasons for its success were threefold. First, women needed smart suits because they were blazing trails in the boardroom and wanted to look professional and practical. Second, everyone was hailing the Chanel ensemble as a 'classic' and it was thought to be

an excellent investment. Third, and it's back to money again, the suit made you look rich. But whatever clothes women were wearing, they were wearing them with jewellery, and loads of it. Over-the-top costume jewellery – gold chains, strands of enormous pearls and big 'button' earrings – were all components of 1980s flash.

Body consciousness, originating from the USA, changed the way we lived and our wardrobes. Films like *Flashdance* and *Fame* fuelled the fire, and exercise and dance clothes became a craze that has never quite gone away. Azzedine Alaïa emerged on the scene in Paris and gave women exactly what they wanted: short, tight, sexy dresses in pretty colours that moulded to the body and showed off the hours put in at the gym. The attitude was, 'if you've got it, flaunt it', which applied as much to money as to lean limbs. Ronald and Nancy Reagan brought a Republican glitz and glamour to the White House that had been conspicuously absent during the homespun Carter years. *Dallas* and *Dynasty* were all part of that ethos and the world lapped it up, much as they did the heavy eye make-up, full hair, shoulder pads and the Nolan Miller appliquéd evening dresses, so beloved of Alexis Colby and Krystle Carrington. John Frieda sums it up nicely when he says, 'Women were going out to work in a man's environment and, subconsciously or not, they armoured themselves with giant shoulder pads and big, stiff hair as a way of saying "take me seriously".' Christian Lacroix was the new kid on the block and French, American and the newly oil-rich Middle Eastern women adored dressing in his brightly coloured tweeds, accenting them with enormous flash jewellery and gold crucifixes. Part and parcel of this love of luxury were the famously hard-hitting perfumes of the time. Giorgio Beverly Hills and Christian Dior's Poison were the most infamous and the perfect products of an age obsessed with itself. The sweet smell of success went hand in hand with the growth in consumerism, and for a few years women loved their scent to scream, 'Look at me!' instead of being as subtle and intimate as before. Attention-seeking and flash were what mattered in the world of perfumery, and

as a result many scents were banned from restaurants and other public places.

Although the big technological break-throughs had not yet occurred in the beauty industry, the cosmetic giants were starting to put money and time into research and development. Antiageing claims were still 'hope in a jar', a term coined by Charles Revson, the founder of Revlon. Research was on the cusp of fruition, but it would take another ten years to make those break-throughs. Consequently, consumers and press still held the belief that all make-up and skincare was basically the same. In British *Vogue*'s 1982 version of More Dash Than Cash, dual-purpose make-up did not exist yet. Excerpts ran: 'baby powder costs far less than translucent powder and ... does the same job', and even, 'vaseline jelly is also multipurpose; it shines and conditions lips, adds ... gloss ... to eyebrows ... gleam to cheeks'. The genuinely fabulous dual-purpose products of the 1990s (think François Nars' Multiples and Nuxe Huile Prodigeuse) were still only twinkles in the eyes of budding make-up artists and a slew of cosmetic chemists.

the 1990s

When the clock struck midnight on 1980s flash and excess, the 1990s dawned as an era of simplicity and minimalism. It was almost inevitable. Women were now firmly established in positions of power and influence and they no longer needed to pretend to be men. The armour of huge shoulder pads and rows of brightly coloured business suits went out of fashion, to be replaced by a softer, simpler and more feminine silhouette. The ubiquitous jacket, the stalwart in every wardrobe and long-claimed 'classic', now became a rare bird. Even the humble button began to look contrived and was swapped for discreet tie fastenings or hidden hooks. Nothing could be soft, feminine or informal enough. Slip dresses, shell tops, floaty skirts and little cardigans now moved seamlessly from the street to the office to the supper party.

But that is still only half the story. The 1990s were all about individualism. For

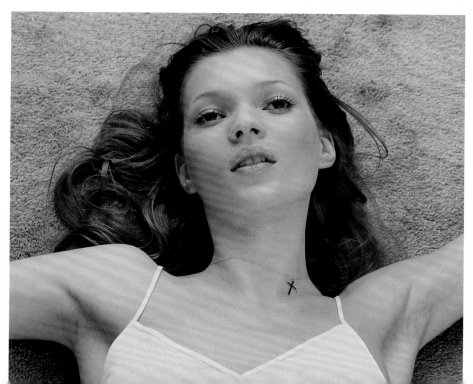

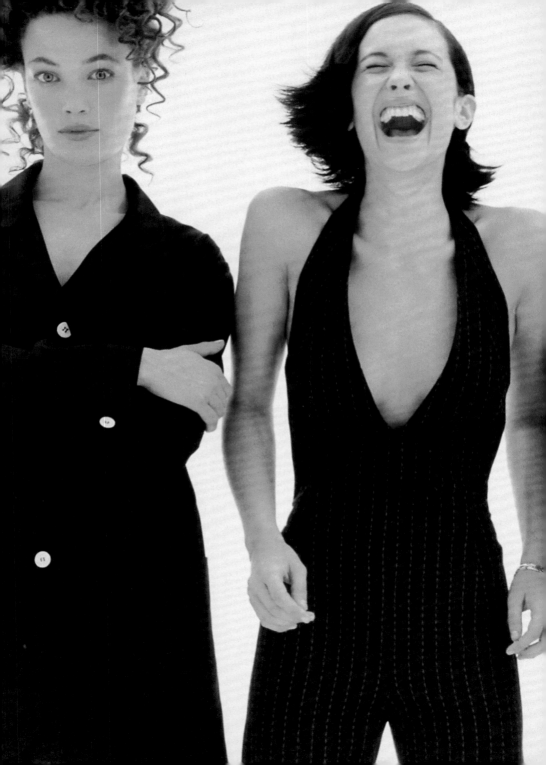

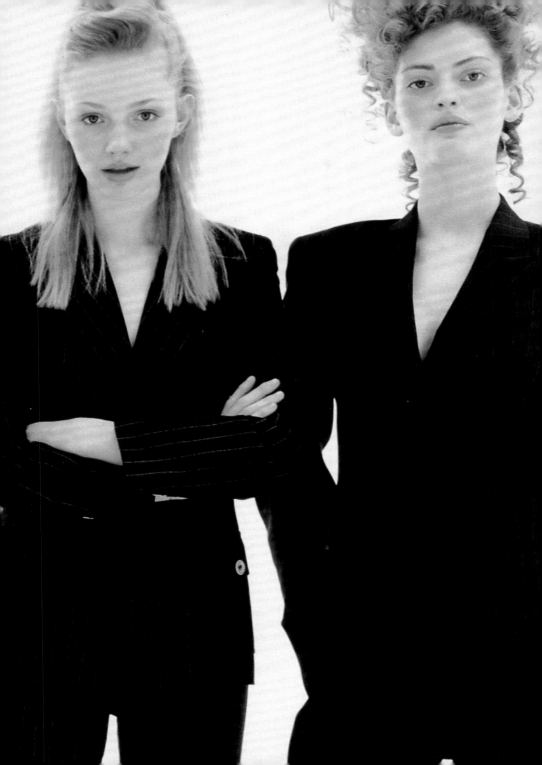

every spaghetti-strap dress, there has been a pair of combat trousers; for every Manolo Blahnik-inspired strappy sandal, a pair of Nike Air Max trainers. At last, it seemed that women could have it all — they could be boys by day, girls by night. They did not even have to choose between long or short hair any more. Hair extensions became mainstream towards the end of the decade, with actresses like Gwyneth Paltrow turning up with waist-length locks one night, a short gamine crop the next. The diversity and ease with which women could choose their looks was so much appreciated that the market happily tolerated Calvin Klein's and Giorgio Armani's simplicity next to the high-glam labels of Versace, Voyage, Galliano and McQueen. There was room for everyone.

An explosion of British design talent took over the runways of Paris — John Galliano at Dior, Alexander McQueen at Givenchy, Stella McCartney at Chloé and Vivienne Westwood. Fresh young blood burst into the beauty industry and changed the whole face of the market. Make-up artists, who clearly knew more about make-up than cosmetic company directors and marketing managers, started to launch their own innovative ranges. First was Bobbi Brown, but soon she was joined by Vincent Longo, François Nars, Janine Lobell at Stila, Ruby and Millie, Laura Mercier, Frank Toskin at MAC, Trish McEvoy and Terry de Gunzburg. If an idea was good and original enough, the beauty market had an ever-expanding desire to lap it up.

The 'trickle down' effect, which had happened in the fashion world, soon applied to beauty. Major technical advances began appearing in cheaper products and everyone could join in the fun. Huge conglomerates bought up many of the beauty companies, big and small, and research was shared, so no sooner had one brand launched the latest and greatest skincare than it was found in another cheaper one. And if the conglomerates were big enough, research was shared between separate industries, with cosmetics and skincare benefiting from breakthroughs in food and textiles. Aromatherapy, fake tanning and designer haircare also moved from niche products to the more affordable mass-market. Suddenly beauty became democratic and the boom had hit.

post-millennium

Fashion and beauty have always been hand in hand until the 1990s changed all that. Genuine technological advances are not something that can be reversed and this is where, finally, fashion and beauty parted company. No one will ever go back to foundation that does not seem like real skin, or hair that is not in glossy, fabulous condition, or fake tan that smells bad and looks orange, or make-up that slides off the minute you put it on. Beauty has been able to move on in a way that fashion never can. Terry de Gunzburg was the brains and beauty behind Yves Saint Laurent make-up, Nuxe, and now heads her own couture make-up line, By Terry. 'New technology has changed the rules of make-up application. Today, without any level of expertise, any woman can make the new products look wonderful on the skin; it's the equivalent of the most complicated video machine being used by a child.'

With the rise of confidence that women now feel and the desire of

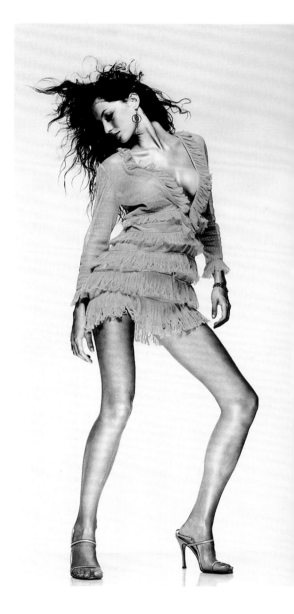

each of us to express our own individuality, the beauty companies are beginning to respond with their own version of personalized 'couture' products, specifically make-up and skincare. No longer is it enough to have to choose between seven shades of foundation from your favourite company's range. As consumers we are becoming increasingly demanding and are no longer happy to be pigeonholed. We all want our own perfect colours, but we require them in every choice of texture, too. Terry de Gunzburg continues, 'Make-up has certainly become personalized and focused on the individual, but trends are still strong. In the future I think that women will be able to choose their favourite colours in whatever texture the trend demands – glossy, matt, creamy, silky, satin or sheer. Multifunction products are another amazing trend that is going to grow and grow, because it is such a natural progression; products that you can use on your face, hair, body and as make-up. I am constantly amazed by the technology. It is giving us so much choice and freedom.'

So if individuality was what the 1990s were all about, versatility and freedom of choice seems to be the future. Already there are amazing cosmetic and surgical breakthroughs out there, waiting for us to take advantage, but no longer do we feel compelled to conform. Take the suntan issue as an example. Now we all know that tanning is bad for us. We are informed, but also free to make a choice. Many of us are going down the pale and protected route, liberated to be our natural colour. Others of us are fake-tanning to our heart's content, happy and confident to know that our healthy, sun-kissed limbs look entirely natural, without streaks or smells. Neither are we forced to buy masses of bottles of sun protection for the beach. Variosun, for example, has one bottle that will do it all. Swivel the dial from SPF2 to SPF30 and it dispenses the sun protection you want. Custom-made scent is now available, and your own lipsticks and skincare are right around the corner, too. And haircare labs are perfecting products that remove dye safely and naturally, so colour can be changed regularly and you need never fear a mistake. Now that is what I call progress.

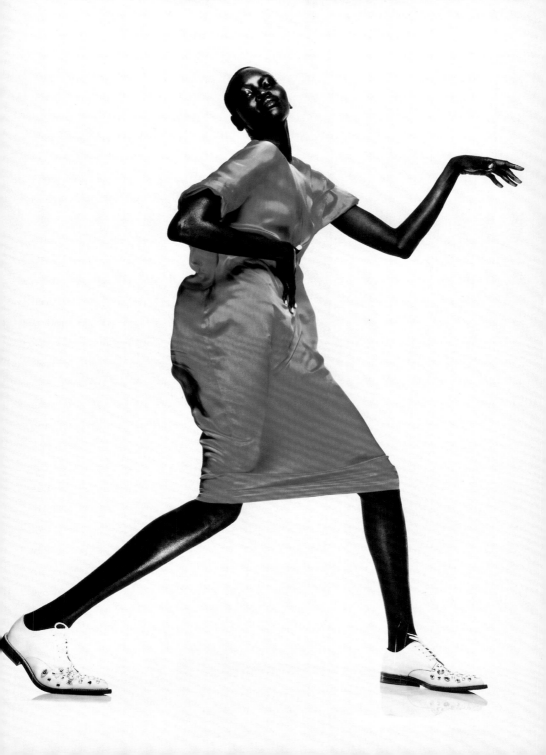

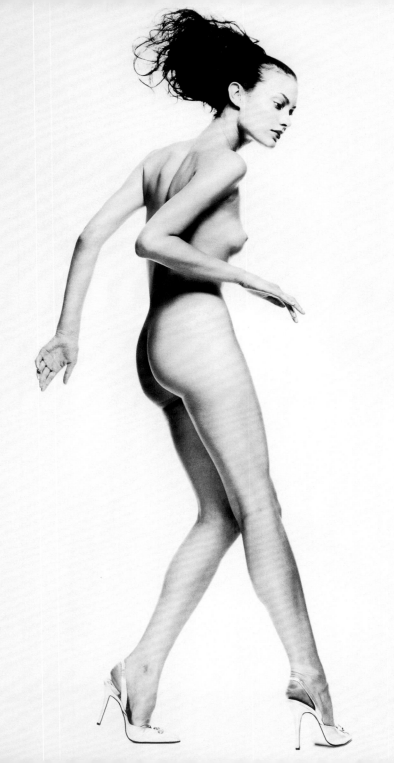

THE BODY

What is vital for every woman is that she loves her body – its size, shape, attributes and imperfections. This is more important than striving to be a perfect dress size or weight, or cultivating a personal sense of style. One study concluded that feeling uncomfortable in your own skin distracts attention away from areas that need focus in life – relationships, work and physical and mental wellbeing. Loving your natural size and features will help you gain more control over your life.

'Women often get so frustrated when they feel they are not at their "perfect shape",' says Teresa Hale, founder of London's Hale Clinic. Hale believes that everyone has a 'natural shape'. That shape may not be supermodel thin, but accepting and working with your body to express your own individuality is important. If you eat healthily and exercise regularly, your natural weight should be easily achieved. 'Love your body,' says Hale. 'A natural part of loving your body is looking after it.'

You may not be the weight you were at 20 years old. The average person, male or female, gains 3 kg (7 lb) between the ages of 25 and 34. Working every day at maintaining a healthy body will help to promote a sense of wellbeing. Physical transformation will not happen overnight, but this chapter will help you get to know your body better and acquaint you with some methods of exercise and therapy that can improve your overall health and sense of wellbeing.

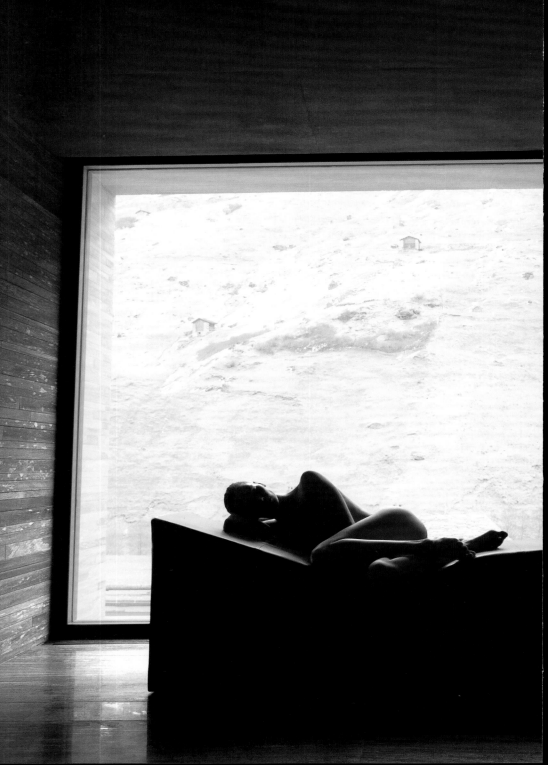

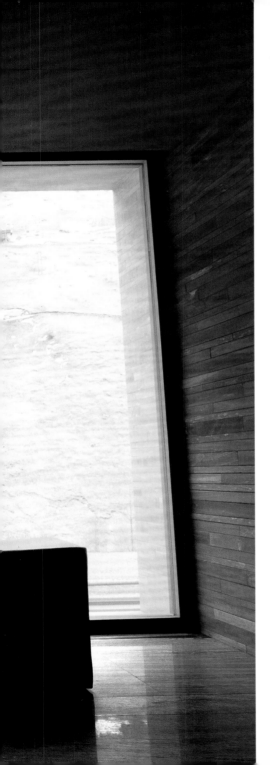

stress &
the body

Everyone suffers from stress, but stress does not necessarily have to be a negative factor. In the form of mental pressure, stress can be a powerful force. It can be a motivator – urging us to carry out tasks or conquer problems and achieve certain goals in our lives. Ignoring stress, however, will lead to feelings of tension and fatigue. Chronic psychological stress can increase the chance of developing a number of harmful conditions, including migraine headaches, digestive disorders and impaired memory. Depression, premenstrual tension (PMT), sleep disorders and weight fluctuations are other possible side effects of unresolved stress.

HOW TO CONQUER STRESS

Overcoming stress should be the first step towards improving the body. Take some time out and begin to think about the sources of any stress and agitation in your life. Before jumping to conclusions or blaming other people or things, think positively. Look for solutions that could help to resolve the stress. Try to approach each day with a positive attitude.

Begin to seek pleasure or pleasant situations rather than crisis or conflict. Think about how much better you look when your face is not expressing tension. Now imagine what a more serene demeanour could do to improve your overall sense of self. Rest is a powerful stressbuster, according to Teresa Hale. 'Society is so geared up,' she says. 'We are living in exciting times, but there is no time to rest. Today people not only work hard, but when they are away from the office, they work more.' Any free time is used to exercise, or perhaps freelance, or work around the house. 'Relaxing,' continues Hale, 'is like leaving a field fallow to renew itself.' If you find winding down quite difficult, seek help from others. 'Have a massage once a week,' Hale suggests. 'It will help balance your mood, and it is good for the skin because it gets the blood circulating throughout the whole body.'

Sleep can be used as another natural form of stress relief. The hours we spend asleep replenish the body's supply of neuro-transmitters – hormones that help produce a positive mood. Those who sleep better tend to be happier and more confident than those who deny themselves rest or suffer from insomnia. A study in the USA discovered that people who only manage to sleep for four to five hours a night felt stressed and more depressed than those who slept for eight hours. A good night's sleep, which experts calculate at an uninterrupted eight hours, will leave the body feeling relaxed and ready to handle the challenges of the day ahead. Although everyone needs different amounts of sleep, experts recommend developing consistent habits by falling asleep and waking up at nearly the same time each day.

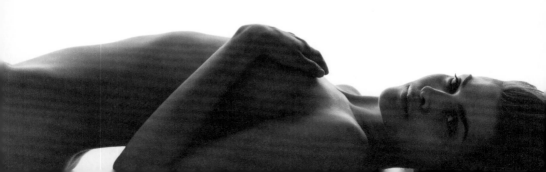

food – the body's fuel

Along with rest and relaxation, a nutritious diet is one of the essential sources of fuel the body requires to maintain optimum health. On the never-ending quest to eat right, most people set out with the best intentions, only to discover that, after weeks of cutting out the foods they love, excess body weight is not disappearing as quickly as desired. Most people have every reason to fear the word 'diet'. 'People equate the word "diet" with deprivation. That's not a good motivator,' says John P Foreyt, author of *Living Without Dieting*. Complicated weight-loss strategies do not work. Nutritionists universally agree that the most effective weight-loss plan, and the most beneficial strategy for the body, is to personally develop lifelong healthy eating habits.

'Trends in nutrition come and go,' adds Teresa Hale. 'What's more, nutritional

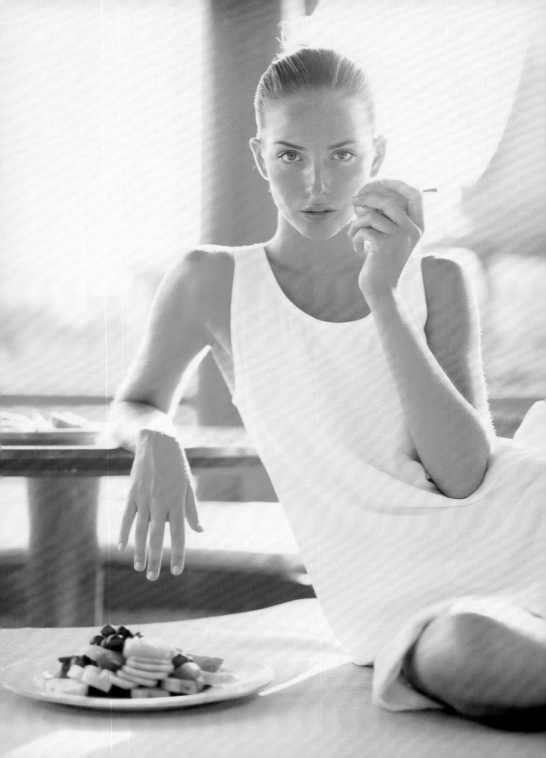

science can often contradict itself.' Hale's advice is sound and simple. 'The important thing to develop is a sense of individual nutritional awareness. Get to know the nutrients that suit your body type and then try to maintain a balanced diet that suits your body best.

To do this, ask yourself a few questions: "What are the best foods for me?" and "What is the best way to combine foods so that I can maintain a healthy, balanced diet?" If the answers prove elusive, consult a trained nutritionist.'

A BALANCED DIET

Nutritional experts at Clinique La Prairie, one of the finest health spas in the world, all advocate a balanced diet that includes something from their seven food classifications, below, every day.

1 Group one: milk, cheese and yogurt

2 Group two: meat and its substitutes, such as tofu

3 Group three: bread, cereal and potatoes

4 Group four: fruit and vegetables

5 Group five: fats, such as butter

6 Group six: sugars

7 Group seven: liquids, such as water and juice

Eating a variety of foods from each of the groups should satisfy all nutritional needs. The key to a balanced diet, La Prairie nutritionists claim, is the right mixture of proteins, carbohydrates and fats. Vegetables should make up the dominant part of any diet, with fish and fruit being the other important components. A number of studies carried out on children prove that eating an early morning meal has beneficial effects on mental and physical functions. Eating breakfast makes sense; the body needs to refuel itself after sleep. Food helps the brain and body to function at its fullest capacity. Breakfast can also be of benefit throughout the whole day. A high-fibre breakfast can help prevent snacking and overeating during lunch and dinner. Whether or not they realize it, people who skip breakfast often make up for it later in the day by overeating. Research has also

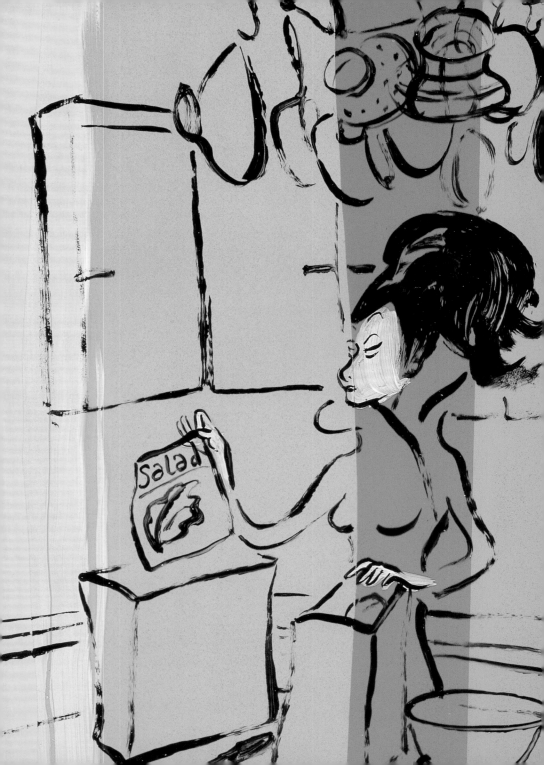

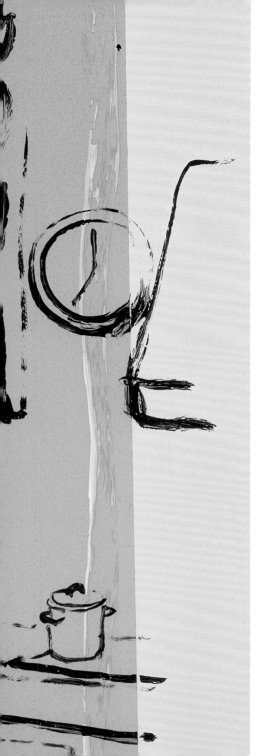

concluded that women who eat break-fast get more out of a workout than those who prefer to skip it. They have stronger concentration levels and can maintain a more consistent level of weight. Breakfast should consist of about 25 per cent of your daily calorific needs. A nutritious breakfast, therefore, should add up to somewhere between 300 and 600 calories. Those calories should then be divided up as follows: 30 per cent are derived from fat, 15 to 20 per cent consists of protein and the remainder is made up of carbohydrates.

Women often have a tendency to feel guilty for thinking about food throughout the day: they shouldn't. Nutritionists frequently urge their patients to feed the body whenever it is hungry. This does not mean that you will be eating all of the time. If you really listen to your body, you will begin to understand the types of foods that fill you up and make you feel good. As Geneen Roth, author of *Feeding the Hungry Heart*, says: '[People think] "What if I'm hungry all of the time?" But when you consciously tune in, you realize, "I'm physically hungry less often than I thought" or "It takes less food to fill me than I thought".'

HEALTHY BREAKFAST FOODS

Oatmeal: Easily digestible, oatmeal is also a good source of fibre.

Cereal: High-fibre varieties of cereal can help to prevent constipation and, according to some doctors, they may also prevent cancer.

Half-fat or skimmed milk: Both types of milk are a rich source of vitamin D, calcium and protein.

Fresh fruit: Low in calories but high in vitamins, fruit contains a good source of soluble fibre. Fruit can also help to satisfy a sweet tooth in place of chocolate.

Juice: Choose tomato and vegetable juices, as they are the best nutritional options. Low in calories, vegetable juice also provides vitamins A and C.

Water: Drinking two glasses of water in the morning before a meal will wake up and rehydrate the body. But try to drink water consistently throughout the day and not just in the morning.

Yogurt: Choose either a plain or low-fat yogurt. A good source of calcium and protein, as well as a natural bacteria, yogurt helps to aid your digestive system.

dietary
supplements

Although most nutritionists explain that the need for supplements is minimal if a diet is balanced, more purport that healthy diets are harder to maintain. Global pesticide pollution and the ever-increasing availability of processed food make it increasingly difficult to acquire nutrition from food. As a result, more women are taking a dietary supplement in the form of a vitamin, multivitamin or mineral to help keep them fit and healthy. While supplements are a daily part of a balanced diet for some people, they are still a subject of curiosity for others. Increasingly, supplements are a topic of conversation and the names of energy-boosting vitamins and minerals are exchanged by models and designers backstage at fashion shows. Some brand names turn up on the pages of fashion magazines and have become as exclusive as the right designer labels. This 'cool factor' can be easily explained. People are working harder than ever and are realizing that supplements can boost their performance levels.

But it is important to take the correct supplement for your needs, and to not expect miracles. 'There is no "magic bullet",' says Teresa Hale. 'A trained nutritionist can help you find the right supplement that will work for your own individual needs.' Vitamins should never replace food but should be consumed along with a healthy balanced diet. One supplement is not going to be the answer to all of your nutritional needs. 'If supplements are used merely to counter bad eating habits, improvements in appearance and energy levels will be negligible,' says Kate Neil, former principal of London's Institute of Optimum Nutrition. Use the following information to help you find a vitamin that works for you.

B VITAMINS

Vitamins B3 (niacin) and B5 (pantothenic acid) are essential in the production of red blood cells, adrenaline and sex hormones. Dairy products and liver deliver these nutrients; consequently vegetarians and vegans are often deficient in these vitamins. Brewer's yeast tablets, which help lower cholesterol levels, provide a potent source of both types of B vitamins.

ECHINACEA

An extract of the cornflower, echinacea can help stimulate the immune system, warding off minor colds and illnesses. It is effective in protecting the body against harmful bacteria and viruses. A few drops of the extract diluted in water can be used as a mouthwash for sore throats, ulcers and infections.

FISH OILS

Fish oils are one of the few fats in which most people are deficient. Research has shown that fatty acids have beneficial effects on those who suffer from heart disease, arthritis, PMT, migraines and diabetes. Currently research is being conducted on the effects fatty acids may have on cancer. Eating fish or taking a fish oil supplement is often recommended to manic-depressives because it can help stabilize mood. Like Prozac, Omega-3 fatty acids seem to increase the brain's production of the feel-good chemical, seratonin. Some doctors believe that everyone can benefit from eating more fish, particularly such cold-water fish as salmon and sardines. Sushi and lightly cooked salmon are also potent sources of fatty acids. If fish oils are not in your diet, consider taking starflower, linseed or hemp oil pills.

FOLIC ACID

Alternately known as pteroylglutanic acid, folic acid is an energy booster. Raw dark green vegetables, such as broccoli and spinach, are rich in folic acid. As with all vegetables, cooking detracts from its healthy benefits. Deficiencies can lead to anaemia and depression, but excessive consumption has been shown to increase the chance of epilepsy.

GINKGO BILOBA

This is an extract of the maidenhair tree, known to help circulation, thrombosis and varicose veins. It can be taken in tincture or tablet form, or as a tea, in which case three cups a day are recommended. The Chinese believe that ginkgo biloba improves memory and concentration levels. Devotees claim it helps them feel calm, yet alert

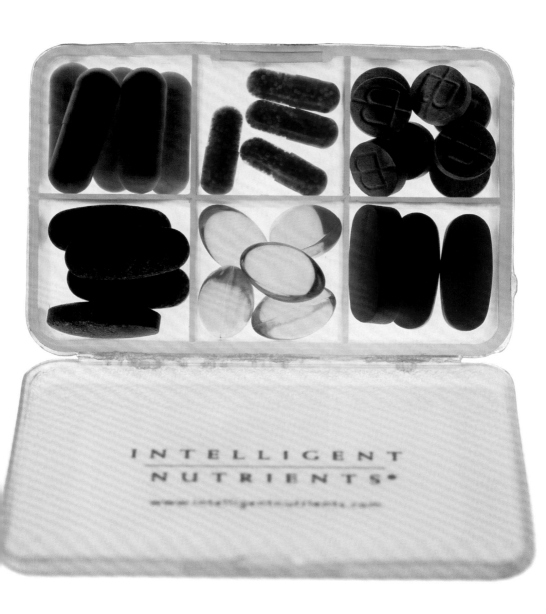

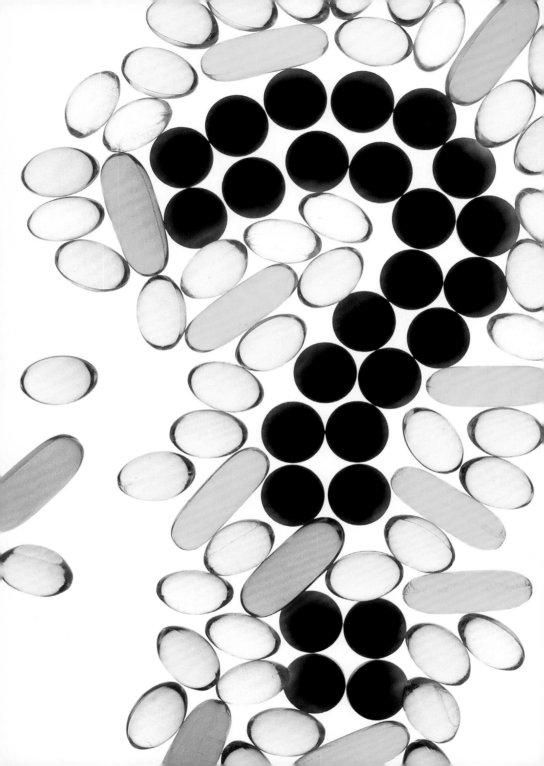

and focused. Along with St John's wort, it has been hailed as a 'New Age Prozac'.

GINSENG

Said to mean 'wonder of the world', ginseng is an energy booster, which can strengthen the immune system and increase concentration. It is often used to treat exhaustion. The root of the plant, which contains ginsenocide, a sugar-like boosting substance, is used as a tonic to help revitalize the body. Nutritionists recommend that ginseng is taken as a 30-day course. Pregnant women and those suffering from acute anxiety or irritability should avoid taking ginseng.

ST JOHN'S WORT

This herbal supplement can help lift mild depression, however it can interact with other drugs and interfere with the effectiveness of birth-control pills, so check with your doctor before taking. Best results follow about a month after taking a daily dose. Regarded as a wild plant in Europe and a weed in many parts of the world,

St John's wort strengthens the nervous system and speeds up healing. Due to its antiviral and anti-inflammatory properties, it can be used in cream form to treat sore skin, calm a rash and heal cuts.

SELENIUM

This helps fight fatigue and premature ageing and can also counteract the groggy effect of a hangover. A trace element that works with vitamin E to prohibit free-radical damage to the cell membrane, selenium is an antioxidant that can protect against damage caused by pollution and stress.

SPIRULINA

Also called blue-green algae, spirulina is composed of 60 per cent protein. An energy booster, it is rich in beta-carotene, vitamin B and minerals. Spirulina also promotes energy, aids digestion and boosts the immune system. It can be taken as a tablet or in powder form.

WHEATGRASS

A super supplement: a dose of wheat grass, which is ingested as a shot of juice, contains seven times the amount of vitamin C than an orange and five times more iron than a serving of spinach. Rich in vitamins A, B and C, wheatgrass helps purify the system, allowing the body to absorb nutrients and eliminate toxins more effectively. However, the taste is harsh and excessive consumption can cause diarrhoea.

ZINC

A protein-rich mineral, zinc is found in every body cell. It stimulates growth and the sex hormones. Vegetables and grains are rich in zinc, as are oysters and red meat, but genetic farming has reduced the amount naturally available in foods. Taking a zinc supplement can help fight fatigue and clear the complexion. If your body is lacking zinc, white spots on the fingernails or a white coating on the tongue may appear. Impotence and halitosis are other signs of a zinc deficiency.

FACTS ABOUT SUPPLEMENTS

When should I take a supplement?

Vitamins are best taken during the day so that they can work to promote the necessary bodily functions. Minerals, however, should be taken at night because they help build up bodily functions. Vitamins should be consumed just before, or with, a meal. Food helps the body to absorb essential vitamins and minerals, and promotes the release of gastric acid.

How many supplements should I take?

A daily multivitamin should suffice, but your doctor, a pharmacist or a qualified nutritionist can help you choose the correct dietary supplement to suit your particular needs. If you're taking medicine that interferes with nutrient absorption, if you're an elderly person with a low calorie intake, or if you're an athlete or pregnant, you may benefit from specific supplements. The US Institute of Medicine lists a 'tolerable upper intake level' for all vitamins and minerals – which is the maximum safe amount that anyone should take – as does the European Food Safety Authority (EFSA).

exercise

Deborah Bull, former principal dancer with the Royal Ballet, admits: 'However many diets I tried, I never managed to lose weight permanently. It was only when I started to work with my body, rather than fight against it, that my personal battle became a thing of the past.' While model Jerry Hall comments: 'Losing weight is not about the things you should not do, it's about the things you should do. You can stay slim without starving yourself, and you don't need expensive gyms or exercise }equipment to keep fit.'

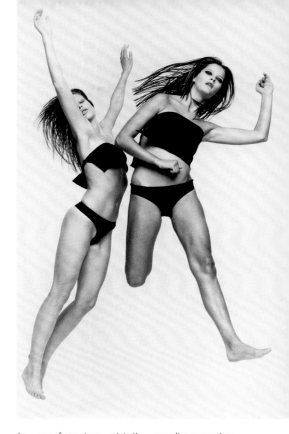

The way we exercise is changing. Why? Because, as Jerry Hall says, the thinking on exercise has changed. More women have now realized what the American College of Sports Medicine discovered in the mid-1990s. Moderate physical exercise, such as walking, cycling or jogging, performed for approximately 30 minutes a day, though not necessarily consecutively, will help balance the mind and reshape the body. Exercise is no longer a quick fix. Going all out − overexerting the body by performing strictly cardiovascular exercise − will not deliver optimum benefits, as so many of us have discovered after enduring injury and feeling exhausted. Today more of us are beginning to realize that exercise should and must become an integral part of our daily routine.

Cardiovascular exercise keeps the heart and lungs pumping and healthy. A regular, vigorous exercise routine that is performed for approximately

20 minutes a day or more will also promote energy levels, help keep you well and promote a strong immune system. Blood pressure and cholesterol levels also tend to be lower in those who exercise than in those who are sedentary.

MOTIVATION

Winter months are often a time when we feel the most sluggish. Adverse climatic conditions, such as driving rain, wind and snow, often reduce our ability to exercise outdoors. However, you can choose the winter months as a time to change your approach to exercise. Some of the best forms of exercise are conducted indoors. Get to know the strength-training exercise machines at your local gym and discover how they can be used to reshape your body. Incorporate a new yoga or Pilates class, or a group programme, into your routine.

Rest is good for the body; quitting exercise is not. What happens to the body when an exercise routine ceases? The muscles become weaker and shrink in size. Muscles will not turn into fat overnight, but weight gain is a distinct possibility, especially if you continue to consume the same amount of calories as you did while exercising. Muscle loss can also slow down the metabolism, thus increasing the chances of weight gain.

Use the gym as a get-away zone. A workout can relax the body and the time after exercising can be used to enhance that feeling. For an ultimate wind-down, spend 15 minutes in the steam room or sauna, though avoid these zones if you are pregnant or feel dizzy. Pack a gym kit with luxury feel-good products to promote a sense of wellbeing. Maintaining a healthy diet helps the body to exercise better. Eating protein-rich food can help you recover from exercise more effectively; leucine, a key ingredient in high-protein foods, helps to build muscle and balance blood sugar levels.

FEELING UNDER-PAR

Illness and exercise do not mix, but do not let a minor ailment keep you away from a workout. Fitness instructors claim that you can still exercise if you have a cold, as long as you are not feverish or taking over-the-counter antihistamines (which speed up the heart). If you do choose to exercise when you have a cold, try to reduce the intensity of the workout to about 60 per cent of your normal level. Remember to listen to your body. If you are feeling really under the weather or have the flu, avoid exercise completely.

HUNGOVER?

Performing a low-impact workout like yoga could help ease the pain. Make sure the body is well hydrated by drinking a few large glasses of water before and after exercise.

JET-LAGGED?

Flying between time zones disrupts the body's internal clock, but exercise can help overcome that sluggish, sleepy feeling that long-distance flying induces. It is best, though, to wait a day for the body to adjust to its new surroundings. Start slowly with light exercise — running on a treadmill at full speed can be dangerous; when the body is tired, coordination decreases.

STRESSED?

Exercise can help fight feelings of agitation. 'There's something about moving rhythmically and repetitively over a period of time that's psychologically soothing,' says Kate Hayes, a clinical sports psychologist, lecturer and the author of *Working it Out: Using Exercise in Psychotherapy*. Researchers are still trying to discover how and why exercise has such positive benefits on stress and mood. Some believe that it alters the body's internal chemistry, boosting mood-enhancing hormones, which in turn reduce the feelings of stress.

TOO TIRED?

Try to exercise after work or when you are feeling sluggish. The evening is actually one of the best times to work out as it can help promote a deeper sleep. An article in the American publication *Medicine & Science in Sports & Exercise* concluded that, contrary to popular belief, exercising in the evening did not keep participants up at night. Researchers do believe, however, that those who exercise in the evening are in better physical shape because their nervous system is more in tune to the intensity and they can recover overnight from any strain induced by their routine.

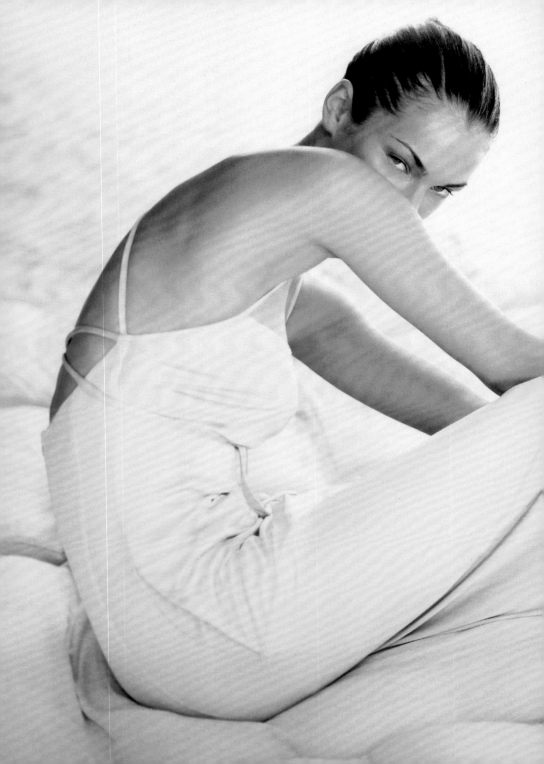

STRETCHING

Stretching is a good way to get to know your body, and is the perfect beginning to every fitness session. Through the physical sensation it delivers you will learn which muscles are tight and tense, as well as which ones are loose and limber. Performed regularly, stretching will lengthen and strengthen the muscles, as well as make them less susceptible to injury. Stretching will also prepare the body to exercise effectively and improves posture, which in turn can prevent back pain. Keep in mind these tips.

1 Stretch mindfully. Perform each stretch slowly, with no bouncing or jerky movements.

2 Breathe deeply. Exhale as you deepen the stretch.

3 Relax your shoulders.

4 Be aware of your stomach muscles. Gently tightening your abdominals will increase the toning benefits of a stretch.

5 Maintain each stretch for no less than 30 seconds.

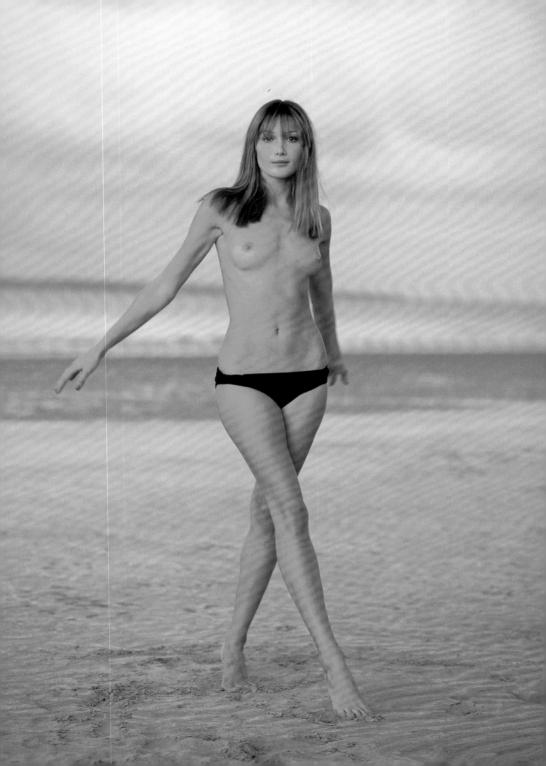

fitness options

Experiment with different disciplines. Aerobics and jogging may be two of the most popular forms of exercise, but trying a new exercise or taking a fresh approach to an old regime can increase the physical and mental benefits. Use the following information as a guide to help you choose a new routine.

HOME GYMS

If the very thought of going to a gym induces fear, consider working out at home instead. Many actors keep fitness equipment in their homes and exercise in their hotel rooms when on location. Although most celebrities work out in the comfort and splendour of their own palatial homes, it is a misconception to think that you have to be rich to afford a home gym. An annual gym membership can be expensive and the money may add up significantly after a few years. Investing a comparable amount in fitness equipment could build a home gym. The essential pieces include a treadmill for cardiovascular work and a multigym for toning. If you are short of space and money, start small by investing in a stomach cruncher or Swiss ball and then make the acquisition of a fitness machine a personal goal by saving up for it. Using equipment properly — always check the manufacturer's instructions — will certainly reap physical rewards.

THE LIFE COACH

Just as the thinking behind exercise has evolved, so has the approach to personal training. Those of us who have worked out in a gym are well acquainted with the old approach to personal training. The scene used to be aggressive: a svelte super-fit trainer pushed a sweaty, panting, out-of-shape gym enthusiast to new heights of physical pain. Times have changed and statistics prove the point. Today in Britain the British National Register of Personal Trainers represents 800 qualified personal trainers, and their numbers are increasing by approximately 100 per year. Why the growing demand? 'Today we are more like life coaches,' says UK-based personal trainer Josh Salzmann. A qualified trainer can provide useful expertise on an array of crucial lifestyle areas – not just exercise, but diet and nutrition, alternative therapies and fitness equipment. Says Salzmann, 'I help my clients get organized.'

Matt Roberts, another top London trainer who offers personal training at his clubs in London's Mayfair and in Mauritius at Le Saint Géran and Le Touessrok, takes a scientific, medical approach to his sessions. A doctor, acupuncturist and physiotherapist are all involved in devising the optimum workout to meet each individual's health and fitness requirements. The main advantage of working out with a personal trainer is that this increasingly customized hands-on approach helps make the most of an exercise routine. Training with a life coach costs money, but most people find it is worth the investment. A trainer can ensure that you are exercising at the right level and intensity for your body, so that the routine performed will render the maximum physical and mental benefits.

LOTTE BERK METHOD

Mixing movements from ballet, yoga, physiotherapy and modern dance, Lotte Berk provides an intense, low-impact workout that focuses on flexibility and pelvic control. Classes last for about an hour, beginning with a series of warm-up stretches and then progressing to upper-body work and leg exercises which are performed at a barre. Deeper, stretching movements are carried out at the end. Participants notice postural improvement as well as elongated muscles, leaner legs and a firmer bottom.

MARTIAL ARTS

The Chinese view martial arts, such as t'ai chi, qi gong and wing chun, as internal exercises, which help focus the mind and develop a sense of inner strength. Once practised, internal exercise develops health and mental harmony.

T'AI CHI: This is like meditation in motion. It is a series of slow, flowing linked movements, which promote inner relaxation and aim to relax the muscles and nerves. There are five types or families of t'ai chi, including chen, wu and sun, but yang – a series of 24 or a longer 108 linked postures that combine to form a 'flow' – is the most popular type in the West.

QI GONG: Qi gong traces its roots back to 200 BC and was first practised by Chinese doctors. During the exercise, attention is focused on posture, and all of the movements are performed slowly. The aim is all in its translation: 'The curing of illness through muscle movement.'

WING CHUN: A form of kung fu that women often learn as self-defence and which includes close-range unarmed fighting. Holding a set, defined position, the aim is to use the least amount of exertion for self-defence and then to 'zone in' on an attack of your partner's (or 'enemy's') acupressure points.

CAPOEIRA: This is a rhythmical, non-contact fighting dance of Brazilian origin. Swift movements, such as front and back flips, cartwheels and handstands, are performed with the intention of outwitting your opponent. Capoeira can provide an intense form of cardiovascular exercise. It tones the buttocks and thighs and, when practised frequently, can increase endurance and flexibility.

METHOD PUTKISTO

Marja Putkisto, a Finnish dance and fitness instructor, developed this deep-stretch, core-strengthing technique involving lunges, front bends and body tilts. The method teaches extremely deep stretch positions, which Putkisto encourages participants to hold beyond the average time of 30 seconds to up to 5 minutes. She claims that holding stretches not only lengthens and strengthens the muscles, but also produces a range of benefits, from improved digestion and circulation to increased lung capacity and flexibility.

PILATES

Pilates has become as popular as yoga. The majority of the A-list celebrities are doing yoga and Pilates, confirms Greg Isaacs, a Hollywood fitness trainer, who says, 'now it's all about the lean, athletic body' that yoga and Pilates can deliver. Like yoga, Pilates is an exercise technique that lengthens and strengthens the muscles.

The two regimes also deliver similar benefits – a lean, toned body and relief from stress and tension – and they require the same high level of concentration. 'What makes Pilates different from other exercise methods is that it involves your mind,' says Brooke Siler, a Manhattan-based instructor and author of *The Pilates Body*. 'You have to concentrate and learn. You are not just coming in to train. You are studying.'

Pilates involves a series of slow, controlled movements (there are 500 in all), which can be performed on a mat or with the help of a spring resistance machine, called the Reformer. Pilates was developed about 85 years ago by Joseph Pilates, who originally called his method 'Contrology'. Some of its earliest disciples were dancers; the late Martha Graham, for example, was a devotee, as was George Balanchine. Today both models and real women are reaping the benefits of the technique. Those who practise it regularly cite a host of benefits, from dramatic weight loss to firmer muscles, better posture and flexibility, and even an increased libido.

YOGA

Since such celebrities as Madonna, Cindy Crawford and Gwyneth Paltrow began preaching the wonders of yoga, the level of awareness in this Indian stretch technique has increased. In Sanskrit, yoga means 'union' and yoga postures, or 'asanas', aim to unite the mind, body and breath. Today class numbers have skyrocketed dramatically: 300,000 people in the UK do yoga. Yoga is not competitive and instructors encourage participants to work at their own level.

Classes are also becoming increasingly accessible. Yoga instructors teach at the blossoming number of yoga centres, health clubs and community centres, with more visiting homes and offices to offer private one-to-one sessions. Yoga may not burn fat but it can tone the body in specific zones, especially the abdomen, buttocks and thighs. There are several different types of yoga but the variations are united in a common purpose: to reduce tension and stress and to induce a deep feeling of relaxation (see pages 330–1 and 370–4 for further information on yoga).

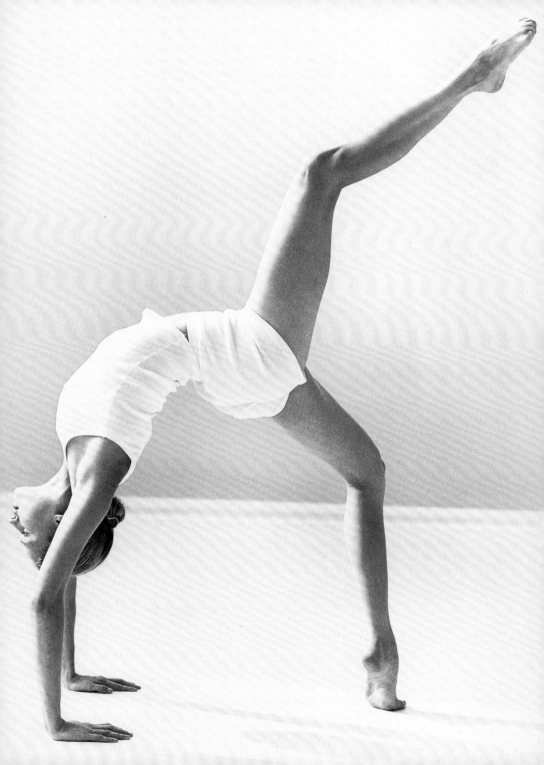

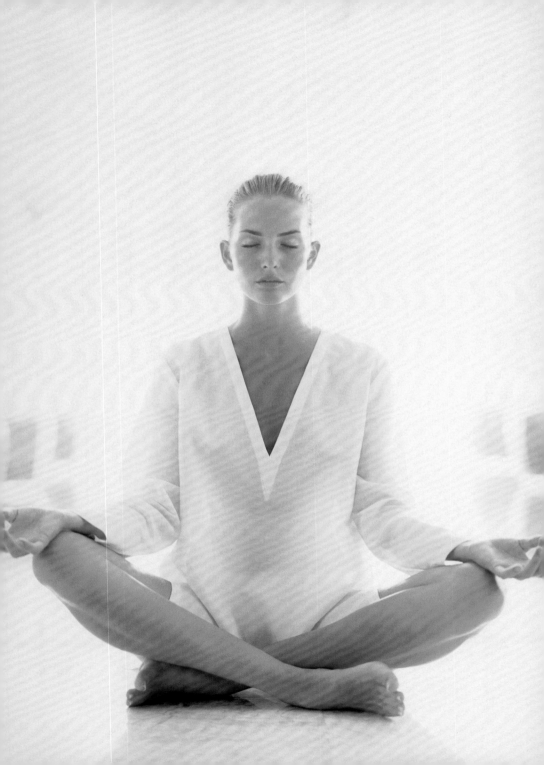

body work – holistic therapies

As beneficial for the body as good nutrition and regular exercise, body work helps promote total wellbeing. A range of hands-on treatments can help joints stay lithe, keep blood circulating through the system and encourage a sense of calmness and relaxation. Body work is an individual process. A treatment that might work for a friend, might not work for you. If you are unsure about undergoing any treatment, research it first to understand the process and the benefits it can deliver. Talk to your therapist; a reliable practitioner, whatever his or her discipline, should offer a consultation first to introduce the treatment. The therapies that are particularly well suited for the body are listed below. For more in-depth information on each practice, as well as other options, refer to the advice on complementary medicine (see pages 324–87).

ALEXANDER TECHNIQUE

Taught as a hands-on therapy, as well as through movement and dialogue, the aim is to re-educate muscles and realign the musculoskeletal system (see also page 374–5).

CRANIOSACRAL THERAPY

The aim of this treatment is to balance the craniosacral system, also known as the body's hydraulic system. An osteopath targets points on the bones and tissue from the head to the bottom of the spine (see also page 365).

HELLERWORK

Hellerwork massage focuses on the myo-fascial tissue, the connective tissue that holds the body together. Sessions involve deep-tissue massage and movement re-education to help realign the body and release tension and stress.

MASSAGE

Swedish massage is a classic backrub based on five main strokes: a gliding hand movement, a kneading of the skin, friction, circular strokes, gentle tapping pressure to aid circulation and hand vibration. Aromatherapy massage usually incorporates movements derived from Swedish massage with specific essential oils to affect mood. Thai massage is a dynamic massage, involving stretching, movement and stimulation of certain body zones. Other beneficial types of massage include sports massage, shiatsu and rolfing (see also pages 353–60).

REIKI

Reiki works almost like a magnetic force to pull the negative energy away from the patient. It aims to generate positive energy, relieve stress and boost vitality (see also pages 368–9).

REFLEXOLOGY

Finger pressure is applied to the parts of the feet connected to specific internal and external body zones to release blocked energy (see also page 237).

MAXIMIZE THE BENEFITS OF BODY WORK

1 Set goals: Know what you want from a treatment. Use the time effectively during your therapy session to relax and concentrate on how the session will enhance your life.

2 Communicate: Express your thoughts and feelings to the practitioner. If something makes you feel uncomfortable, say so. Conversely, remark on that which makes you feel good.

3 Spread out a sereis of sessions: Allow the effects of the bodywork to settle into the system before returning for more. Ask the therapist how often you should undertake a treatment. If you are unsure about the answer, seek a second opinion.

4 Do not expect miracles: Some treatments offer immediate benefits while others require a more lengthy commitment. Be patient: everyone reacts differently to body work.

5 Abstain: Avoid alcohol and stimulants prior to a treatment. It is also best not to eat before a session. If you are hungry, eat a light, healthy snack that will not challenge the digestive system.

6 Prepare mentally beforehand: If you are travelling some distance, leave yourself 15 minutes before the treatment to wind down from the journey. Allow relaxation time afterwards, too.

detoxifying

'Detoxifying is a great way to wake up a tired body, lift the lethargy caused by too many late nights or compensate for a period of overindulgence,' explains health writer Kathryn Marsden. So often women resort to extreme measures to purify their system. There is nothing harmful in wanting to detoxify or cleanse the system, but proceed cautiously. Fasting and water diets – two common methods women often choose to quickly detox and lose weight – are dangerous and drastic, and could result in dizzy spells, exhaustion or illness. Cutting down on the intake of alcohol, sugar, salt, caffeine and processed foods, all substances that cause the build-up of toxins in the body, is a good start.

COLONIC HYDROTHERAPY

Another option towards detoxifying the body is colonic hydrotherapy. Jane Waterman, the colonic hydrotherapist at Balance, a London-based complementary health and beauty clinic, provides the facts and dispels a few myths.

Q: WHAT IS COLONIC HYDROTHERAPY?

Jane Waterman: Colonic hydrotherapy is the gentle infusion of water into the colon. The actual process of colonics dates back to around 1500 BC. Today it is administered under the guidance of the therapist, who monitors a gentle process in which water under low gravitational pressure flows and expels from the colon. This process is repeated many times, during what is usually a 40-minute treatment.

Q: WHY AND WHEN SHOULD SOMEONE CONSIDER HAVING A COLONIC?

JW: People consider colonics for many different reasons. A colonic may help relieve constipation and irritable bowel syndrome. Those people who are intolerant to wheat and yeast have also found relief from a colonic hydrotherapy. They are often administered to someone who is starting a detox programme.

Q: HOW SHOULD
I PREPARE MYSELF?

JW: There is no special preparation beforehand.

Q: WHEN SHOULD
ONE NOT HAVE COLONIC
HYDROTHERAPY?

JW: Consult your doctor if you are unsure about the process. Certain bowel conditions can be irritated by colonic hydrotherapy. Also, avoid the treatment if you are pregnant or suffering from heart problems. A detailed medical history should be taken during a consultation prior to the treatment, so all of the necessary information is known.

Q: ARE COLONICS SAFE?

JW: Yes, the treatment is absolutely safe. The water is introduced at a low pressure so there is no danger of bowel perforation. All equipment involved in the treatment is either disposable or disinfected using hospital-approved disinfecting solutions, which kill all viruses, bacteria and fungi. Colonic hydrotherapy, unlike taking laxatives, is not habit-forming and actually improves the tone of the colon.

Q: A LOT OF PEOPLE
FEAR THE TREATMENT –
WHY?

JW: There are conflicting views about colonic hydrotherapy and, as a result, confusion about its benefits. A good therapist is aware that patients may feel nervous and embarrassed and will soon have one feeling relaxed and confident.

Q: IS THERE A LIMIT
TO HOW MANY COLONICS
ONE SHOULD HAVE IN
A LIFETIME?

JW: It can vary from one to a number of treatments spread over a period of time, after which preventative measures or a maintenance treatment may be considered. Each specific case is individual and advice on a limit should be given during a consultation.

Q: WHAT SHOULD
I DO AFTER THE
TREATMENT?

JW: Give yourself a big pat on the back. You have taken a big step into really detoxifying your body and achieving maximum health and energy.

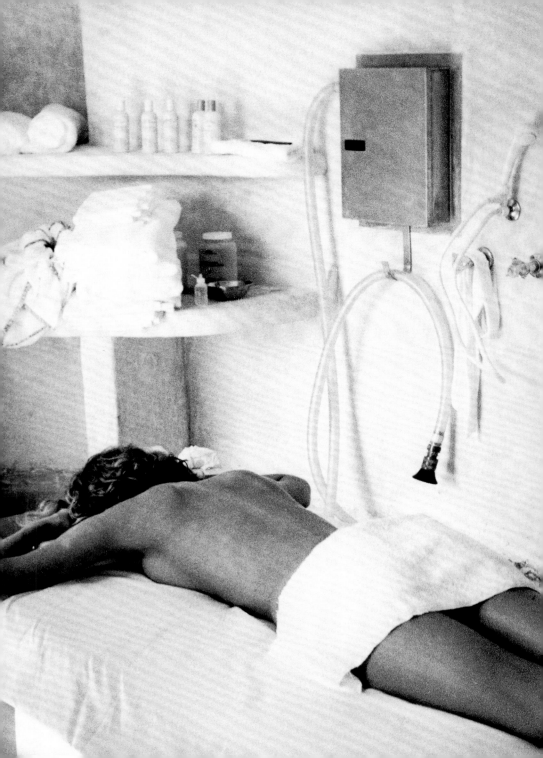

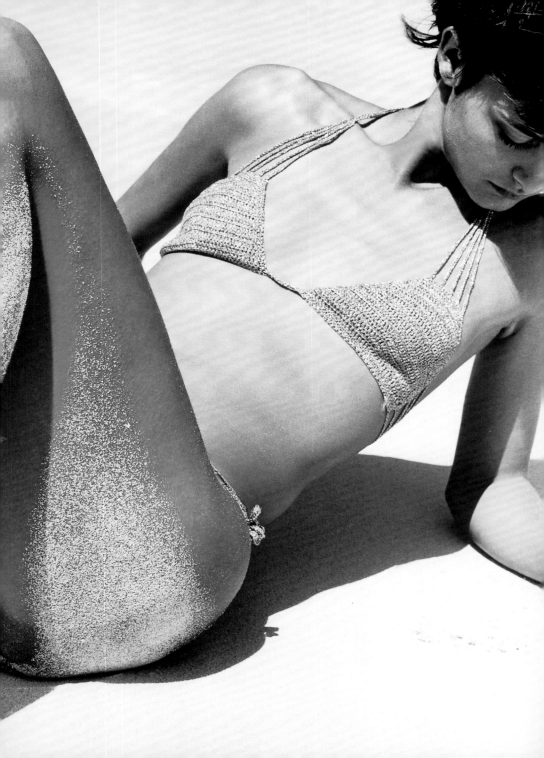

smooth skin

CLEANSE: Clean skin glows, but baths and showers — whether you use soap, gel or liquid cleanser — rob the skin of its natural moisture, so always use a lotion or body oil after either. Hydrotherapy is beneficial to maintaining an even skin tone, as well as stimulating your energy levels, blood and lymph circulation, nervous system and immune system. When you take a shower, simply alternate the temperature from hot (not scalding) to cold.

EXFOLIATE: Youthful skin renews itself every 28 days, but as we grow older this process slows down. Exfoliating once a week will help it to maintain this cycle of renewal, so the skin will have a smooth texture and even tone. A body exfoliator should have rougher granules than one formulated for the face. Those that contain sea salt work best. Work on the body zones where dry skin develops first, such as the knees, elbows and feet.

MOISTURIZE: A cleansing routine should be followed by moisturizing. Creams, oils and gels all work effectively. You may prefer an unperfumed moisturizer because scent can often irritate the skin. Always test a moisturizer before you make a purchase.

MAINTAIN: You are what you eat, drink and do. If your system is sluggish, the signs will show up as uneven skin tone or blemishes. A balanced diet, a hydrated system (dehydration can increase conditions like eczema or psoriasis, so if you are prone to these, drink approximately 2 litres/$3\frac{1}{2}$ pints of water a day) and regular exercise will ensure your system functions to its optimum potential.

HAIR REMOVAL

A regular chore for most women, hair removal can be particularly necessary after menopause and during pregnancy when hormonal changes can trigger an increase in hair growth. There are several methods and your choice depends on personal preference.

BLEACHING: This method works best for facial hair, forearms and body hair. Always adhere to the instructions that accompany a bleaching product when preparing the formula. For best results conduct a patch test by applying a sample 24 hours before your treatment. If you note any sensitivity or a rash develops, do not use it.

DEPILATION: This is a hair-removal treatment for the legs, arms and underarms, and should not be administered to the face. Depilation treatments are available as powders, gels, creams or sprays and work by dissolving the hair shaft. As the treatment does not affect the root of the hair, it will not prevent regrowth. The treatment takes 10 to 15 minutes, but if you normally shave, it could take longer. Repeated use weakens the hair and slows down regrowth. A patch test should be conducted before you proceed.

ELECTROLYSIS: Although expensive, this method is one of the most effective, especially for removing hair from the face or tender areas. A fine wire, steel or platinum needle is applied to the opening of a hair follicle. A 40-second low-voltage electric current transmits down the needle to destroy the papilla, loosening the hair shaft to allow for removal. While a slight burning sensation may be felt, the pain varies from person to person. Success depends on the therapist, so be sure to consult a reliable practitioner. Electrolysis is not a quick fix; several sessions may be necessary.

SHAVING: Quick and effective, shaving is probably the cheapest and most convenient way to remove hair from underarms and legs. Never shave on dry skin and always use a shaving foam, gel or lotion.

TWEEZING: Using tweezers is the best way to remove scattered hairs and hair from facial zones like the eyebrows. Before tweezing the eyebrows, wipe them with a cotton pad soaked in astringent.

WAXING: Once a layer of melted wax is applied to the skin, cooled and stripped off, hair is removed, skin is smooth and regrowth is often not noticeable for months. The bad news is that it can hurt, although how much depends on your pain threshold. Waxing can be done at home, but salon treatments are quicker and safer.

body zone problem areas

Certain areas of the body need more attention than others. A regular check-up with a doctor, plus an annual visit to a gynaecologist for a cervical smear, will ensure that the body is healthy. Listen to your body; notice the way it feels under pressure, such as during intense exercise or when suffering from a cold. Does your body bounce back? If minor aches and pains due to a tough session at the gym are gone in a day or if cold symptoms disappear rapidly, congratulate yourself. You are probably treating your body well by exercising regularly and effectively, eating the proper foods and drinking plenty of pure fluids.

If recovery takes far more time than it should, consult your doctor, then if his or her answer does not satisfy you, always seek a second opinion.

BONES

Osteoporosis affects many women worldwide. Osteopenia is a condition that develops when bone density is 10 to 25 per cent below optimum levels; when left untreated, it can lead to osteoporosis. A bone density test can help prevent osteoporosis by determining the health of the body's vital zones, such as the hips and spine. Taking some form of exercise on a regular basis, increasing consumption of calcium, avoiding stimulants such as caffeine and alcohol, and not smoking are all good preventive measures to consider. Maintaining a good posture can help to keep the body healthy, too. Slouching increases the risk of minor body ailments such as neck pain and headaches, so try to remember to stand straight. Standing tall projects a much more

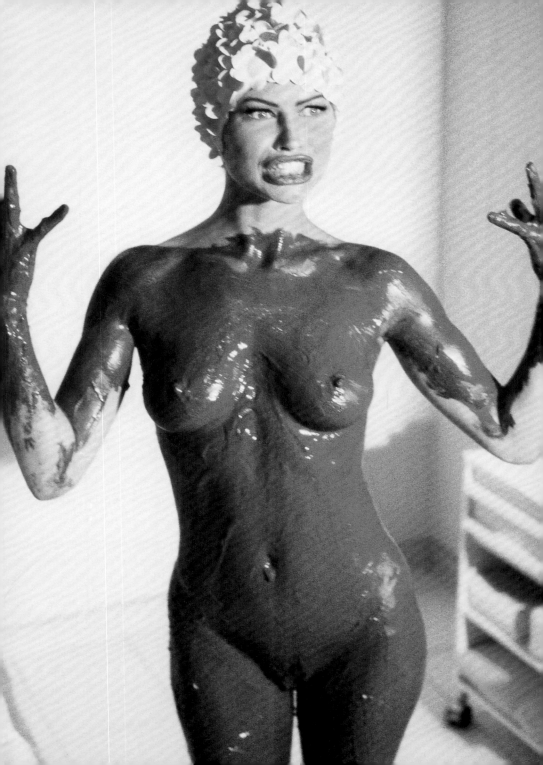

positive body language; in addition, posture studies reveal that men find women who stand up straight more appealing.

BREASTS

Approximately one in nine women in the UK and one in seven in the USA develops breast cancer. One-fifth of those women are under the age of 40. While nine out of ten breast lumps are actually benign, being 'breast aware' will help you to understand your body and alert you to any changes. Observe your breasts while you are in the bath, shower or in front of a mirror. Probe and press them with the tips of your first three fingers. Perform the examination throughout the month rather than simply monthly, and if you're over 50 or have a family history of breast cancer talk to your doctor about getting regular mammograms. If you are unsure, pick up a leaflet at a pharmacy.

CELLULITE

The thighs are probably a woman's least favourite body zone. 'Eighty per cent of women have cellulite,' says Noella Gabrielle, aromatherapist for Elemis, who believes that cellulite develops for a few main reasons. Stress is a huge factor, she claims. Processed food can take another part of the blame, as the body cannot eliminate it. Medical experts classify cellulite as being rippled, dimpled skin around the hips, buttocks and thigh area. They claim that cellulite is not a body disorder, but hereditary and that it starts to form on women after they reach puberty. Cellulite develops when the body's fat storage areas become blocked – due to ingesting toxins from sources such as nicotine, alcohol and caffeine. Once these storage areas are blocked, the skin above them stretches and an orange-peel effect develops. Although cellulite is commonly associated with women who are overweight, it is not linked to obesity. We all get cellulite, but an excessive amount should be a signal that you need to take more care of your body. No amount of massage or specifically blended cream can banish cellulite, but you can reduce it.

Approximately seven to eight weeks are needed to break down cellulite. There are three stages: break down, build up and smooth out. Break down involves body brushing, massaging the skin and introducing spirulina into the diet. For the build-up stage, use a skin-tightening cream and eat a healthy diet. Eliminate processed foods and toxins such as caffeine and alcohol.

EXERCISE: Cellulite is rare in female athletes because women who exercise frequently, whether or not they realize it, are preventing its formation. Exercise replaces body fat with muscle. It will prevent the fat cells from becoming blocked because exercise improves circulation and encourages the elimination of toxins. Activities that tone the hips, buttocks and thighs, such as swimming, walking, cycling and jogging, are all excellent ways to fight cellulite. Yoga and Pilates are also beneficial because they stimulate circulation and encourage elimination.

EXFOLIATION & CREAMS: To smooth the skin and revitalize the texture, exfoliate regularly. Massaging an exfoliator containing granules such as sea salt into the cellulite-prone zones can help to break up fatty deposits under the skin. Although a cream will not prevent cellulite, it will help to build up collagen and elastin, substances that encourage

the body's skin-firming cells. 'Don't scrub the skin,' Noella Gabrielle advises. 'Use a gel-based exfoliator containing a natural particle like phytoplankton. Exfoliate the elbows, knees, the feet and the bum. Exfoliation will activate the body's oil glands, which encourage the skin to moisturize.'

BODY BRUSHING: Most experts advise dry-skin brushing to restore cellulite-prone skin to its natural smooth texture. Work with a body brush made of natural fibres, such as horsehair. Using a long, stroking motion, brush along the backs of the legs, then concentrate around the thigh area, where cellulite is most pronounced. Apply circular strokes around the buttocks area.

MENSTRUAL CRAMPS

Exercise is one of the best ways to alleviate menstrual cramps, although if you are experiencing severe pain and bloating, doctors advise that it is better to give the body a rest. If symptoms persist, consult a gynaecologist. Cycling or a fast-paced walk — either outside or on a treadmill — will release endorphins, the feel-good chemicals in the body, thus elevating the mood and easing the

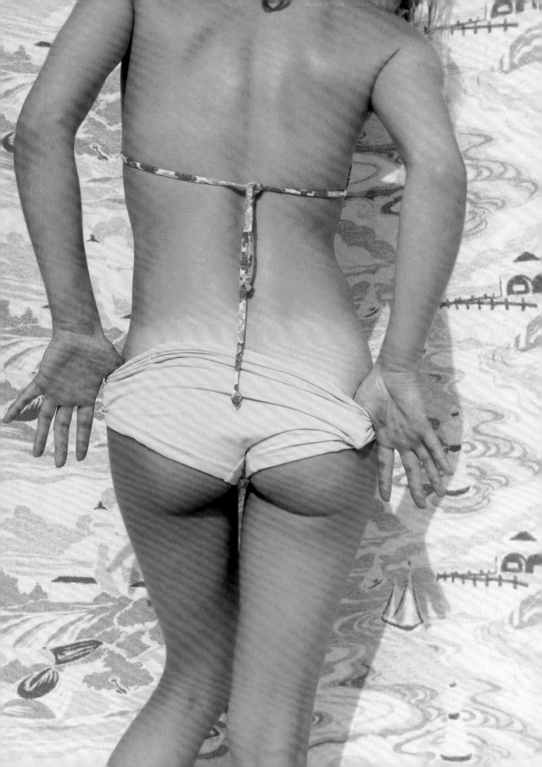

pain of cramps. Gynaecologists advise swimming because water pressure can help to reduce the bloating caused by water retention. Stretch-based exercises, such as Pilates and yoga, can also help relieve physical symptoms and control mood swings.

Aromatherapy is another option to consider. 'Menstrual cramps are often a result of congestion in the body,' says Noella Gabrielle. 'Cramps are a sign that the system is blocked. Blood is not flowing through the body as it should.' Clary sage oil can help to decongest the body. Three drops of the oil can be added to a bath. Alternatively, mix a few drops with the same amount of a carrier oil, such as evening primrose oil, then inhale the mixture or apply it to the stomach with smooth, gentle strokes.

VARICOSE VEINS

Surgery used to be the one fail-safe cure for varicose veins – those bulging, sometimes painful leg veins. The process requires general anaesthesia, incisions in the legs, knees and groin, as well as an overnight stay in the hospital. A newer procedure, endoluminal radiofrequency elimination (ERFE), is available in the USA and Europe, and is becoming popular as a faster and more effective method of treating the condition. It is less invasive and involves fewer complications. During this process a wire-like electrode-enhanced catheter is inserted into the troublesome vein and the resulting intense heat causes the vein to collapse. A local anaesthetic is used so patients can be treated as outpatients. There is no pain, nor are scars a side effect.

Varicose veins can be hereditary or the result of poor circulation. Noella Gabrielle recommends massaging the legs to encourage circulation. Start at the ankle and slowly move up the leg to the knee. Circulation will also be improved by relaxing in a warm bath that has been infused with ten drops of geranium and cypress oils. While in the bath, drink peppermint tea sweetened with honey.

HANDS

Today nail bars are as popular as coffee bars. Women who make time for manicures should not be considered vain. Not only do groomed nails

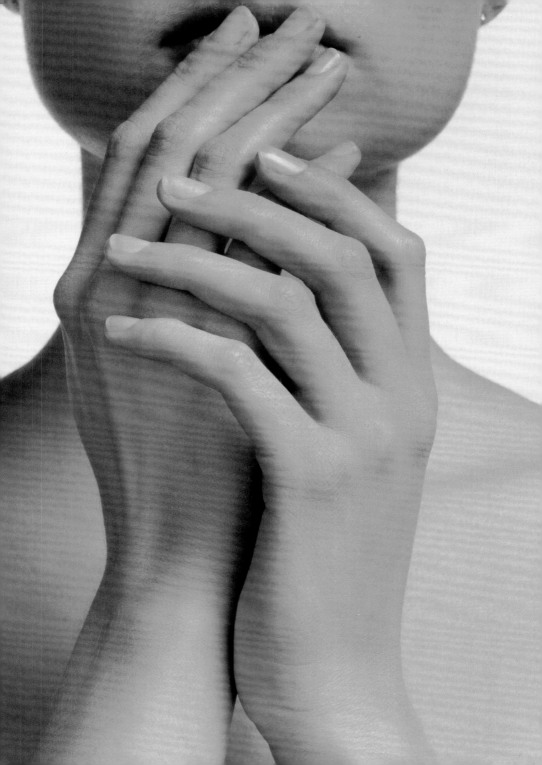

MANICURE KIT

A manicure does not have to be performed in a nail bar. At home, use a nail kit with all the right accessories to help keep both your nails and your hands healthy. The following tools should be included in it:

Nipper: This is a useful tool for trimming hangnails and should feature a pointed tip to enable a precise trim.

Nail brush: Use a nail brush in the morning and in the evening when cleaning the hands, nails and cuticles. Replace the brush when the bristles lose their density – before the bristles bend or break.

Nail scissors: Gentler on the nails, scissors are often preferred to clippers for ultimate precision.

Nail stone: A nail stone is a pumice that is shaped like a pencil. The stone will extract dead skin surrounding the cuticle area and on the surface of the nails.

White pencil: Gently drawing the pencil under damp nails will simulate the look of a French manicure.

Cuticle oil: Vitamin E-enriched oils and sweet almond oil, applied regularly, will condition the cuticle area and maintain it at optimum health.

Cuticle cream: Smoothing a specially blended cream around the cuticle zone will soften the area and prevent hangnails from developing.

Orangewood stick: Use an orangewood stick wrapped in a piece of cotton wool to push back the cuticles. To prevent yellow stains, dip a cotton wool-tipped stick in nail polish remover to extract excess polish. The orangewood stick can be used as an alternative to a nail brush to clean underneath the nails.

Emery boards: A coarsely grained, double-sided emery board works best to shorten or smooth the nails. Use a fine-grained version for the final smoothing.

Nail buffing stick: Used gently in a swift back-and-forth manner, this tool will smooth, shine and buff the nails to give an excellent finish.

Cuticle remover: The cream or gel remover formula will dissolve dead skin from the cuticle area, but should be applied sparingly and left on only for the recommended time.

look more appealing than unsightly uneven nails, but cared-for hands are also healthier. A regular manicure can also reduce the chance of nail afflictions. The nail guide below can help you solve problems before they become emergencies.

PROBLEM: SPLIT NAILS

Solution: Try to resist using your nails as a substitute for tools. Moisturize them as you would your skin. Rub sweet almond oil into the nails and on the fingers and toes before bed to help prevent splitting. Apply a vitamin E-enriched oil or cream onto the cuticles to keep the zone healthy and hydrated – this will also help to prevent painful and unsightly hangnails.

PROBLEM: THIN NAILS

Solution: Like good skin and thick hair, strong nails are a hereditary trait. Vitamin A and nail-strengthening supplements can help firm thin nails. Regular grooming, as well as brushing on a nail-strengthening formula, can also prevent breakage. Clippers can bend and break the nails, so use manicure scissors for trimming.

PROBLEM: RIDGES OR IRREGULARLY SHAPED NAILS

Solution: Irritating or injuring the bed of the nail can cause ridges. Buffing the nails smooths the surface and applying a ridge-filler can encourage them to form a more natural, smoother shape.

PROBLEM: YELLOW STAINS

Solution: Experimenting with nail colour, particularly dark shades, can leave light, yellowish stains on the surface. Before applying any colour, brush on a transparent base coat. Soaking clean nails in warm water and hydrogen peroxide will remove nail stains.

PROBLEM: FUNGUS

Solution: Poor hygiene can cause nail fungus to develop. Sterilize the tools in your nail kit using an anti-bacterial spray. Bring your own kit to a manicure if you are concerned about hygiene conditions. If a fungus problem is persistent, consult a dermatologist. Avoid biting the nails as this can increase the risk of infection.

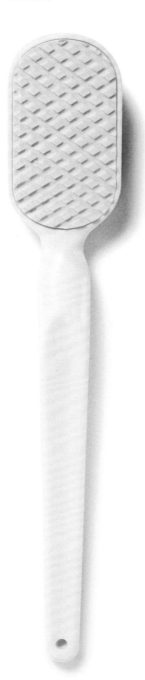

FEET

Women are four times as likely to suffer from foot problems as men. Why? For centuries we have insisted on wearing shoes that not only constrict, but also contort the foot into unnatural positions. Add to that the pressure we put on our feet daily: an average day of walking exerts the equivalent of several hundred tons of pressure. But there are simple, straightforward cures for common problems.

AILMENT: VERRUCA

Cause: A verruca or wart is a benign tumour, which could be caused by a virus that forms in a cut in the skin. The cut is often tiny and quite difficult to detect.

Solution: In time, some verrucas will vanish without any treatment, but others are more stubborn. Consult a pharmacist for an over-the-counter treatment. Those that work best contain salicylic acid. Alternatively, consult a chiropodist. If you are a keen swimmer or take showers in public places, wear shower sandals. Often, verrucas are picked up if you go barefoot in damp environments.

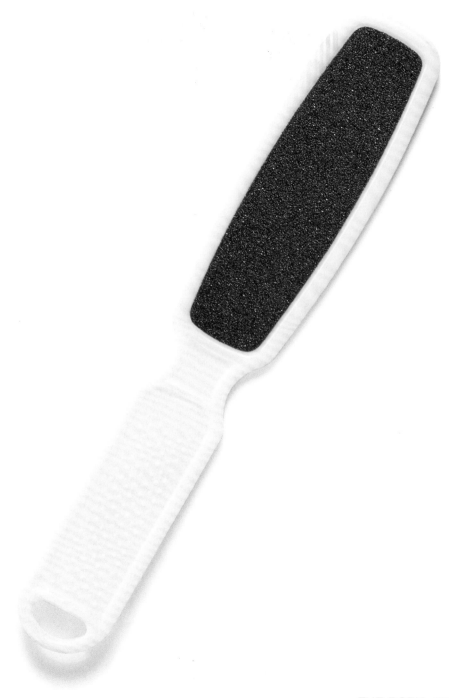

AILMENT: INGROWN TOENAIL

Cause: Ingrown toenails will result whenever a nail grows directly into the skin of a toe. Tight-fitting shoes, nail infections or even cutting the nail roughly using clippers or scissors can cause this problem. The surrounding skin can become inflamed, infected and very painful.

Solution: Always clip your toenails straight across and never cut them too short. If the nail starts to become painful or pus begins to build up, you need to consult a chiropodist or your doctor immediately.

AILMENT: BUNION

Cause: Bunions form as a tender bump at the joint nearest to the big toe. The two main causes of the condition are: hereditary factors or wearing tight or ill-fitting shoes.

Solution: If one of your parents suffered from bunions and you suspect you may also be prone to them, avoid wearing stilettos or any shoes with narrow or pointed toes. If necessary, a surgical procedure can be carried out to remove bunions.

AILMENT: CORNS

Cause: Corns are small layers of dead skin that have thickened and hardened due to pressure or fiction.

Solution: Footwear that is comfortable and also supportive can help to prevent corns, and should always be worn if corns start to develop. Avoid shaving or cutting corns away from the feet. They should be exfoliated and can also be thinned out by using a washcloth after a bath or shower. There are also many over-the-counter ointments and plasters available, but if problems persist, seek further advice from a chiropodist.

AILMENT: STRESS FRACTURE

Cause: Orthopaedic surgeons say that stress fractures tend to develop in women who are physically active, especially those performing a repetitive, high-impact activity, such as running or aerobics. Tiny fractures develop when more weight is placed on the bone than it can support.

Solution: Vary your routine by jogging one day, then doing yoga the next, for example. When building up endurance levels, do so slowly.

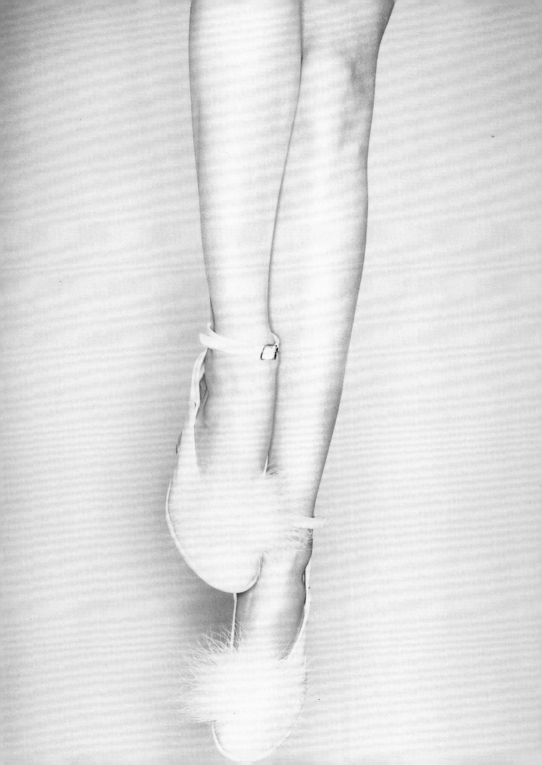

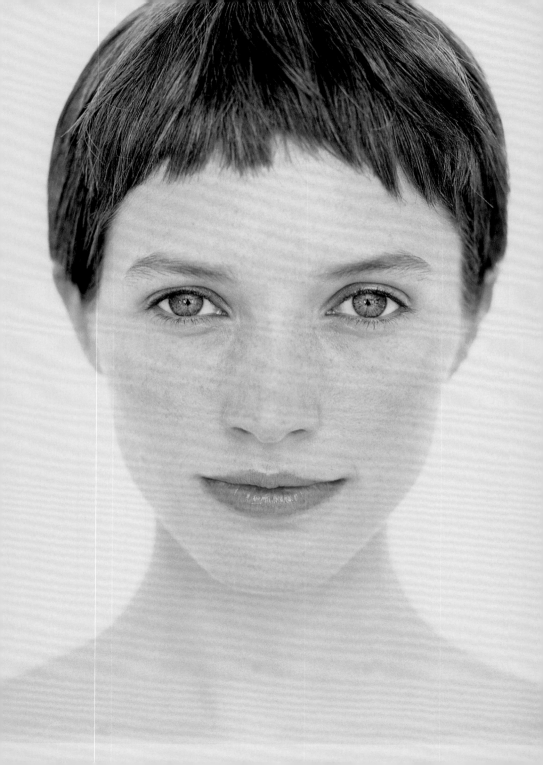

SKINCARE

The search for beautiful skin is universal, as, all too often, the appearance of skin defines our perception of others and ourselves. A rash, wrinkles, eczema, even one untimely blemish, can cause an astonishing degree of anguish because, let's face it, sometimes beauty is skin-deep. The good news is that you do have some degree of control over your skin, but how much control is up to you.

Skincare technology has moved forward in leaps and bounds over the last few years, allowing us to manipulate our skin in ways never before possible. Today mattifying agents can conceal oily skin, retinoids can literally erase the years and full-spectrum sunscreens signal the advent of the year-round porcelain complexion. While the twenty-first century demands nothing less, the proliferation of beauty products and sheer range of choice has led to increased awareness and, simultaneously, confusion when it comes to skin. Bathroom cabinets around the world are brimming with every kind of cream and corrector, and yet complaints and problems persist. Perhaps it is time to go back to basics: you may be fluent when it comes to translating the ingredients listed on every jar, but do you really listen to your skin? In ancient Eastern medicine it was understood that, like the pulse, the skin tells the story of the human condition. For this reason, taking time to understand your skin and the effects that lifestyle, diet, skincare routines and just plain old time can have on its appearance is paramount. Only then can you make informed choices and reap the benefits.

the facts

The skin is the body's largest organ. If we stepped out of our skin and put it on a set of scales, it would weigh just under 3 kg (6 lb). Its total surface area is almost 97,000 square cm (15,000 square in). Skin is dynamic and made up of cells and tissues. It is designed to act as a protective barrier against the environment and impedes the penetration of microorganisms. Skin absorbs and blocks radiation, as well as the shock of physical blows. It also acts as a thermostat. When the body needs to lose heat, the blood vessels dilate and sweat glands secrete moisture, which cools the body as it evaporates; when the body needs to conserve heat, the blood vessels constrict and the pores close. Skin secretes sebum and oil to protect its smooth surface. It reproduces young cells to replace old ones. Skin drinks, breathes, gives off carbon dioxide and, in short, lives. But unlike our internal organs, it ages right before our eyes. Fortunately, skin is magical in its ability to care for and repair itself. Our skin, with its scars, stretchmarks and laughter lines, tells the story of our lives. The skin is made up of multiple layers; the three most relevant to skincare are the epidermis, dermis and subcutaneous layer.

THE EPIDERMIS

The epidermis is the transparent top layer that covers the entire surface of the body. Numerous nerve endings that make the skin into one large sense organ, detecting warmth, cold, light, taste and touch, reside here. The epidermis is incredibly thin, about as thin as a piece of paper, and it is made up of five distinct cell layers. From top to bottom, they are: stratum corneum

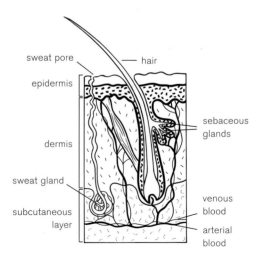

sweat pore

hair

epidermis

sebaceous glands

dermis

sweat gland

subcutaneous layer

venous blood

arterial blood

(horny cell layer); stratum lucidum (clear cell layer); stratum granulosum (granular cell layer); stratum spinosum (prickle cell or spinous cell layer); stratum germinativum (basal cell layer).

Basal cells make new skin cells called keratinocytes that continually push older cells towards the skin's surface. As the new cells move upwards, they become flat and scaly squamous cells. When cells reach the surface, they are composed primarily of keratin – the same protein that makes up hair and nails. These cells remain briefly on the skin's surface, then flake off in a process called desquamation. It takes about a month for a newly formed skin cell to reach the surface and slough off. At the bottom layer are melanocytes, the cells responsible for producing the melanin that gives skin colour. A person's natural colour and ability to tan is dependent on melanocyte activity. Also present in the epidermis are Langerhans cells that provide immune protection from bacteria, viruses and cancer.

THE DERMIS

The dermis is 20 to 40 times thicker than the epidermis. Collagen and elastin fibres that contribute to the skin's appearance, plumpness and firmness are found here. This skin layer provides a flexible support structure and encloses blood vessels, nerves, and skin appendages, such as sweat glands, hair follicles and sebaceous glands. Blood vessels in the dermis provide nutrition for the skin, maintain body temperature, and provide white blood cells that circulate to defend against infection and foreign substances. Sebaceous glands are located deep in the dermis and they secrete sebum, which lubricates the skin. Normal functioning of the sweat and sebaceous glands is essential for well-balanced skin. Together, these glands provide the 'acid mantle', a natural film that protects the skin from outside attack.

THE SUBCUTANEOUS LAYER

The subcutaneous layer is a layer of fat that lies beneath the dermis and acts as an insulator and shock absorber. These tissues also store energy in the form of calories as a reserve nutritional source. The thickness of the subcutaneous fat varies from body area to body area, tending to be thickest at the waist and practically nonexistent at the eyelids.

skin types

Your skin is constantly changing. Not only does it alter with the passage of time but also with hormonal, dietary and environmental changes. So while it is important to know your skin in order to care for it properly, you must also appreciate that your particular skin 'type' is also dynamic and may change at any time throughout your life. Even more important than knowing your 'type' is to recognize the appearance, complaints and causes of 'dry', 'sensitive', 'oily' and 'combination' skin and learn how to treat and remedy the skin accordingly.

DRY SKIN

For the skin to look normal and healthy, water content in the upper layer of the epidermis, the stratum corneum, should be above 10 per cent. Water constantly evaporates through skin into the air at a rate of about 600 ml (1 pint) per day. The evaporation may vary depending on genetics, climate and age. When water is lost faster than it can be replaced by underlying tissue, the outer layer of skin can dry out.

If you are dehydrated, then your skin will also be dry; if you have normal hydration, then additional water will not help your skin any more. To remedy dehydration, drink plenty of water. If you have a centrally heated or air-conditioned home or office, then investing in a humidifier will slow down the evaporation of water from your skin. Dry skin may feel tight and itchy, and look flaky and dull.

OILY SKIN

All healthy skin produces sebum, a natural oil that moisturizes the skin. Oily skin is a result of overactive sebaceous glands and can lead to spots and acne if the pores become blocked. Excessive sebum production can be a result of stress, hormonal disorders or a genetic predisposition.

COMBINATION SKIN

This is a term developed by cosmetic companies and not by dermatologists. All skin is effectively combination skin, as the T-zone (the central face, forehead and chin) is always oilier than other parts of the face. No one product has yet been developed that can moisturize one area of the face while absorbing oil from another, so products for 'combination skin' are meaningless. If necessary, treat the oily and dry parts separately.

SENSITIVE SKIN

Like combination skin, everyone has sensitive skin in that we are potentially reactive to cosmetics, pollution or sunlight. Sensitivity levels can also fluctuate depending on internal and external factors. Skin may appear red, irritated and uneven or patchy.

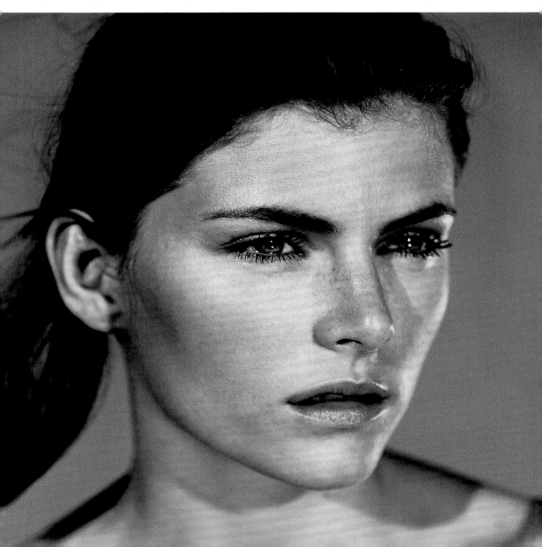

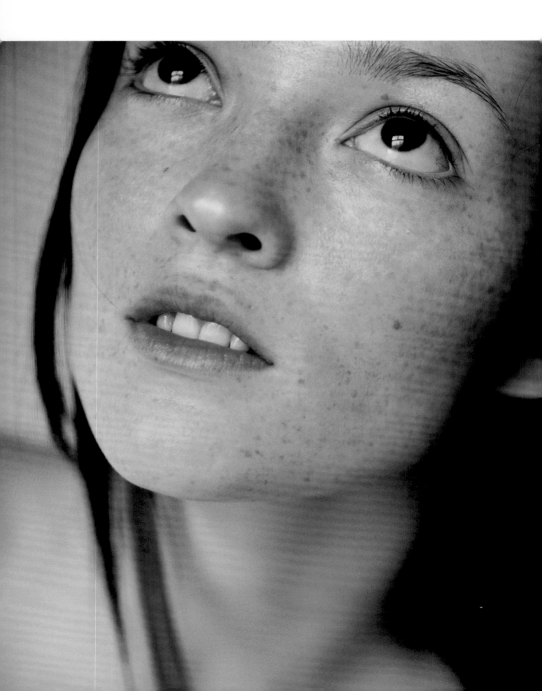

the ins & outs
of skin

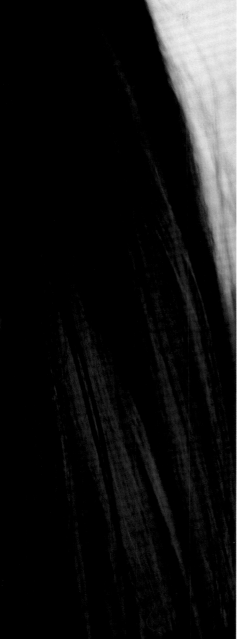

The appearance and health of skin, while largely determined by genes, are not immune to internal or external forces. A prime example of how the environment affects the skin is illustrated by the fact that Australia, with a population of fair-skinned people, has the highest incidence of skin cancer in the world. Other influential factors are diet, mood and hormones. Depression and anxiety are associated with psoriasis flare-ups, while acne break-outs around menstruation are par for the course.

THE ENVIRONMENT

Skin is greatly affected by external factors. Excessive exposure to ultraviolet (UV) rays leads to sun damage, broken blood vessels and a leathery, dry appearance. Cold weather creates windburn and broken blood vessels, and dry weather contributes to dry, flaky skin. Premature ageing has nothing to do with dryness, but is a result of sun exposure. Cigarette smoke and chemicals in the air all

FREE RADICALS & ANTIOXIDANTS

Free radicals are unstable high-energy molecules that attack cells in our bodies, damaging the DNA, proteins and fats within them on a daily basis. It is believed that the damage caused by free radicals is cumulative and leads to the physical deterioration we call ageing. In response to these attacks, our bodies call upon antioxidants, or free-radical scavengers, to repair the damage – with a 99 per cent success rate, according to research. Supplementation of antioxidants through consuming 5–8 servings of fruits and vegetables a day or by taking vitamins is a good idea and can help fight free-radical damage, assist healing and make skin appear younger. The most powerful antioxidants are vitamins A, B, C and E and essential fatty acids.

deprive skin of oxygen and generate harmful free radicals.

NUTRITION

When it comes to 'feeding' the skin, an unusual rule applies: it is both what you eat and how you eat it. The facialist Ole Henrikson refers to the skin as 'the third kidney' and facialist Eve Lom refers to it as 'the body's waste disposal' because of the skin's function as an elimination system. An interesting analogy, but while doctors unanimously concur that a diet low in saturated fats is important for the maintenance of a healthy heart, they generally dismiss processed and devitalized foods as having zero

negative effect on another vital organ, the skin. Some dermatologists argue that eating greasy food like french fries with your fingers and then rubbing the face is the cause of break-outs, not the actual ingestion of the greasy food. As for chocolate, Marcia Kilgore, facialist and founder of the Bliss spa in New York City, believes that a lot of women crave sweets when their hormones are fluctuating, a time when they would naturally tend to break out anyway.

Each person reacts differently to foods, but eating well is critical for healthy skin. A diet rich in vitamins and fibre helps skin repair itself and the most important vitamins are A, B, C and E – all of which are antioxidants. Vitamin A helps skin cells develop normally and gives skin its structural integrity. It stimulates immune activity, helps fight infection and reduces the damage caused by environmental pollutants. Lack of vitamin A results in rough, dry and scaly skin. Since vitamin A is stored in the body and not secreted, toxicity can occur from overdosing. Dry skin is a feature of insufficient vitamin E, which is also known as tocopherol, and vitamin B, particularly niacin. Vitamin C is another excellent antioxidant, especially in terms of ultraviolet radiation. Vitamin C is needed for healing wounds, as it enables the production of enzymes that stabilize collagen fibres. A shortage of the vitamin can compromise collagen production. Excessive alcohol consumption robs skin of nutrients and dilates the facial blood vessels, putting a strain on the collagen and elastin supporting the dermis. Eventually the blood vessels are no longer able to resist the pressure and dilated capillaries become apparent on the cheeks and the sides of the nose. Sufficient daily water intake is vital to keep skin hydrated from within and replace the moisture lost through evaporation.

HORMONES

Hormones are probably our worst enemy, as we only really notice them when they are badly out of balance and we can do little to regulate them. In teenagers hormonal changes are responsible for an increase in sebum production, which often leads to mild or severe cases of acne. When a woman goes through menopause, decreased oestrogen production causes the skin to lose some of its plumpness and tone. The monthly hormonal surge in women causes those big 'under-the-skin bulges' and pregnant women often suffer from acne break-outs during the first trimester of pregnancy.

High stress levels or an inadequate amount of sleep can also lead to a number of hormonal disruptions. Marcia Kilgore, of Bliss spa, says: 'I recommend staying as stress-free as possible. I always ask my clients, "What's the worst-case scenario here?", whereupon they realize that anyone forking out for a facial really doesn't have it all that bad. A reality check now and then is never bad for the hormones.'

ACNE

Close to 100 per cent of people have the occasional spot. Most are able to manage acne with non-prescription over-the-counter treatments. For some, however, acne is more serious. Acne usually starts between the ages of 10 and 13, and lasts for five to ten years; however, it can persist into the late 20s, 30s or even beyond. Some people get acne for the first time as adults. Acne is a disease of the sebaceous hair follicles. Under normal circumstances, sebum travels up the hair follicle and out to the skin's surface. In acne, however, the sebum is trapped within the follicle. Acne develops on those areas where sebaceous glands are most numerous: the face, scalp, neck, chest, back, upper arms and shoulders. Blackheads are called comedones. Red, swollen, pus-filled lesions are called papules, nodules and pustules. Four basic factors work together for the development of acne: hormones (androgens); increased sebum production; changes inside the follicle; and bacteria (specifically *Propionibacterium acnes*).

TREATING ACNE

There are many cleansers and other products widely available and advertised for acne. Most special cleansers are unnecessary if the acne is being treated properly with a medicated topical preparation and some may even aggravate acne. Benzoyl peroxide works by destroying the bacteria associated with acne. It must be used continuously as it does not affect sebum production or the way skin follicle cells are shed. Salicylic acid, a beta-hydroxy acid, helps correct abnormal shedding of cells. For milder acne, salicylic acid helps unclog pores to resolve and prevent lesions. It does not affect *Propionibacterium acnes* or sebum production, so its effects stop when you stop using it.

POMADE ACNE

It is a phenomenon: greasy hair products like pomade and wax can leak down onto the face during the day and cause acne. If you have regular break-outs around the hairline and forehead, consider changing your hair products.

SCARRING

Scarring occurs because the skin responds to acne by trying to repair itself. The process can produce a scar that looks like a pit in the skin. But not every mark left on the skin by acne is a scar and scarring can sometimes be avoided when acne is treated and cleared. There are several methods available now that minimize scarring (see Cosmetic Dermatology, pages 134–51).

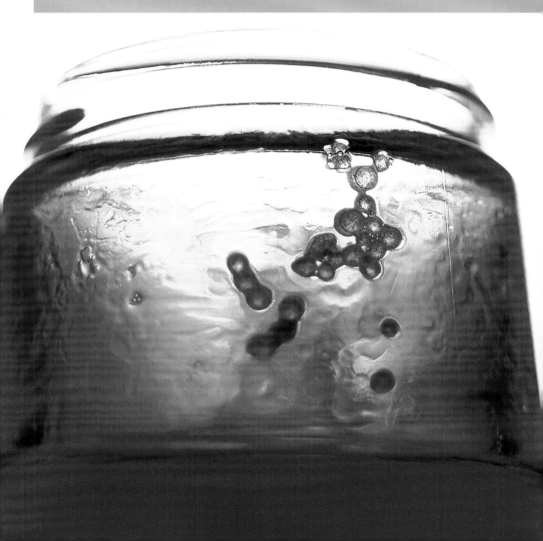

SKIN COMPLAINTS & POSSIBLE CAUSES

COMPLAINT	EXTERNAL CAUSES
Dryness	Dry weather or a lack of moisture in the air; dehydration
Redness	Windburn or sunburn
Oiliness	Humid climate

Antibiotics work by clearing the skin of *Propionibacterium acnes* and may be used topically or taken systemically (orally). Topical antibiotics are limited in their ability to penetrate the skin and clear more deep-seated *Propionibacterium acnes*, whereas systemic antibiotics circulate throughout the body and into sebaceous glands. Systemic antibiotics often cause more side effects than topical treatments, but they can be used for more severe cases. They should not be used during pregnancy, and some may reduce the effectiveness of oral contraception pills. Retinoid preparations, vitamin A derivatives, help unclog pores to clear up moderate-to-severe acne by normalizing the way the skin grows and sheds. Oral retinoids (roaccutane) reduce sebum output, improve the shedding of skin and reduce the spread of *Propionibacterium acnes*. It is the only medication that intervenes in all the causes of acne. Although the product can have long-lasting results, it can cause significant side

INTERNAL CAUSES	ADDITIONAL CAUSES
A genetic propensity to dryness or eczema; a diet lacking in nutrients; ageing	Fragranced products and soaps; excessive washing
Inflammation of the skin; an underlying disease, such as acne rosacea	Steam or heat can cause flushing; products that irritate can cause a red, scaly rash
Hormones; overactive sebaceous glands; stress; a genetic predisposition; the T-zone naturally tends to be oilier	Products that are too emollient

effects, including depression. It has also been shown to cause birth defects if taken during pregnancy. Past treatment has no effect on future pregnancies, but a woman who believes she may become pregnant should not use the drug. A person taking oral retinoids should follow the dermatologist's directions and never underestimate their strength.

Oral contraceptives may also help to counteract the effect of male hormones (androgens) on acne. But because the pills include female hormones, their use is strictly limited to female patients. In the USA the Food and Drug Administration (FDA) has approved Ortho-Tri-Cyclen to treat acne, and in the UK doctors can prescribe Dianette. Be aware that some brands of pills contain androgen, the hormone that causes acne, and that the contraceptive pill carries its own health risks. Other medications for the treatment of acne include anti-inflammatories called corticosteroids, which may be injected by a dermatologist into inflamed lesions to aid healing.

AGEING

You can fight it as much as you like, but unfortunately, whatever you do, it is inevitable that you will age. How well you age, however, is something that you may have some control over if you understand the process itself. Skin ages by two biologically independent processes: intrinsic and extrinsic. Intrinsic ageing refers to the changes that result from the passing of time and it occurs at a genetically predetermined rate. Extrinsic ageing refers to changes caused by exposure to the elements and pollution, some of which you have more control over than others. Damage caused by exposure to the sun (photo-ageing) accounts for most of this type of ageing. There are actions we can take to help reduce the effects of extrinsic ageing, such as wearing sunscreen, staying away from cigarette smoke and environmental toxins, and using only gentle skincare products, but intrinsic ageing is inescapable. The effects of ageing on the skin are:

DRYNESS: The production of sebum drops significantly as your skin ages. Increased exposure to ultraviolet damage from sunlight means that the melanocytes become weaker and fewer. This in turn causes uneven pigmentation, such as age spots, and reduces the skin's ability to protect itself from the harmful and damaging effects of the sun.

THINNING OF THE SKIN: The dermis and subcutaneous layers begin to thin, leading to sagging skin. Loss of fat in the subcutaneous layer also leaves the skin more fragile.

LOSS OF FIRMNESS: As the years go by, the fibroblast cells in the dermis that replenish the skin's collagen and elastin slowly cease functioning, resulting in loss of elasticity.

DIMINISHED IMMUNE RESPONSE: A drop in the number of Langerhans cells in the epidermis layer of the skin leads to a corresponding drop in the skin's immune system, lowering its defence against viruses and bacteria.

DIMINISHED ABILITY TO REPAIR DAMAGE: The skin's ability to repair free-radical damage is reduced over time.

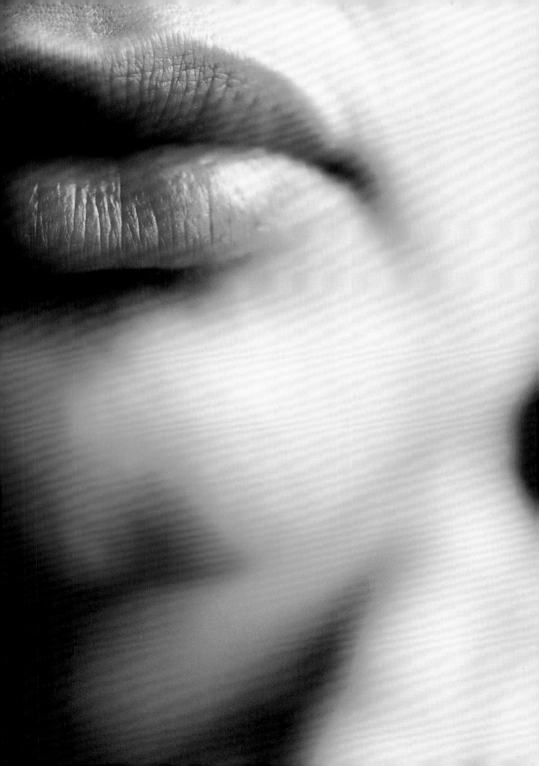

WRINKLES

Wrinkles are big business. Facialist Eve Lom estimates that 99 per cent of her clients are primarily concerned with facial wrinkles. Wrinkle creams are in no short supply on cosmetic counters, though few things applied topically have any effect. Wrinkles are a result of scarred and damaged collagen, a process that occurs naturally as a result of ageing. Applying collagen on top of the skin will not do anything for wrinkles, but all is not lost.

If ageing gracefully is not your style or you feel you are looking old before your time, there are now several anti-wrinkle options that have undergone studies for safety and effectiveness. Two of these are Renova and the CO_2 and YAG lasers, both of which have been approved by the Food and Drug Administration (FDA) in the USA for treating signs of sun-damaged or ageing skin.

Retinova or Renova (tretinoin cream): This vitamin A derivative, available by prescription only, can reduce the appearance of fine lines and wrinkles, mottled darkened spots and roughness of facial skin (see also pages 113–14).

Carbon dioxide (CO_2) and Erbium (YAG) lasers: Laser resurfacing involves the layer-by-layer removal of facial skin. A doctor in an outpatient surgical clinic performs the treatment under anaesthesia (see also pages 143 and 145–7).

Oestrogen and testosterone: Recent research has shown that the levels of oestrogen in women and testosterone in men may influence some of the visible effects of ageing. The levels of these hormones decrease over time, possibly resulting in the thinning of the skin as well as the decreased growth of body hair. Anti-androgens, available in systemic and topical formulations, help maintain the level of androgens circulating throughout the body. In a small, unpublished study of Ethocyn, one such topical formulation, elastic tissue, was found to increase over 50 per cent in aged facial and wrist surface skin.

caring for
your skin

In an ideal world, without dehydrating central heating or ultraviolet radiation, we would have great skin all the time and never need to think about 'skincare' or buy a single product. In reality we need to reach an achievable level of happiness with our skin.

Like all of our organs, skin can use a helping hand. The best thing you can do for your skin is nourish it from the inside with good nutrition (see pages 96–7) and protect it on the outside with a full-spectrum sunscreen. The worst thing you can do is to continually interfere with your skin by assaulting it with a gamut of products that have either no effect, or worse, a negative one. Skin performs its job extraordinarily well — on the whole. The purpose of skincare products should be to promote, aid and supplement the skin's natural function — not replace it. When it comes to healthy, beautiful skin, the fewer products the better.

THE RULES OF
SUCCESSFUL SKINCARE

1 Knowledge — educate yourself. If you understand your skin and how it functions, you will make more informed skincare decisions and achieve better results.

2 Realism — face the facts and do not expect anything more than your personal best. You will never look like you did 20 years ago, or indeed, like an entirely different person — Christy Turlington, for example. Good skin requires commitment, so be honest about the level you can maintain. Understanding your own habits and lifestyle is essential. Do not buy products or adopt a skincare routine that requires more time than you are willing to take or are capable of giving.

3 Holism — health and beauty are inextricably linked. You cannot lead an unhealthy lifestyle and expect your skin to look good. Diet, exercise, bad habits like smoking and drinking, and the environment must be taken into account.

4 Patience – Rome was not built in a day and damaged skin needs time to repair. Maintain a routine to get the best from it.

CLEANSING

Washing your face is refreshing and beneficial. However, too much cleansing, even with just water, can wash away the skin's naturally produced oils and cause dry, itchy and irritated skin. Choosing the right cleanser for your skin is, therefore, the first important step in a daily skincare routine.

THE SOAP VERSUS SOAP-FREE DEBATE: WHICH SHOULD YOU USE?

Soaps contain surfactants that allow oil and water to mix so that sebum can be rinsed off the skin. Too much surfactant can irritate the skin and cause dryness. Despite the notion that soap strips all oils from the skin, many soaps contain lards and fats that can leave oil on the skin and block pores. Soap is alkaline with a pH of about 8; skin is slightly acidic with a pH of 5.5. Soap, therefore, changes the composition of good bacterial flora and the activity of enzymes in the upper epidermis. In addition, soaps do not remove make-up very well. Those with very oily skin may like using soap, but if your skin still feels tight and dry an hour after washing, you should use a gentler product.

Although synthetic detergents or soap-free cleansers may not sound very

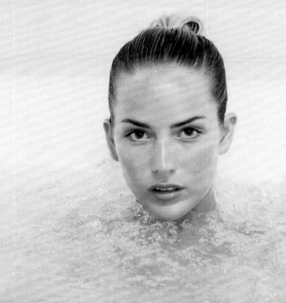

appealing, they are kind on the skin and effective at removing make-up, excess oil and dirt. Their pH is closer to that of the skin and they seldom leave the skin feeling as tight and dry as soap does. It is even better to use a cleanser that is water-soluble, since rinsing a cleanser off with water is gentler on the skin than rubbing it with tissues or cotton wool. Furthermore, if you stop using cold cream or a creamy make-up remover, you will no longer need to use toner or astringent to wipe off the residue. For extremely dry skin, wipe-off cleansers or oils leave the skin feeling supple. However, the residue could block pores and a 'refreshing' toner or astringent may dry out skin even more.

ACNE SOAPS: These types of soaps contain strong drying ingredients, such as sulphur and benzoyl peroxide, and such exfoliants as salicylic acid. They can cause skin irritation.

SUPERFATTED SOAPS: These include 'fatty' substances like cocoa butter, lanolin, paraffin and added moisturizers. Although less drying than regular soaps, they are inclined to leave behind a residue and block pores.

TRANSPARENT SOAPS: These contain fats and glycerine which is a humectant. They are less drying but do not lather very well and tend to melt quickly. Transparent soaps can also leave a residue and block pores.

SOAP-FREE CLEANSERS: These contain synthetic detergents and may or may not lather. Although they do not remove oil as effectively as soaps, soap-free cleansers do remove dirt and make-up well. They are suitable for sensitive skins, since they are very gentle.

CLEANSING MILKS & CREAMS: Cleansing milks and creams are based on water and oil emulsions, which makes them heavier than water-soluble cleansers and therefore more difficult to remove. They remove make-up effectively and are not drying, but they may leave a greasy residue that blocks pores. For this reason it is advisable to use a toner or astringent afterwards.

CLEANSING OILS: Containing mineral or vegetable oil, these are heavy and oily cleansers. They remove make-up well but leave behind an oily film on the skin that can block pores.

EXFOLIATION

There is a lot to be said for exfoliation, as it can alleviate the problems of both dry and oily skin. By removing the top layer of dead skin, dry skin appears less dull and flaky, and oily skin will not have as many blocked pores and spots. Moderation, however, is the key. The top stratum corneum layer defends the skin, so skin should not be completely stripped and left exposed and raw. There are several ways to exfoliate the skin. Physical exfoliants, such as sponges, brushes, washcloths and pads, are generally too abrasive and provide a breeding ground for bacteria. Facial scrubs can contain natural abrasives, such as ground apricot pits and walnut kernels, or synthetic particles.

The synthetic option is the best because the particles are smooth and spherical, and will not cut or scratch the skin. Formulations containing alpha-hydroxy acids (AHAs) dissolve the protein bonds that bind dead skin cells together, thus allowing cells to be shed. This is the best way to exfoliate if you do not find AHAs too irritating, as the acid concentration, and hence the level of exfoliation, can be controlled.

TONERS & ASTRINGENTS

Unless you have very oily skin or use a cleansing oil, milk or cold cream, there is little need for a toner or astringent. Skin does not need to be 'toned'. Toners can be refreshing and smell pleasant but they are basically a dressed-up alternative to water for removing excess oil. Unlike water, however, they can also irritate and dry the skin. Toners, astringents, clarifying lotions, refreshing mists, and so on, all contain solvents, such as alcohol, witch hazel, resorcinol, salicylic acid or propylene glycol, which essentially remove oil from the skin's surface. They cannot affect the production of sebum, nor can they shrink pores. There are very few dermatologists who recommend these products. If you cannot live without a toner, choose one that does not contain alcohol or witch hazel.

MOISTURIZERS

Cosmetic companies would have us believe the very life of our skin is dependent on our moisturizer. This is simply not true. Skin should have a moist appearance. If you have dry patches, apply moisturizer only to those parts. If your skin feels fine in the summer

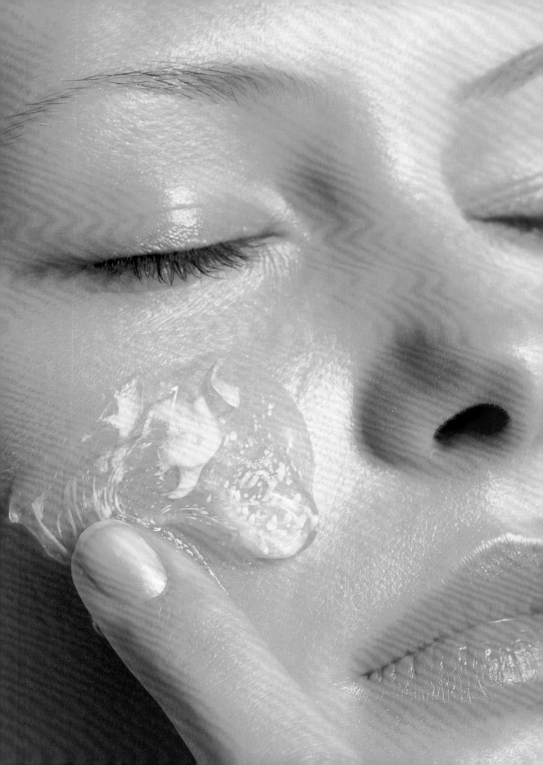

months but dry in the winter, only use moisturizer in the winter. There are no hard and fast rules, so use your own judgement and do not worry – failing to use a moisturizer will not cause wrinkles! Moisturizers are available in oil-based and oil-free forms, so choose one to suit your skin type.

OIL-IN-WATER & WATER-IN-OIL EMULSIONS

These contain five main oils: vegetable, animal, mineral, silicone and vitamin E. Vegetable oils include jojoba, olive, soy, almond, avocado and wheat germ, to name a few, and many can be absorbed through the epidermis. Animal oils include fish oils, lanolin and such lipids as cholesterol and can be absorbed into the skin. Mineral oils, derived from petroleum, are heavy and stay on the skin's surface to provide a barrier against water loss. Silicone oils, derived from sand or rock, are lighter than mineral oils but have the same effect. Vitamin E, known as tocopherol, is also a good moisturizing oil but it cannot nourish skin topically as well as it can systemically. Do not open vitamin E capsules and use them on the skin. They often contain other oils, such as mineral, palm or coconut oils, that may cause break-outs.

OIL-FREE HUMECTANTS

Humectants, such as hyaluronic acid, squalene, urea and glycerine, attract moisture from the air and form a water-binding film on the surface of the skin.

MASKS

Face masks are more of a luxury than a necessity. Masks can act as an exfoliant, a moisturizer, a cleanser or a cooling skin-soother. Separate products formulated specifically for these purposes could probably perform the actions more efficiently, but masks are a relaxing means to an end. The most important considerations to keep in mind when choosing a mask are:

1 Choose a mask formulated for your skin type. A clay mask could further dry out and irritate dry skin, while a moisturizing mask could aggravate acne-prone skin.

2 A mask that stings should be removed immediately.

3 A twice-monthly mask application is usually sufficient.

LIPOSOMES

These are microscopic sacs that allow a cream's active ingredients to penetrate the skin more efficiently by sustaining the release of water-soluble chemicals and other water-binding agents. Liposomes are good, but it is what is in the liposomes that counts. If the active ingredient is irritating, you do not want more efficient penetration. Make your decision about a cream on its active ingredients, not the delivery system.

THE EYES & NECK

Skin around the eyes and on the neck is thinner than on the face. As it has fewer sebaceous glands, it could need extra moisturizing. Those with oily skin may even wish to use a moisturizer on the eyes and neck, if not anywhere else. The skin around the eyes is also a little more sensitive so you might not want to use alpha-hydroxy acids, beta-hydroxy acids, retinoids or other irritating ingredients on this area unless they are specifically formulated for such use. To avoid irritating the eyes, be sure to use a fragrance-free product.

NATURAL VERSUS CHEMICAL INGREDIENTS

Despite the popular opinion that natural is always best, this is not necessarily true with skincare. Natural ingredients tend to be either foodstuffs that need to be preserved or botanicals that can irritate the skin or cause allergic reactions. Chemical formulations have the advantage of extensive research followed by rigorous testing. Ironically, those with sensitive skin should stick to lab-tested and dermatologist-prescribed products.

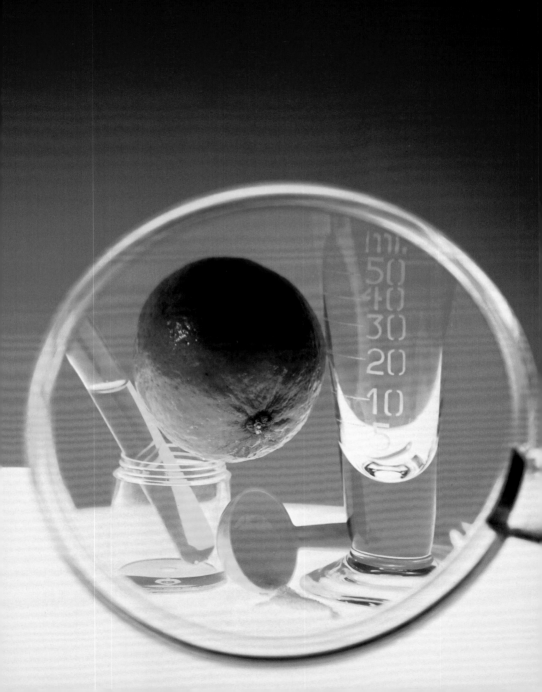

miracles in a jar

Moisturizers no longer just moisturize: they multitask, performing several different functions at the same time. While searching for a suitable moisturizer, consider whether you would like any of the following ingredients included in the formula.

RETINOIDS (VITAMIN A DERIVATIVES)

These include tretinoin (Renova, Retin-A, Retinova and Avita), retinol and retinyl palmitate. Vitamin A creams have been shown to have a truly amazing effect on the skin. Topical application speeds up cell activity and unclogs pores, allowing sebum to flow freely up towards the skin's surface.

Tretinoins are used primarily to treat oily, acne-prone skin; however, some patients treated with topical tretinoin have also shown improvement in skin texture, wrinkling, pigmentation and sallowness. This is because vitamin A improves the skin's structure and increases collagen production. Recent data suggests that tretinoin may even prevent damage to skin's collagen and elastin fillers that occurs during sun exposure. Topical tretinoin also appears to reverse the chronological ageing process at the cellular level by altering protein production and growth kinetics. If you have sun damage and fine wrinkles, tretinoin is a highly effective treatment, but needs to be prescribed by a dermatologist and visible results can take up to six months. Retinol cream is weaker than tretinoin cream and is available without prescription. It can also reduce fine lines and skin discoloration, but to a lesser extent.

There are a few side effects. Most people experience a stinging sensation on applying retinoid creams, but this should only last a few seconds. Skin may appear flaky and dry for the first few weeks of use but this too should subside. When using retinoids, skin may become photosensitive, so the creams are best used at night and sunscreen is necessary during the day. Because vitamin A impairs the skin's wound-healing process, no one using tretinoins or isotretinoins should undertake any kind of body waxing, dermabrasion or laser resurfacing.

ALPHA-LIPOIC ACID

Alpha-lipoic acid is a powerful antioxidant and anti-inflammatory that occurs naturally within the body's cells. Currently the most powerful antioxidant we know of, alpha-lipoic acid is both water- and lipid-soluble, making it able to fight free radicals in any part of a cell and even enter the space between cells. It is also the only known antioxidant that can increase a cell's metabolism, boosting its energy production and capacity to heal. Alpha-lipoic acid is highly effective at reducing edema (under-eye puffiness), so it makes an excellent addition to eye creams.

ALPHA-HYDROXY
ACIDS (AHAS)

These include: glycolic acid, derived from sugar cane; lactic acid, derived from tomatoes and sour milk; malic acid, derived from apples; tartaric acid, derived from grapes

and wine; and citric acid, derived from citrus fruits. Although traditionally based on natural acids, synthetic acids are now being manufactured, too.

Alpha-hydroxy acid acts as a mild exfoliant and produces a slight stinging sensation on the skin. It penetrates the stratum corneum and dissolves protein bonds that hold the skin cells together. The dead cells are then shed, which increases cell turnover and allows healthy new cells to come to the surface. The process gives skin a healthier

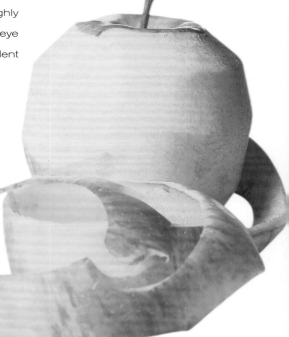

appearance, improves its texture and colour, and unclogs pores, thereby decreasing the build-up of blackheads and spots. Long-term AHA use has been shown to prevent skin irritation and increase the skin's moisture-retaining abilities. The effects are seen immediately but once you stop using AHAs, all the benefits stop, too. At high concentrations of 25 per cent, AHAs increase epidermal thickness, improve elastin fibre quality and increase the density of collagen. AHAs are water-soluble, so they work well in products like facial washes. AHA moisturizers can be worn during the day or night. In many cases, however, AHAs can cause irritation, especially to sensitive skins. Wearing sunscreen when using AHAs is vital, as the shedding of the top layer of cells can leave the skin more exposed to sunlight.

BETA-HYDROXY ACIDS (BHAS)

Beta-hydroxy acids are organic carboxylic acids. Like AHAs, they act as an exfoliant. The primary difference between them is that BHAs are less irritating. The most commonly used BHA is salicylic acid and at high concentrations of 30 per cent it has been shown to fade pigmented spots, decrease surface roughness and reduce fine lines. Newer formulations of BHAs, called beta-lipohydroxy acids or beta-LHAs, appear to cause epidermal thickening and improvement of the signs of ageing. BHAs are lipid- (oil-) soluble, which allows them to loosen oil in the pores. As a result, BHAs are commonly used to treat acne, blackheads and blemishes, and lend themselves well to on-the-spot treatments and toner-type lotions. As with AHAs, BHAs can cause irritation and wearing sunscreen is essential.

VITAMIN C (L-ASCORBIC ACID)

Vitamin C has powerful antioxidant effects, stimulates collagen production and aids healing. For many years scientists were unable to find a stable, trans-epidermal form of the vitamin until the discovery of L-ascorbic acid. Studies have shown that the topical application of L-ascorbic acid effects antioxidant and collagen stimulation. For the skin, this means a reversal of the ageing process and wrinkles. In addition, several studies have shown that topical applications of vitamin C can decrease the effects of sun exposure and UVB radiation. It may also help reduce the damage caused to the cutaneous immune system by sun exposure, leading to a reduction in the development of skin cancer. Because topical vitamin C does not absorb light in UVB/UVA range, it is not a sunscreen; instead, it exerts its effects by neutralizing oxygen free radicals.

Vitamin C is being touted as the most exciting advance in skincare, but inevitably scepticism comes with the hype. The jury is still out on the benefits of topical antioxidants and the use of ascorbic acid on collagen formation. Be aware of this when buying vitamin C preparations, as they are very expensive and must also contain L-ascorbic acid at a concentration of no less than 10 per cent to be effective. Vitamin C cream is best used under a sunscreen before going out in the sun to boost the skin's resistance to UV damage. Side effects are irritation and a stinging sensation on application.

COENZYME Q-10

Coenzyme Q-10 is considered essential for the body's cells, tissues and organs. As age leads to deficiencies in these areas, taking a supplement of Q-10, along with using a topical preparation, is a good idea. In a cream, Coenzyme Q-10 is oil-soluble and an excellent antioxidant. It is very stable, greatly beneficial to the immune system and helps fight off free-radical damage. It is usually delivered in a liposome system to prevent irritation. Q-10 is a popular antioxidant alternative to retinoids and vitamin C because it is not as irritating. However, the results are less striking.

KINERASE OR KINETIN

Both these formulas contain a naturally occurring plant-growth factor, N6-furfuryladenine, which keeps plant leaves moist and healthy and slows the ageing of plant cells. N6-furfuryladenine reduces the appearance of wrinkles, fine lines, hyper-pigmentation (sun spots) and moisture loss, and improves skin texture. Like Coenzyme Q10, these are popular antioxidant alternatives to retinoids and vitamin C for the same reasons.

A FEW OTHERS

CERAMIDES: These are lipid components of skin, which are deficient in dry skin. While there is currently no evidence that

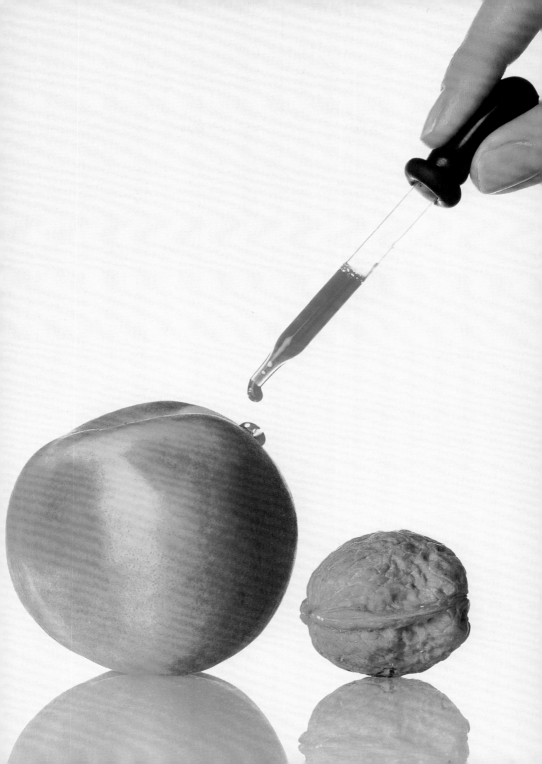

topical application can perform the same function as that which occurs naturally, ceramides act as good water-binding agents.

COLLAGEN: Collagen is vital to the skin's youthful, plump appearance. As an ingredient in moisturizers, collagen attracts moisture and can absorb up to 30 times its weight in water. It cannot influence collagen production, and the only way to put collagen back into your skin is to inject it.

KERATIN: This is a protein component of skin. Similar to collagen, it attracts moisture but cannot influence keratin production in the skin.

THE PLACENTA: The placenta is an organ that provides nutrients to the fetus during pregnancy. Although ongoing studies of its use in skincare are being conducted, there is no proof that the placenta can enhance blood circulation or stimulate cell metabolism when applied topically to the skin.

OXYGEN: Although oxygen boosts cellular activity and turnover, there is no evidence to show that blasting oxygen at the skin or applying it via a topical preparation has any benefits.

NIGHT CREAMS

Studies have confirmed that the skin's temperature increases during sleep and that warmer skin absorbs more of a skincare product's active ingredients. Choose a 'treatment' night cream that is packed with vitamins and reap the benefits while you sleep.

COSMECEUTICALS

This buzz-word of the beauty world has little legal meaning as yet. Consider the word to refer to drugs and skincare products that require a prescription or a visit to a dermatologist.

BETTER BOTANICALS

Grapeseed extract, pycnogenol and green tea extract all contain polyphenols, which are not only potent antioxidants in their own right but also support and enhance the effects of other antioxidants. Look for them in moisturizers and other skincare products.

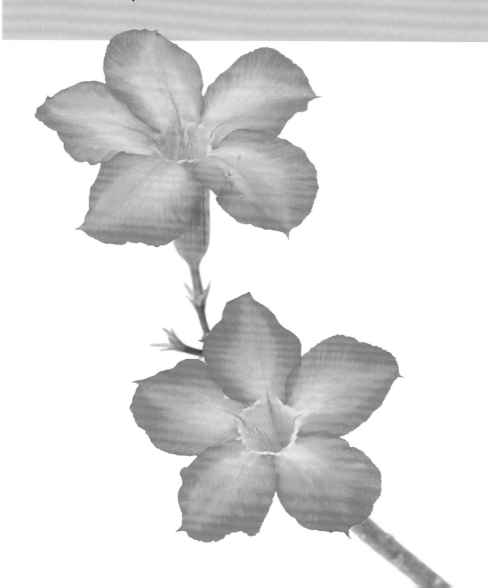

SPA & SALON FACIALS

Facials are a great way to pamper yourself and care for your skin, especially if you are not as devoted to a skincare regime as you would like to be. They are also an opportunity to get some advice from a professional skin 'carer'. So how do you spot a good facialist? We asked the experts. 'An A-list facialist can eliminate any type of clogging in a very gentle manner, with no or hardly any redness visible after the treatment,' says facialist Ole Henrikson, 'and a good facialist educates her or his clients in all aspects of skincare, including dietary guidance.'

'Shake their hand. If they've got a firm grip and large hands that's a good sign,' says Eve Lom, another facialist. 'Also, look for someone who sees life as a bit of a mystery and follows their gut instinct.' Marcia Kilgore of Bliss spa advises, 'Tip-offs include cleanliness, a willingness to listen, pre-facial questions about your skincare regime, and concern.'

To get the most from a facial consider what you want. Is it a serious cleanse using steam and extraction or just a pampering mask and soothing massage? Many facialists now offer light peels, lymphatic drainage massage, aromatherapy and scalp massages as part of the package or as an extra. Do not be afraid to ask questions, refuse a treatment or leave without a bagful of products. If you feel the suggestions offered are wrong for you and your skin, go with your gut instinct.

SKINCARE ESSENTIALS

INGREDIENTS	CHEMICAL CLASS
SKINCARE STAPLES	
Alpha-hydroxy acid (AHA)	Natural (fruits, sugar, milk)
Alpha-lipoic acid	Chemical
Beta-hydroxy acid (BHA)	Chemical
Co-Enzyme Q10 (Ubiquinone)	Chemical
Kinerase or Kinetin	Natural (plants)/chemical
Retinol	Chemical/alcohol/organic
Vitamin C (L-ascorbic acid)	Natural (fruits)/chemical

FUNCTION	SKIN TYPES	RECOMMENDED USE LEVEL
Anti-wrinkle; exfoliation; skin-smoothing	Dull; dry; damaged; flaky	5.0%–12.0%
Antioxidant; anti-inflammatory	Damaged; puffy	1%
Antioxidant	Oily; acne-prone	0.5%–2.0%
Antioxidant; anti-wrinkle; skin-conditioning	Mature	0.5%–2.0%
Skin-conditioning; antiageing	Mature; damaged; discoloured	0.1%
Windburn or sunburn	Mature; damaged	0.5%–2.0%
Antioxidant; collagen stimulator	Mature; damaged; discoloured	2.0%–20.0%

sun & skin cancer

Basking in the sun's rays may feel great and a glowing tan may make you feel more attractive, but there is nothing more detrimental to the skin than exposure to the ultraviolet radiation that is sunlight. Unfortunately, it is that simple. You do not have to spend your life indoors or covered up like a mummy when you do venture outside, just wear sunscreen – always.

Solar radiation hits the earth in three ways: infrared (heat), visible light and ultraviolet light. Ultraviolet rays are classified into UVA, UVB and UVC. Out of these three, only UVA and UVB hit the earth (UVC is filtered out by the atmosphere) and it is these rays from which we have to protect our skin. Sun works like a powerful X-ray, making its way through the epidermis and down to the dermis, where it gradually breaks down the spider-web formation of collagen and elastin and damages cells. Ultraviolet light has different effects: UVA rays penetrate the dermis and cause wrinkles, a loss of elasticity and skin cancer; UVB rays penetrate the epidermis and cause an immediate reaction in the form of redness, sunburn and, eventually, skin cancer.

SKIN DAMAGE

Skin damage from sunlight builds up with continued exposure, whether sunburn occurs or not. By the age of 18 most of us have already accumulated 80 per cent of our lifetime sun exposure and at least 80 per cent of what we consider normal skin ageing is really sun damage. Pale skin suffers more UVB damage than dark skin, so is most at risk. Mediterranean, dark brown and black skins can usually tolerate more sun, but ageing UVA rays are still able to penetrate.

According to dermatologists, the worst kind of sun damage occurs when skin is given a large dose of exposure after months without any at all. So, regardless of how fair or dark the skin, use a high-protection full-spectrum (UVA and UVB) sunscreen with a SPF of at least 15 (see pages 127–31) from the beginning of a holiday. Remember

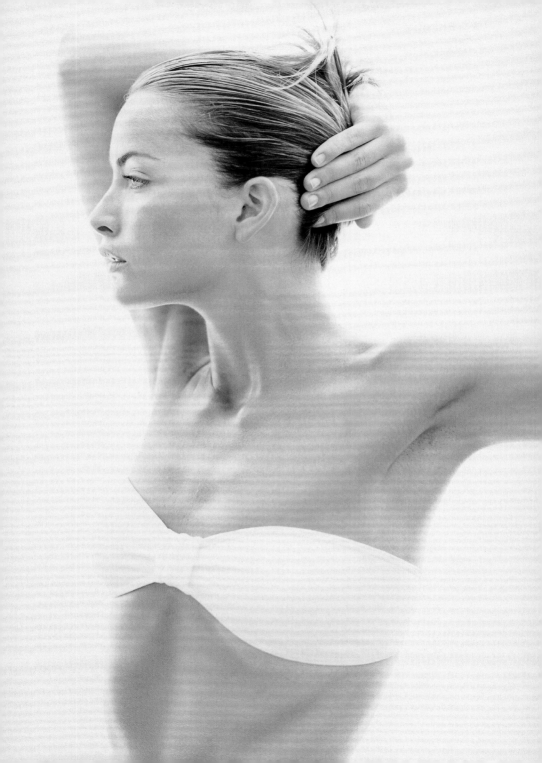

that incidental exposure to damaging rays occurs every time your skin is in the sun, whether you are driving in a car with the windows closed on a cloudy day or out on the ski slopes.

SKIN CANCER

Skin cancer is on the increase in the UK, with approximately 85,000 new cases and around 2,300 deaths every year, and it is striking at increasingly younger ages. The way it develops is like this: the sun changes the nature of the skin's melanocyte cells (the cells that cause tanning), making them abnormal and, in rare cases, malignant. Skin cancer is a disease in which the abnormal cells grow uncontrollably in the outer layers of the skin. There are three main types:

1 Basal cell carcinomas are easily treated and rarely fatal. The areas usually appear as raised translucent lumps on the skin that are pearly in appearance.

2 Squamous cell carinomas are also unlikely to lead to death and sometimes appear as nodules or red, scaly patches.

3 Malignant melanoma is the least common, but most aggressive, form of skin cancer. It is generally irregular in shape, sometimes in or around a mole, and has black, tan or brown shading. Early treatment is vital as it accounts for the vast majority of deaths from skin cancer.

Skin cancer is more common in people with light-coloured skin who have spent a lot of time in the sun. It can appear anywhere on the body, but it is most likely to occur on those areas exposed to the most sunlight, such as the face, neck and arms.

A combination of factors determines whether you get skin cancer. People with a family history of the disease are probably at greater risk. Altitude and cloud cover will affect the sun's intensity. The sun's rays are most intense on the equator, but recent concern has centred on countries in the extreme south and north where ozone depletion allows greater penetration of ultraviolet wavelengths. That said, the sunshine over the UK is more than capable of triggering a skin cancer.

SUNSCREENS

These are available in an amazing range of lotions, gels, oils and other products. Whatever type you choose, the ingredients to look for are: titanium dioxide, zinc oxide or avobenzone (also Parsol) and octyl-methoxycinnimate (OMC). Titanium dioxide and zinc oxide are UVA and UVB blocking agents, meaning that they block ultraviolet rays from penetrating the skin by reflecting the light off the skin's surface. In the past these agents often left the skin looking white and powdery, but modern micronized formulas leave only the faintest white hue. Both titanium dioxide and zinc oxide are natural ingredients so they do not irritate the skin.

Avobenzone and octyl-methoxycinnimate are ultraviolet filters, which means they absorb and minimize the harmful rays

ANTIOXIDANTS & CAROTENES

Antioxidants are free-radical scavengers that help limit and then repair the damage to the skin's cells incurred during ultraviolet exposure. For this reason suncare products often include antioxidants in their formulas. There are even some pre-sun antioxidant treatments, including supplements, on the market that can be used before and after a day on the beach to give skin a helping hand. Antioxidants, however, are a complementary therapy, and not photo-protective agents.

Carotenes are being included in more and more suncare products and serve two purposes. First, certain carotenes, including lycopene and beta-carotene, have the ability to increase growth-regulatory signals between cells, which can help prevent damaged cells from becoming cancerous. Secondly, when carotenes are exposed to the sun they oxidize, thus giving the skin an orange hue. This not only makes skin appear tanned more quickly, but also makes the colour more even. Look for carotenes in the ingredient listing when choosing a sunscreen.

THE GOLDEN RULES OF TANNING

• Avoid the sun between 11 am and 3 pm.

• Apply sunscreen 20 minutes before going out in the sun.

• Apply at least a shot-glass's worth of lotion all over to adequately protect the skin, and at least a teaspoon-worth to adequately protect the face.

• Use a high SPF sunscreen that includes both UVA and UVB protection.

• Build up your sun exposure time gradually.

• Apply sunscreen liberally every one to two hours and also make sure you apply immediately after swimming.

• When applying sunscreen, pay particular attention to the nose, cheeks, forehead, backs of ears, neck and shoulders, as these areas are first to catch the sun.

• Wear a sun hat, cover-up clothing and UVA/UVB protection sunglasses in the hot midday sun.

• Never expose babies under six months old to the sun and take extra care with children.

• At the first sign of burning, get out of the sun immediately.

• If you develop any new moles or freckles after burning in the sun, have them checked by your dermatologist.

before they can penetrate the skin. Avobenzone is organic and absorbs UVA rays, while octyl-methoxycinnimate absorbs UVB rays. Without both of these ingredients, you are not protected from UVA and UVB radiation.

Be aware, however, that the SPF number on sunscreens relates to UVB rays only, not UVA. The letters SPF stand for sun protection factor and relate to the skin's natural protection time. So, if you can usually stay in the sun for up to 10 minutes without burning, an SPF15 will keep skin protected 15 times longer ($15 \times 10 = 2\frac{1}{2}$ hours) than if no sun protection was used. The higher a product's SPF, the

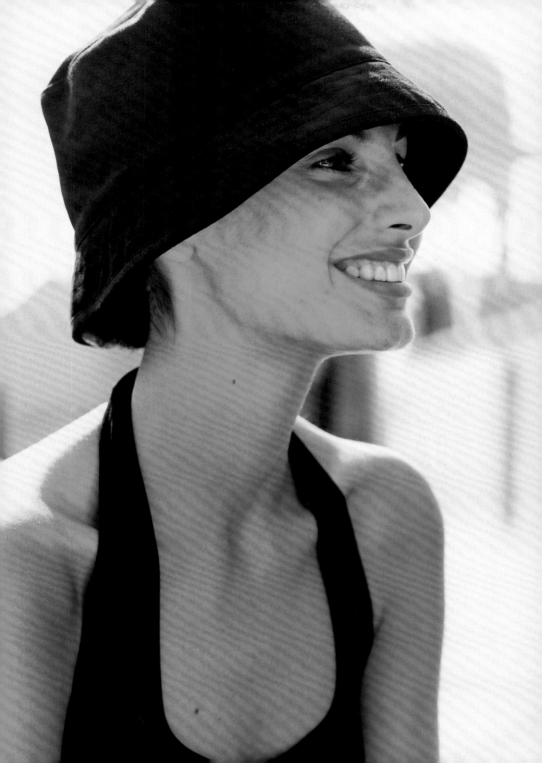

SUNSCREEN GIVES YOU CANCER

This is a theory that pops up every now and then and has a couple of different meanings. Some dermatologists have argued that sunscreens, in effect, cause cancer because the majority of people believe that, as long as they are wearing a sunscreen, they are protected. In fact, most of us do not wear a high enough SPF, apply enough or reapply it sufficiently to protect ourselves fully from the risk of skin cancer. We also spend longer in the sun than is healthy because there seems to be no risk if we are not burning. A paper entitled 'Sunscreen Gives You Cancer', published in *The Journal of Chemical Research in Toxicology* in 1999 claimed that phenylbenzimidazole-5-sulfonic acid (PBSA), an ingredient in some sunscreens, could damage DNA and lead to skin cancer. The paper did not present evidence showing that PBSA applied topically could penetrate human skin cells, nor did it argue that the benefits associated with PBSA sunscreens outweighed the risks. The paper's claims have largely been discounted by newer studies; PBSA is on the positive list in EU legislation and when the CTPA reviewed it in 2006 they gave it a clean bill of health. However, if you are concerned, choose a sunscreen that does not list PBSA among its ingredients.

more defence it offers against damaging UVB rays. As yet, there is no universally recognized UVA rating system, though the European Commission has now recommended the use of a logo (the letters UVA in a circle) which signifies that the product complies with its minimum level of UVA protection. Certain brands have their own systems that indicate the protection a sunscreen offers from UVA rays, but the only way you will be assured of safety is by reading the label carefully.

SUNBEDS

Tanning beds are worse than tanning on the beach for several reasons. The light tubes emit bursts of UVA rays that are three times more concentrated than those emitted by the sun. In terms of ultraviolet exposure, a typical sunbed session is equivalent to one full day at the beach. While you will not burn on a sunbed, as they do not emit UVB rays, you will sustain the kind of damage associated with ageing. Furthermore, most people do not use sunscreen on tanning beds, making them even more dangerous. A study in Sweden has shown that people who use a tanning bed more than ten times a year have a seven times greater risk of melanoma.

REPAIRING SUN DAMAGE

Treating sun-damaged skin is not all that different to treating ageing skin, as the problems are the same. Studies have shown a reversal of sun damage in patients using tretinoin Retin-A creams. Glycolic acid, chemical peels, micro-dermabrasion and laser resurfacing have all been shown to remove fine lines and wrinkles, even out pigmentation and fade brown spots. Fresh elastin and collagen production can be stimulated by topical applications of L-ascorbic acid (see also pages 115–6 and 122–3). Finally, remember skin can repair itself if you give it a chance by staying out of the sun and using a full-spectrum sunscreen.

WHEN IS THE SUN GOOD FOR SKIN?

There are certain medical conditions for which sunlight is beneficial and UV light treatment is prescribed, including psoriasis, acne, vitiligo and eczema.

Statistics show that the incidence of skin cancer has greatly increased in people who have undergone light treatment. However, as dermatologist Laurie Polis says, 'These cases are a matter of risk-benefit ratio. If your life is disrupted by a severe skin condition, have the treatment. We can take precautions against skin cancer by prescribing a short course of UV and covering the unaffected areas.'

TANS IN A TUBE

Today self-tanning creams are becoming increasingly more sophisticated. They are less greasy and heavy on the skin, and actually offer a colour similar to a natural tan. The active ingredient in self-tanners is dihydroxyacetone (DHA), which interacts with the proteins in the epidermis and temporarily darkens the skin. Self-tanners are available in a variety of forms, including gels, creams and sprays, many of which instantly deposit a non-permanent colour on the skin so you can easily see any missed spots. Sprays are handy for those hard-to-reach spots, but use the product that you find easiest. Apply the self-tanner smoothly and evenly and use a shade suited to your skin tone. For oily or acne-prone skin, choose gels or oil-free formulas.

If possible, apply the product before going to bed and leave it overnight, or apply it on a lazy Sunday. Despite their greatly improved quality, self-tanners can still smell unpleasant and discolour clothes, although the dye usually washes out. Try not to wash your hands too frequently or eat and wipe your face directly after applying the product, or else you may end up with pale hands and a light ring around your mouth.

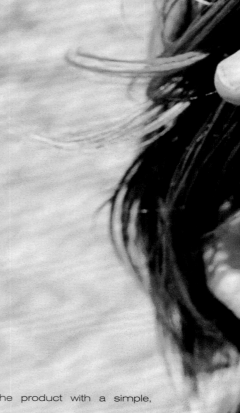

HOW TO FAKE IT

1 Exfoliate by using either an exfoliating mitt or a scrub in the shower, or an AHA product (see pages 114–15 and 122–3). Pay special attention to the knees, elbows and feet.

2 Wash thoroughly and rinse yourself well. If a soapy alkaline residue or toner is left on the skin, you could turn an unattractive shade of orange or green.

3 Apply the product evenly and rub it in well. Be meticulous, or the colour will look splotchy and streaky when it develops.

4 Separate products do not need to be used for the face and body, but dilute the product with a simple, unperfumed moisturizer on the face and ears, around the hairline and eyebrows, and on the elbows and knees.

5 Wash the hands or brown palms will give the game away. Wait at least three hours until showering, or shower immediately to wash off some or all of the colour. If you accidentally turn your palms brown, apply a coating of whitening toothpaste for several minutes to remove all traces of the discoloration.

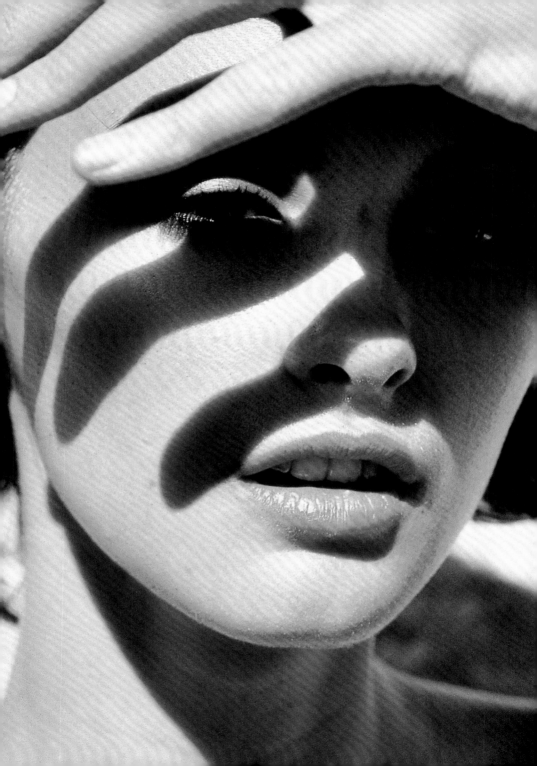

cosmetic dermatology

In the USA cosmetic procedures such as dermabrasion and peels are largely under the aegis of dermatologists, and in the UK and the rest of Europe they are now available at many beauty and skin clinics. The fact that these procedures can be performed in an office, or increasingly in spas and salons, sometimes in a matter of minutes, does not mean that they should be treated casually. While very effective (often miraculous, in fact), many are actually quite invasive and not without risk. Wherever you choose to undergo a treatment, and with whom, do your research – the experience and the results will be better.

CHEMICAL PEELS

Chemical peels are a more aggressive form of exfoliation and are very effective at correcting sun damage and mild scarring, removing wrinkles and pre-cancerous growths, and evening out irregular pigmentation. They are best performed by a cosmetic surgeon or dermatologist, both for safety reasons and because those offered at salons or spas remove only a little more skin than can be achieved by using AHA or BHA creams at home.

Chemical peels involve the application of a caustic solution onto the skin with a cotton swab or brush to remove layers of the epidermis and dermis, depending on how deep the peel. The caustic solution basically burns off your skin – and all flaws along with it. The level of improvement and the downtime (time spent recovering) of a peel depends again on how deep it is: a lunchtime peel means you can have it at lunchtime and be back at work with your colleagues none the wiser, a deep peel can leave you in bandages for several days and looking red for weeks. While the solution is on the skin you will experience a stinging sensation, the degree of which increases with the level of peel. Ask for a fan to blow cool air on the area being treated if you find it

FINDING A QUALIFIED PHYSICIAN

The procedure may be tried and tested, but is your physician? Finding a qualified and competent cosmetic surgeon is imperative. Do not select one from the telephone directory or the classified section of a magazine; instead get names and recommendations from your doctor, dermatologist, local hospital and friends who have had similar procedures. Also, contact such organizations as the British Association of Dermatologists, the British Association of Plastic Surgeons, the American Society of Plastic Surgeons or the Australian Society of Plastic Surgeons and ask them to provide a list of members. Once you have a short list of names, make appointments to see several different physicians. During the initial consultation, keep the following in mind:

- What are the doctor's credentials? Is he or she a board-certified dermatologist or other appropriately trained surgeon? Ask to see their credentials.
- How many of the cosmetic surgery procedures has the physician actually performed him- or herself?
- What results can be expected? How long is the recuperation period? Ask to see before and after photographs of the physician's previous patients.
- What are the risks and side effects?
- Where is the cosmetic surgery usually performed? Who will the cosmetic surgery be performed by?
- What is the cost of the treatment and might there be any hidden extras added on?

Finally, ask yourself: do you feel comfortable with the physician you have seen? If they avoid answering any of the above questions, or are evasive or sketchy in their reply, it is likely to be a sign of untrustworthiness or unprofessionalism. Also, do not choose someone you feel is qualified but seems unapproachable.

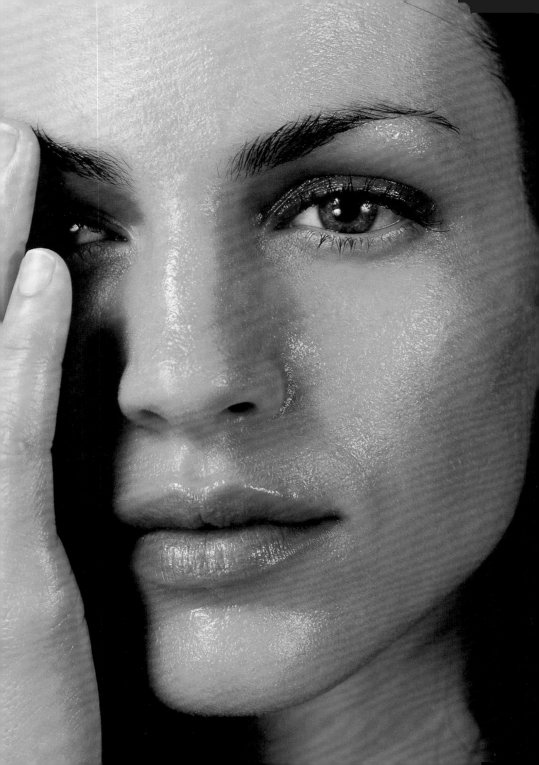

particularly unpleasant, or have a general anaesthetic or sedative for a deep peel. The time the solution is left on the face varies with the type of peels. When the time is up, the solution is washed off with water or another neutralizing wash.

The skin that grows back after a peel is without sun damage, wrinkles, superficial scars and so on. A miracle, yes, but one that is not without a price – namely pain, downtime and possible loss of pigmentation, meaning you can never go into the sun again. You might, therefore, consider opting for dermabrasion or laser surgery rather than a deep phenol peel. If you are concerned about possible adverse reactions, ask for a patch test of peel solution to be applied on the neck behind the ear a couple of weeks before you plan to have the treatment. Always tell your dermatologist if you are using any active products like retinoids or vitamin C cream; they should, however, ask you these questions as a matter of course. You cannot have a peel if you are sunburned or taking oral retinoids. Light and medium peels can also be performed on the neck, hands and back to reduce the signs of ageing or treat acne.

LIGHT PEELS

ALPHA HYDROXY ACID PEELS

Glycolic Acid and other AHA treatments are light, exfoliating, superficial peels that remove the upper layers of the epidermis. Light peels can be repeated every ten days to two weeks; a series of three to five peels is usually recommended as the results are cumulative. This means that repeated peels have been shown to stimulate increased cell and collagen production. Light peels help 'dry out' active acne, dislodge blackheads, reduce shallow wrinkling and scarring, and lighten hyperpigmentation spots. Your complexion should appear brighter and your skin feel softer. Most people experience no side effects or visible peeling, making it a perfect 'lunchtime' treatment, but some experience temporary side effects that include mild stinging, swelling, redness, flaking and peeling. Apply a full spectrum non-irritating sunblock like zinc oxide or titanium dioxide before going outside, as the skin will be more sensitive to UV radiation.

BETA HYDROXY ACID PEELS

Although less common, a beta hydroxy peel is a good alternative to an AHA peel for those who find AHAs too irritating. The effects are similar, but a beta hydroxy peel is particularly good for those with active acne, as BHAs are lipophilic (fat soluble), so they get down into the pores where the lipids are. While a BHA peel is less irritating, the down side is that most people experience some visible peeling for a few days. Apply a full spectrum non-irritating sunblock like zinc oxide or titanium dioxide before going outside as the skin will be more sensitive to UV radiation.

LIGHT TO MEDIUM PEELS

TRICHLOROACETIC ACID (TCA)

Trichloroacetic acid (TCA) can be used in many concentrations, but it is most commonly used for medium peels to remove the epidermis and the upper layers of the dermis. Fine surface wrinkles, crow's feet, superficial scars, pigment problems and pre-cancerous growths are commonly treated with TCA. Two or more TCA peels spaced out over several months may be needed to obtain the desired result. Because TCA penetrates more deeply than AHAs there is a downtime of five to seven days. Skin will appear white immediately after the peel, then turn red and look

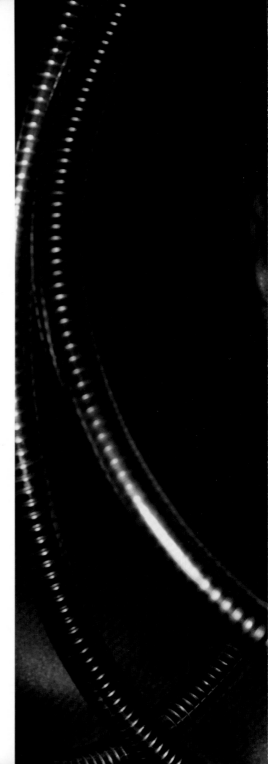

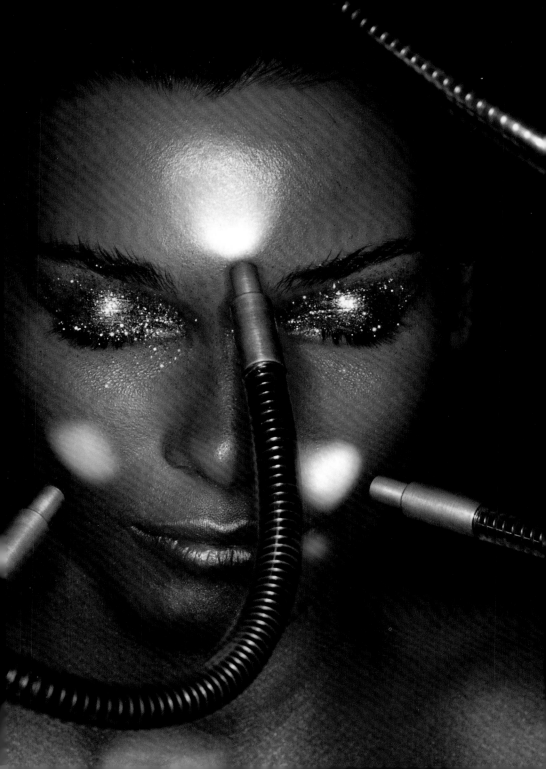

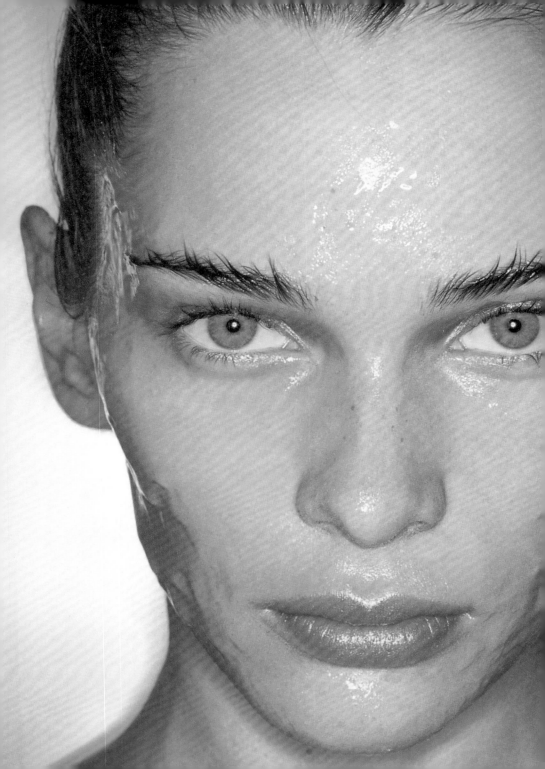

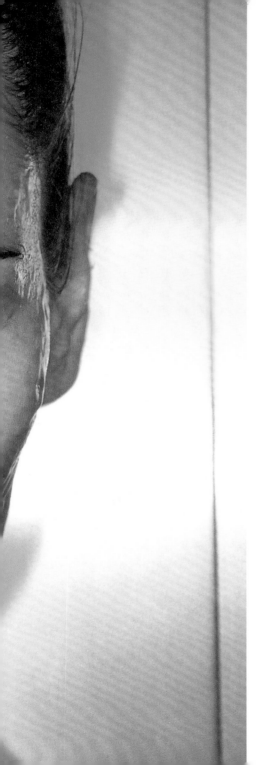

swollen. A few days later you will develop a scab all over your face, which cracks and peels after several more days to reveal new, smooth skin underneath. A full-face TCA peel takes about 15 minutes and it hurts. Afterwards your doctor may prescribe a mild pain medication to relieve any tingling or throbbing you may feel. Unlike a deep phenol peel, a TCA peel will not bleach the skin but it can cause irregular pigmentation. TCA-peel patients are advised to avoid sun exposure for several months after treatment to protect the newly formed layers of skin.

JESSNER'S SOLUTION

Named for its creator Dr Max Jessner, Jessner's solution is a mix of lactic acid, salicylic acid and resorcinol. It is increasingly being seen as a rather old-fashioned peel, but it is not yet obsolete. A Jessner peel is often used on really stubborn brown spots. There is some visible peeling for several days.

DEEP PEELS

PHENOL

Phenol is the strongest of the chemical solutions and is used for deep peels to remove the epidermis and a large part of the dermis. It is used mainly to treat patients with coarse facial wrinkles, areas of blotchy or damaged skin that have been caused by sun exposure, or pre-cancerous growths. Since phenol sometimes lightens the treated areas, your skin pigmentation will be a determining factor as to whether or not this is an appropriate treatment. With a phenol peel, the new skin frequently loses its ability to make pigment, so not only will the skin be lighter, but also you will always have to stay out of the sun. Black and Asian skins should never have deep peels (see CoolTouch non-ablative laser, opposite).

Phenol is dangerous: there have been reports of it causing irregular heartbeats when absorbed through the skin, so it poses a special risk for patients with a history of heart disease. Phenol peels should therefore always be performed in a location where medical equipment is available. Phenol is only used on the face because scarring may result if it is applied to the neck or other body areas. A full-face phenol peel takes between one and two hours to perform and really hurts. Fortunately, a single treatment usually suffices.

Deep peels come with a downtime of several weeks. Your face will initially turn totally white and then become swollen and crusted. Later, it will peel and even bleed. Your eyes could also swell and temporarily close. For obvious reasons you will have to wear a mask or dressing for several days. Arrange for someone to drive you home and help you out for a day or two, as you will probably be on a liquid diet and not able to talk much during the first few days of recovery. To help your face heal properly, it is essential that you follow your doctor's specific post-operative instructions. It is especially important that you use a sunblock, otherwise blotchy, irregular skin colouring may result.

POWER PEELS – THE TOAST OF LA

Power Peels, which are also known as microdermabrasion, are not chemical peels but the 'lunchtime' equivalent of dermabrasion. Like chemical peels, power peels are effective at treating problems like rough skin texture, uneven pigmentation, acne, sun damage, fine wrinkles and acne scars. If you don't like the idea of putting a caustic solution on your face or your skin is too irritated

COOLTOUCH – THE LUNCHTIME LASER

The CoolTouch laser is a non-ablative (non-surgical) neodymium:YAG laser. It has several advantages over traditional lasers: the procedure is painless and takes less time; there is no reddening of the skin and no downtime; it can be used to treat darker skins without incurring pigmentation problems. With CoolTouch a hand-held laser gun shoots pulses of concentrated red light into the dermis where the fibroblasts are situated. Just before the laser fires the gun shoots a jet of freezing spray onto the skin to stop burning and protect the sensitive nerve endings. Meanwhile, the cells are heated, briefly, to 80°C (180°F) causing them to start manufacturing new collagen and elastin.

The treatment is particularly effective at removing fine lines and wrinkles, and works best on people in their thirties and forties who have not yet lost too many of their fibroblasts. Men are said to respond especially well. The treatment is used to help reduce acne scars, stretchmarks and sun damage. Usuallytwo treatments are given about six weeks apart, followed by a 'top-up' treatment once every six months to a year after that. CoolTouch has elicited rave reviews from patients and dermatologists alike.

A clinical trial in the USA, conducted by Dr Gregory Chernoff, the clinical assistant professor of the division of facial plastic surgery at Indiana University, showed significant effects after just two 15- to 30-minute sessions of CoolTouch. Four months later the skin had plumped out and a large proportion of fine lines and wrinkles had vanished. In the trial, two-thirds of a group of 212 patients saw positive results after only one treatment. The remaining third saw an improvement after a second or third session. Analysis of surgically removed sections of skin showed a packing together of collagen in the upper dermis, as well as the formation of new collagen.

by AHAs and the like, power peels are a great alternative. Again, they should be performed by a dermatologist or cosmetic surgeon, both for safety reasons and to attain the best results.

Microdermabrasion involves stripping off very thin, superficial layers of the skin using a vacuum-like device and sterile aluminium oxide 'sand'. The 'sand' is blasted onto the face, sloughing off the top layers of the epidermis, and then sucked off. By varying the airflow and sand, microdermabrasion creates only the most superficial wounds – 10 microns, or ten-thousandths of a millimeter in depth – so anaesthesia is not needed. You should experience a mild redness for a few hours after the procedure, which can be easily covered with make-up and a broad-spectrum sunblock, of course. Power peels can be performed once a month, but four times a year should do the trick.

DERMABRASION –
THE ULTIMATE PEEL

Dermabrasion, or surgical skin planing, is a more aggressive procedure than microdermabrasion, or chemical peeling. It is mainly used to smooth out acne and chicken pox scars, remove tattoos, treat age spots and chronic sun damage, and it is particularly effective at smoothing out wrinkles above the upper lip. The procedure involves using a high-speed sanding wheel or rotating steel brush to scrape away all of the epidermis and most of the dermis. Patients are given a local anaesthetic and a sedative, so pain should not be felt. The procedure takes 30 minutes to an hour to perform. Afterwards, the skin may be covered with bandages or left open to heal.

As in a deep peel, a lot of swelling occurs after dermabrasion, followed by the formation of a crust, which later falls off to reveal red or pink skin. The downtime is about three weeks, but skin can look pink for up to 12 weeks. Make-up can be used to conceal this as soon as the skin is healed. Patients are instructed to avoid unnecessary sunlight, both direct and indirect, for three to six months after the procedure and to use a sunscreen regularly whenever they go outdoors. The procedure can be repeated every six months. Although dermabrasion does not destroy all skin pigment, it can cause hyperpigmentation. Because of its gruesome nature, laser treatments are increasingly replacing dermabrasion, though it is still very useful for 'spot' treatments on specific scars or wrinkles, rather than for the whole face.

LASER SKIN RESURFACING

Sometimes called 'laser peeling', laser resurfacing has been a scientific breakthrough in skin rejuvenation. One of its most significant advantages over conventional peels is that it is relatively bloodless. The procedure also offers more control in the depth of penetration and allows a degree of precision and safety in treating delicate areas, like the lips and around the eyes. Laser resurfacing can be done on the entire face or just on specific problem areas.

The two types of laser used in skin resurfacing are the carbon dioxide laser (CO_2) and the erbium:YAG laser. Both lasers generate infrared radiation that is absorbed by the water within the skin's cells. The water heats up and vaporizes thin layers of skin. Each laser can remove 20–100 microns of skin at one pass over the skin (by way of comparison, a sheet of paper is about 100 microns thick). The difference between the two lasers is that the erbium:YAG vaporizes less skin, so it can be used for more intricate work and it is more versatile. It also causes less surrounding tissue damage, so there is a shorter healing time. However, the CO_2 laser is better at treating wrinkles because it removes the epidermis layer of skin, thus stimulating new collagen production in the dermis.

Although lasers are touted as one of the safest forms of cosmetic surgery, all surgical procedures carry some degree of risk. With the CO_2 and erbium:YAG lasers the risk of scarring is low, but side effects may include redness or brown discoloration. Some patients may require bleaching creams to help regulate skin pigmentation following treatment. There is always a downtime of a few days.

A topical anaesthetic cream with a mild sedative, local anaesthetic or intravenous sedative may be given, making both procedures relatively painless. The resurfacing usually takes between one and two hours. As with peels, the treated areas are usually kept moist with ointment or bandages for the first few

LASERS & HAIR REMOVAL

Laser technology is now being utilized for hair removal. Although experts remain uncertain as to how, precisely, the treatment works, it appears that the laser energy causes thermal injury to the hair follicles, thereby 'killing' hair. Several laser hair-removal systems are currently being tested by dermatologists, with promising results. In preliminary clinical trials, test sites remained hair-free for up to three months. That said, there have been no confirmed reports of permanent hair removal – 'permanent', in this case, being defined as no regrowth of hair for two years after treatment.

While the application of lasers for facial and body hair removal is still in its infancy, the Epilight hair removal system is gaining in popularity. If you decide to try Epilight, expect a minimum of three, and perhaps up to six, sessions to remove hair. This is because hair grows in three cycles and the lasers will only respond to hair that is in the growth phase. Also, you will not be a suitable candidate if you have tanned or dark skin because the laser picks up on pigment and can damage the skin. In the same way, if your hair colour is very light, then the laser cannot treat it. Do not shave, pluck or bleach hair for a week prior to photo-epilation. Epilight claims that its machine can be calibrated to your precise skin type, hair colour and target area, so your dermatologist will assess the area and programme the machine accordingly.

During the treatment, the dermatologist should give you a pair of protective glasses to wear. The length of the session depends on the area being treated – five minutes for the upper lip or 15 minutes for the underarms, for example. Epilight is not pain-free: it burns. You can ask the dermatologist to apply a topical anaesthetic 30 minutes or so before the treatment. Epilight can burn hair, making the area look as if it is covered in black spots, and the laser can cause swelling. In other words, do not make any plans afterwards.

days, after which the skin turns red or pink and may be covered with a fine crust. Treated sites must be fully protected from sunlight after the procedure, and, once healed, sunscreen should be applied over the entire area. Fractional lasers, such as the FDA-approved Pixel, treats only tiny dots of skin, allowing for faster healing.

COBLATION RESURFACING

At the March 2000 annual meeting of the American Academy of Dermatology, Tina S Alster, the clinical assistant professor of dermatology at Georgetown University, presented the case for electrosurgical resurfacing. Electrosurgical resurfacing, or coblation, an abbreviation for 'cold ablation', delivers saline to the skin, through which a cool electric current, rather than heat, is passed. The reaction that follows then heats and vaporizes the top shallow layer of skin. The procedure is highly specific and can achieve precise tissue removal. It also appears to minimize any damage to other areas of the skin. A local anaesthetic is administered during the procedure, which lasts approximately 30 to 60 minutes. Immediately afterwards, the skin appears pink and there is moderate swelling and redness for a few days. Within a week, the skin is only slightly pink

and make-up can usually be applied. In most cases all visible signs of the treatment have disappeared after two weeks. Coblation, like CoolTouch, can be used on all skin types as pigmentation does not block the transmission of energy to the treatment area. FDA-approved, coblation is preferred by many cosmetic surgeons over laser resurfacing.

FILLERS

One of the inevitabilities of intrinsic ageing is the breakdown of the collagen and elastin that plumps out the skin. The solution to this problem is a no-brainer: replace the plumpness of youth with a 'filler'. When it comes to fillers, Europe is the leader. There are ever-multiplying varieties of wrinkle fillers available, synthetic and natural, injectable and non-injectable. So many, in fact, it is hard to keep up with the technology. Essentially, however, they all perform the same function. Fillers are generally used to reduce wrinkles, furrows and hollows in specific areas of the face, such as around the lips and mouth, nose, eyes and the forehead. Some treatments hurt more than others; a Dermologen injection, for instance, hurts more than a collagen injection because it requires a thicker needle. Some swelling or bruising usually occurs, which varies from procedure to procedure, but in most cases this lasts only a few days. In every instance, the results are immediate and usually highly gratifying.

COLLAGEN

Collagen has been on the market for more than 20 years but has now been largely replaced by more advanced manmade 'animal-free' fillers, such as Restylane, Hylaform and Juvéderm (see Hyaluronic Acid Gel, page 149). It is most often used for lip augmentation and to plump out laughter lines, frown lines and acne scars. Derived from bovine collagen (specifically, from the hides of specially reared cattle), it is manufactured into three injectable forms: Zyderm, Zyplast and, most recently, Resoplast, the first European-produced implant. Collagen is highly effective and has an established safety record. The only downside is that bovine collagen has a 4 per cent allergy risk, so patients must be tested before being injected. Collagen injections last between three and six months before being absorbed into the body.

ALLODERM & DERMOLOGEN

Both Alloderm and Dermologen are processed from donor human cadaver skin and are used mainly for lip augmentation and to plump out laughter lines, frown lines and acne scars. Alloderm is not injectable but it is available in solid sheets that can be rolled; Dermologen is a viscous fluid that is injectable. Because they are made from human tissue, Alloderm and Dermologen do not usually cause allergic reactions. Alloderm is cut to size depending on the area being treated, then implanted under local anaesthesia. A few fine sutures are placed, which are removed several days later. In the case of lip augmentation, incisions are made at both corners of the mouth and the implant is threaded through. Alloderm becomes permanently incorporated into the graft site after about six weeks. Dermologen is simply injected into the area being treated and although it is temporary, it is longer lasting than collagen. Current estimates average at about six months before the implant is absorbed into the body.

AUTOLOGEN

If you do not like the sound of cadaver skin, Autologen is a 'natural' alternative.

Autologen is an injectable collagen derived from your own skin. Skin that has been removed in other procedures, a facelift for example, is kept in a BioBank until you are ready to use it. Autologous collagen injections last for two to three months. Because Autologen is derived from your own skin cells, there is no chance of an allergic reaction.

HYALURONIC ACID GEL

Hyaluronic acid gel is most often used for dermal fillers and lip augmentation in patients who are looking for a temporary implant and cannot tolerate collagen. It is a viscous gel derived from a hyaluronic acid compound and does not usually elicit allergic reactions because it has the same chemical and molecular structure as hyaluronan, an enzyme that is present in humans and helps keep the skin moist and elastic. Both Hylaform gel and Restylane are absorbed into the body after three to six months. Juvéderm, one of the newest injectable fillers, lasts for up to one year.

FAT TRANSFERS

Fat transfer, also called autologous fat transplantation or microlipo-injection, plumps up the skin using your own fat. It is possible to have the fat liposuctioned from your thighs, abdomen or back and transferred to any area of your body, or the fat can be harvested (taken from another area) specifically for a trans-plant. Fat transfer can be used for deep lines, acne scars and lip augmentation; however, re-injected fat lasts longer in areas of non-movement, such as in sunken cheeks. While fat transfers are highly effective, the disadvantage is swelling and inflammation, so there is a downtime of a couple of weeks. The fat is reabsorbed after about two years.

SOFTFORM

SoftForm is a polytetraflouroethylene hollow implant that comes in a tubular form. Mostly used for lip augmentation, it can also be used for smile or frown lines. SoftForm is implanted beneath the skin under local anaesthesia, and a few fine sutures are placed, which are removed several days later. In a lip aug-mentation, two incisions are made at both corners of the mouth and two dif-ferent pieces are inserted. Because SoftForm is hollow, the body's fibrous tissue grows through it, helping to 'anchor' the implant. Although considered permanent, SoftForm can be removed. Allergic reactions are unusual.

POLYLACTIC ACID

Known by the names New-Fill and Sculptra, this temporary, injectable filler is made of a synthetic polymer manu-factured from lactic acid. It is claimed to stimulate new collagen growth.

RISKY FILLERS

You may think you have found a good physician but what about your filler? Some have better records than others. Whatever your physician says, research your fillers and injectables, and get sev-eral different opinions – from patients, if possible. Some of the less popular ones are listed below.

FORMACRYL/ARGIFORM: Permanent but removable, this filler is made of water and a synthetic polymer. When injected, a thin, natural physiological capsule is formed that acts as an endo-prosthesis and actually encloses the substance so that it can be removed.

DERMALIVE: This semi-permanent injectable contains acrylic hydrogel, which cannot be absorbed into the skin, and hyaluronic acid. It has not been approved by the FDA in the US and granuloma reactions have been reported.

GORTEX: Used mainly in lips, Gortex is a permanent thread-like material that is implanted beneath the skin to add soft-tissue support. The drawback is that it often moves under the skin, requiring either removal or repositioning. Patients have also complained that the implant can be felt when they run their tongue along the inside of their mouth.

ARTECOLL: Permanent and injectable, Artecoll is composed of bovine collagen and micronized acrylic beads of PMMA, a material used in dental implants and bone cement. Detractors say Artecoll can feel hard under the skin, is impos-sible to remove and one Los Angeles surgeon even likened the end result to 'lips resembling a bag of marbles'.

GOLD & COPPER: Semi-permanent and big in South America, gold and copper wire is the bargain basement of cosmetic surgery, and has been in use in Europe. The wire is threaded under the skin to plump it out. The results are reported to be disastrous.

BOTOX – THE FRIENDLY POISON

Botox is the abbreviated term for botulinum toxin A, a liquid injectable used to treat lines between the eyebrows, on the forehead and around the sides of the eyes. Many dermatologists believe Botox should not be used to treat frown or smile lines for the simple reason that it is a neurotoxin, which effectively paralyzes muscles. This can present a problem when speaking or eating, for example, so an off-target Botox injection is really not worth the risk.

Unlike fillers, which simply fill in lines, Botox actually reduces the cause of dynamic facial lines – the repeated contractions of the underlying facial muscles. Botox blocks the signal from the brain to the muscle (to frown, for example) at the neuromuscular junction site. This effect can last between three and eight months. However, there is increasing evidence that Botox treatments are cumulative. In other words, treating dynamic lines with a series of Botox injections may help retrain the muscles used in facial expression. As a result, the treatment is both corrective and preventative.

Botox works like this: the inactive muscles paralyzed by Botox become atrophied and weakened, so are less able to act. Subsequently, the lines produced by these muscular actions become less apparent. Botox is injected using an electromyography (EMG) instrument connected to the delivery needle, an instrument that ensures the accurate delivery of Botox to specific areas. Pre-treatment with a topical anaesthetic cream will render the injection essentially pain-free. Occasionally mild bruising may result in the area.

Complications that can arise from Botox injections are mainly tied up with the skill of the physician – a droopy eye or unnaturally frozen eyes and forehead are not uncommon. Injections need to be well distributed to avoid creating facial disharmonies. Among cosmetic surgeons, Botox treatment is seen as an art form, so choose a surgeon who knows a Picasso when they see it.

cosmetic surgery

There comes a point when Botox and retinoids are no longer doing the trick. With age, skin thins and sags; so if you are determined to reverse the passage of time, you are looking at the knife. The good news is that, contrary to some opinions, 'Thou shalt not have cosmetic surgery,' is not among the Ten Commandments. But the bad news is that cosmetic surgery is no less invasive, traumatic or risky than any other kind of surgery, and there is always downtime. For these reasons, a great deal of thought should go into deciding whether to have a procedure and, if so, the type to have and with whom to have it.

Whatever the pros and cons, one thing is certain: cosmetic surgery has become more common, more accepted and more affordable. Research from the American Society for Aesthetic Plastic Surgery (ASAPS) in the USA reported a 44 per cent increase in cosmetic surgery procedures from 2003 to 2004 alone. Increased competition among surgeons has led to stable prices. Less

invasive techniques and quicker recovery times are also making cosmetic surgery a more attractive option.

According to research, those aged 65 and older make up the fastest-growing segment of the population having cosmetic surgery, followed by those aged between 51 and 64. The age group getting the most cosmetic surgery, however, remains 35 to 50. The reasons for undergoing plastic surgery are varied and always personal, but on the whole most people simply want to look like 'themselves' again – something they feel ageing has robbed them of. While there are still a few who walk into the doctor's office waving a picture of this month's cover girl, most people simply come bearing a picture of themselves 10 or 15 years earlier. Remember that if you start going under the knife at too early an age, you will limit the amount of work you can have done at a later date when you might feel you need it more. Although you need not defend your reasons for embarking on surgery, you do need to

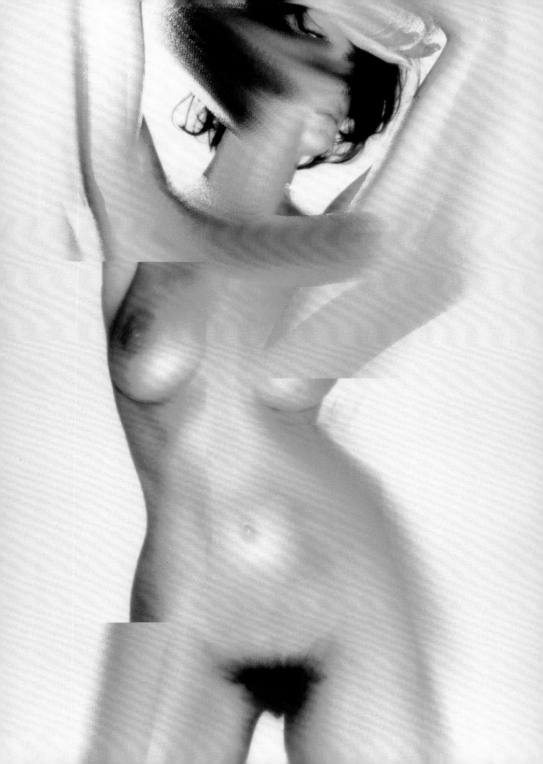

defend yourself against injury. The most important factor in the success of any type of plastic surgery procedure is the surgeon you choose.

THE CONSULTATION

Once you have narrowed a list down to two or three surgeons, visit all of them for an initial consultation in order to compare their personalities, opinions, fees and the ways in which they answer your questions. Keep in mind that the consultations will probably have to be paid for, whether or not you eventually choose that surgeon (see also Finding a Qualified Physician, page 135).

DURING THE INTERVIEW, THE PLASTIC SURGEON SHOULD:

1 Answer each of the questions you pose thoroughly and in an understandable and knowledgeable way.

2 Discuss your motivations and expectations, and solicit your reaction to recommendations.

3 Offer alternatives, where appropriate, without pressurizing you to consider unnecessary procedures.

4 Welcome any questions about professional qualifications, experience, costs and payment policies.

5 Make clear the possible variations in outcome, as well as the risks of surgery. If the surgeon shows photographs of other patients, or uses computer imaging to show possible results, they should make it clear that there is no guarantee that your results will match.

6 Make sure that the final decision is yours alone.

SMOKING

If you are considering cosmetic surgery, it is wise to give up smoking. Smokers have a much higher risk of complications during surgical procedures and take longer to recover. Also, some clinics and surgeons may simply refuse to perform cosmetic surgery on smokers.

cosmetic surgery procedures

LIPOSUCTION, TUMESCENT LIPOSUCTION & SUBMENTAL LIPECTOMIES

LIPOSUCTION

This is the removal of excess fat with a small, straw-like instrument called a cannula, which is attached to a suction machine. It is the most popular form of cosmetic surgery on the market. First developed in the late 1970s, liposuction was designed to remove undesired fat from the face, neck, chin, abdomen, hips, inner and outer thighs, buttocks and knees. More recently, however, a major advancement that completely revolutionized the procedure, tumescent liposuction, was developed by an American dermatologist. Tumescent liposuction allowed surgeons to remove deep and superficial layers of fat under local anaesthesia in areas that were previously considered off limits, such as the arms, ankles and calves. Because liposuction is highly effective at removing fat that does not respond to dieting or exercising, the best candidates are patients in their thirties, who lead a healthy lifestyle but who have pregnancy-related or inherited genetic fat. Unfortunately, even a lifetime on the StairMaster may not be able to shift those saddlebags — a fact confirmed by an exposé in the *New York Magazine*, revealing that a host of the city's top fitness trainers, unable to get rid of certain fat pockets, had undergone liposuction. Liposuction should not be viewed as a substitute for weight loss but, rather, a contouring procedure. Contrary to popular belief, skin is not left sagging after liposuction; it appears to retract and redrape itself naturally.

TUMESCENT LIPOSUCTION

This procedure is safer than the traditional method as it does not require a general anaesthetic. Instead, a solution containing dilute lidocaine (a local anaesthetic) and dilute epinephrine (a drug that shrinks capillaries and prevents blood loss) is injected directly into the areas being treated. Once the liquid is injected, a small incision is made in the skin and a tube, connected to a vacuum, is inserted into the fatty layer. Using to-and-fro movements, the fat is drawn through the tube into a collection system. The method is credited with removing fat more uniformly, with fewer skin irregularities and less bleeding and bruising than conventional liposuction.

There are potential risks with any type of liposuction. The most serious complications, although rare, include bowel perforation in abdominal procedures, shock, blood clots, decreased circulation, and tissue death and infection. The more common side effects are minor indents or irregularities in the skin.

SUBMENTAL LIPECTOMY

This is liposuction of the neck, chin and jowl area, along with a surgical tightening of the underlying neck muscles. An ideal alternative to a facelift for younger patients with good skin elasticity.

EYELID SURGERY

An eye job, technically called blepharoplasty, removes fat, excess skin and muscle from the upper and lower

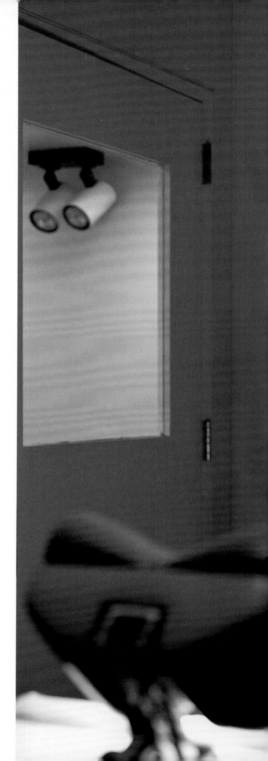

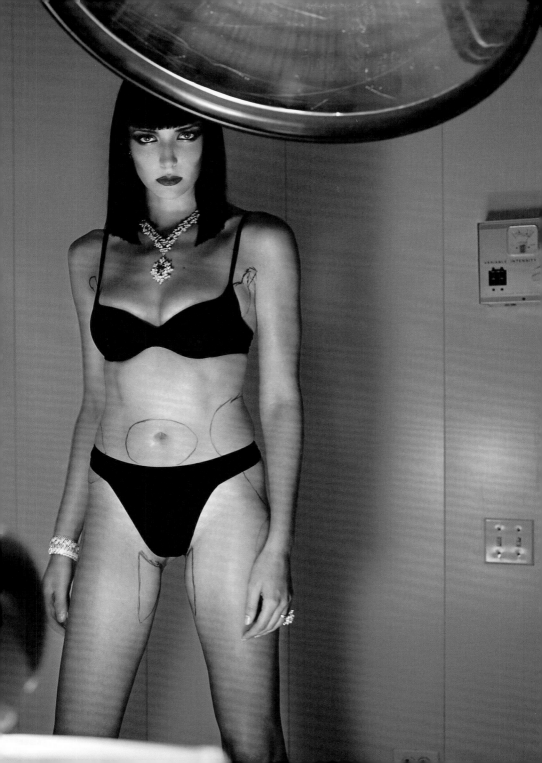

eyelids. The procedure is performed under local anaesthesia and takes between one and three hours. Eyelid surgery can correct drooping upper lids and puffy under-eye bags. However, it will not remove crow's-feet or other wrinkles, eliminate dark circles or lift sagging eyebrows. After the surgery, the sutures are covered with small bandages for several days. Expect blurry vision and weepy, itchy eyes during this period. Bruising should subside after two to three days and the redness around the incision sites will fade after several months.

Fortunately, blepharoplasty lasts forever. Once you have had upper-lid blepharoplasty, however, a browlift cannot be performed, as there is not enough skin left on the eyelids. You may, therefore, want to consider having a browlift first.

THE BROWLIFT & THE ENDOSCOPIC BROWLIFT

A forehead lift, or browlift, corrects drooping brows and upper eyelids, and improves frown lines and furrows that can make you look angry, sad or tired. The procedure is performed under a general or local anaesthesia and takes no more than two hours. Patients can go home the same day.

In a forehead lift, the excess skin is removed and the nerves to the muscles that cause frowning are cut, thus smoothing the forehead, raising the eyebrows and minimizing frown lines (almost like permanent Botox, see page 151). The surgeon may use the conventional method, in which an incision is made across the top of the head from ear to ear and hidden just behind the hairline, or employ an endoscope, a viewing instrument that requires only minimal incisions.

Unfortunately, a conventional browlift usually leads to permanent numbness of the top of the scalp, higher eyebrows, a scar and a permanently 'surprised' look. There may also be some hair loss along the scar. When the endoscope is used, very small incisions are needed, so the method is less traumatic, does not leave a telltale scar and requires a shorter recovery period. Endoscopy works best on patients under 40 years old with relatively elastic skin. Bruising and swelling usually subside after a few weeks.

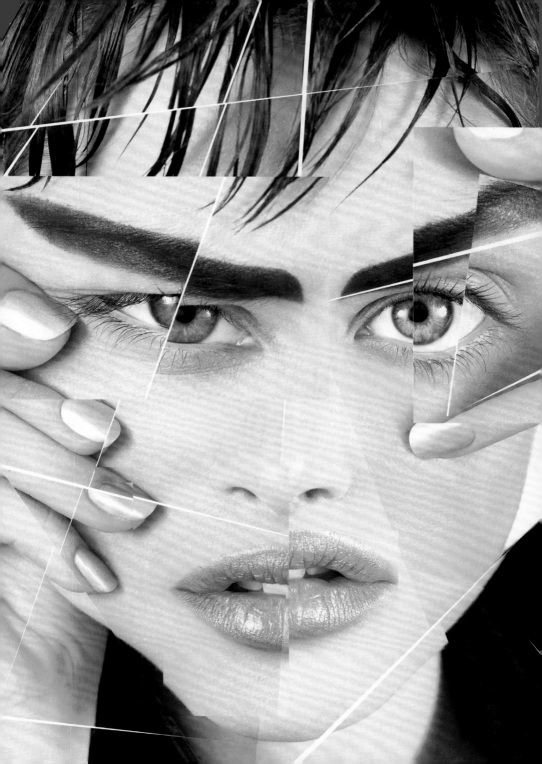

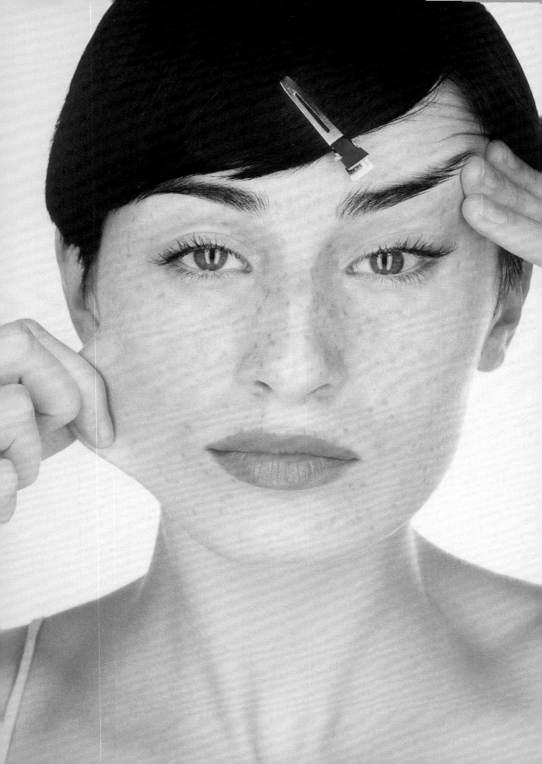

THE FACELIFT

A facelift procedure, technically called a rhytidectomy, is nearly always performed simultaneously with a necklift, because changes due to ageing in the face usually have accompanying changes in the neck. A facelift aims to tighten and smooth the appearance of the skin on the face and neck; it does little for the forehead and eye area, however. The surgery is performed under local anaesthetic with intravenous sedation and takes about three hours.

The incisions are made in existing skin creases and in the hairline around the ear (minimal or no hair is trimmed from the scalp along the incisions). The surgeon then retracts and advances the skin and its underlying tissues to give a smoother and more defined contour to the neck and jaw line. If necessary, the surgeon will trim or suction fat along the jaw line or under the chin (this occasionally requires an incision under the chin). The surgeon may also tighten tissue by moving both the skin and the deeper subcutaneous tissues and muscles. Excess skin is excised and discarded, and the incisions are closed with sutures and staples.

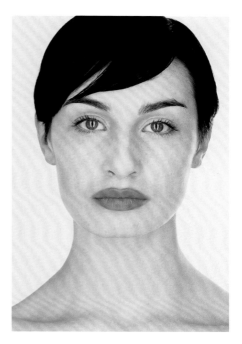

After surgery the face is wrapped in bandages, which nearly cover the entire head, for 24 hours. Swelling and bruising is inevitable. Bruising takes about a month to subside but the swelling can last for three to four months. A good neck job should last for ten years and a good facelift should last for five years. There is some permanent hair loss with a facelift, and repeated facelifts can result in an unnatural-looking hairline.

HIRING A CONSULTANT

Good information is essential in the maze that is cosmetic surgery. As the practice has become more and more popular, so the field of surgery advisors has boomed. A consultant is an independent expert who guides you through the surgical and non-surgical procedures available, helps locate a surgeon and manages your recovery. Consultants are usually former nurses or patients and should have some form of accreditation. Wendy Lewis was among the first to offer this type of service and she is definitely among the most reputable (see Directory, pages 391–7).

MAKING IT LAST

Even cosmetically altered skin is at the mercy of ageing, so once you have had surgery, make it last as long as possible.

1 Stay out of the sun whenever possible and always wear a full-spectrum sunscreen.

2 Feed the skin with antioxidants and a healthy diet.

3 If you stopped smoking, do not start again.

THE INTERNET

There has been a dramatic growth in medical information posted on the Internet. While some information is conflicting, and not all is reliable, there is no denying that the Internet provides a convenient and useful starting point for researching cosmetic surgery and surgeons. But how do you sift the good from the bad?

When it comes to medical information, however, it is safest to rely on that which is posted by reputable medical organizations. The American Society of Plastic Surgeons (ASPS) has maintained a website since 1996 that includes a wealth of information on procedures and the history of plastic surgery. Unfortunately, the website of the British Association of Plastic Surgeons (BAPS) is not quite as consumer-friendly, but there are some good websites that offer information on government standards and regulations, such the Healthcare Commission (www.healthcarecommission.org.uk).

the future
of skincare

As science seeks to enhance the quality and prolong the span of life, so we can rest assured that skincare technology will develop in leaps and bounds. Skincare continues to be at the forefront of science, simply because there is no better gauge for ageing than the skin. That is not to say, however, that products are incorporating more high-tech ingredients. On the contrary, the latest take on skin is a 'return to nature', albeit with a twist. This time technology works with the body.

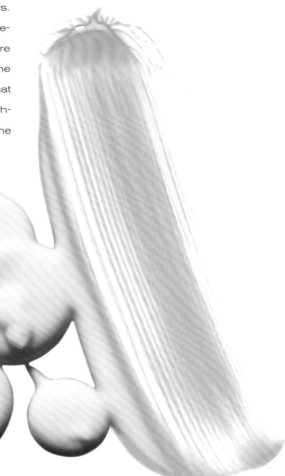

Mere moisturizers, mattifiers and exfolia-tors are no longer enough. Skincare products are now expected to help the skin repair more quickly, regenerate more efficiently and function impecca-bly. Antioxidants, chemical exfoliants and collagen stimulators all boost, rather than replace, skin's natural activity. Simultaneously, there is a welcome increase in customization. Because everyone's skin is different, the terms 'dry', 'oily' and 'combination' skin are old-fashioned and restrictive. Products need to be more specific to individual needs. There was a time when only a select few could have skincare prod-ucts mixed for them by their dermatolo-gist or facialist. Now skincare gurus and major industry players (like Chanel with their Precision line), have brought tailor-made skincare to the masses.

Efficacy is under pressure, as con-sumer savvy means that most of us now know our AHAs from our Retin-As and we want noticeable results. The future of skincare, therefore, seems to be inextricably tied up with knowledge: know your skin and what it needs. And the only way to know your skin is to care for it properly.

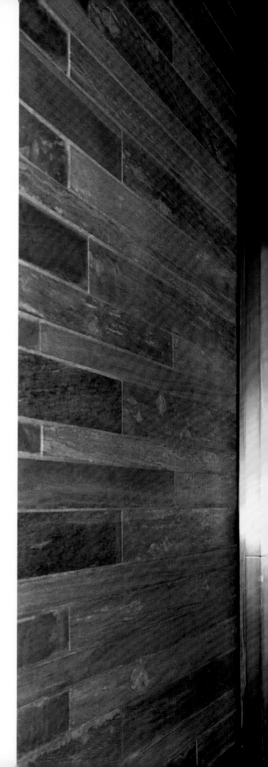

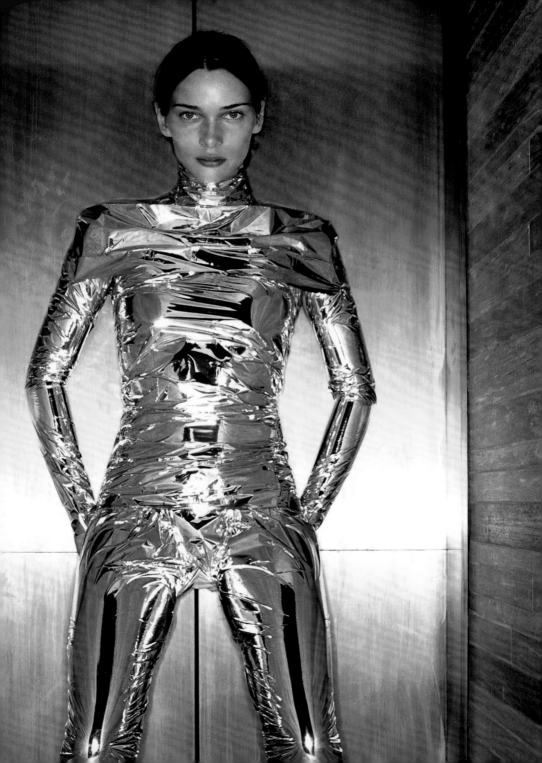

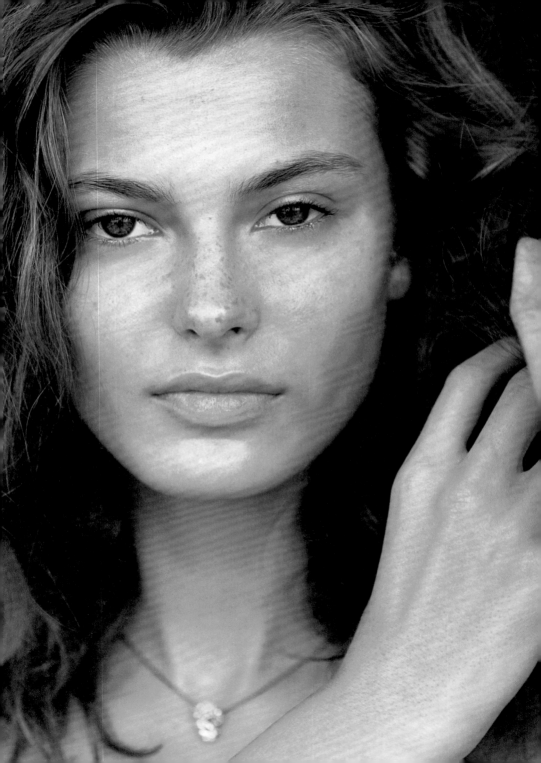

HAIR

Hair is loaded with meaning. It speaks volumes about who we are, our health, our wealth, how we live and how fashionable we are. Throughout history, women have cut, shaved, contorted, twisted, powdered and dyed their hair; some following the social norms of the day, others forging ahead in their quest for what is new, flattering and eye-catching. Whatever the intention, hair has the ability to express what words never can; it can be subtle, sexual, political and powerful — and it is a barometer of social change. In London in the 1780s, for example, women's emergence in politics coincided with the fashion for increasingly high wigs, until the already-huge doors of St Paul's cathedral had to be raised by 1.2 m (4 ft) to accommodate the enormous hairstyles. The wigs, parted in the middle with masses of curls and ringlets falling over the shoulders, became so big that a contemporary satirist described the face as looking like 'a small pimple in the midst of a vast sea of hair'. Almost 200 years later, in the 1970s, Black Power became a political movement in the USA. Men and women stopped feeling the pressure to conform to white ideals of beauty and stopped 'relaxing' their hair. By the beginning of the twenty-first century cornrows and dreadlocks crossed over to catwalks and sidewalks to be worn by all ethnicities.

As much as clothes, the hair we wear is a badge of identity. Close your eyes and imagine four very different styles of female beauty. First, the girl from South America: tanned and honed, with rich chestnut curls falling over her shoulders. Second, the epitome of French chic: classic and pared-down, with short, glossy dark hair. Third, the society hostess with her picture-perfect coiffure: her hair shows her status – she is rich, in control and has time to take care of herself. And last, the hard, anarchic punk of the 1980s: a rebel against the

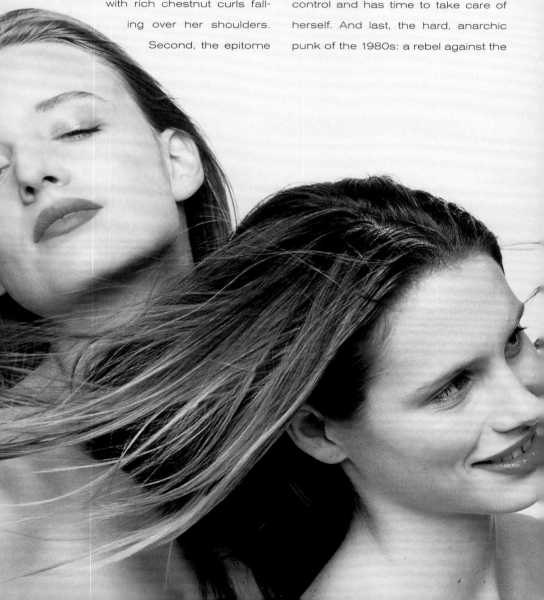

high shine of the 1970s and deliber-
ately anti-beauty. Whatever you think
of the looks, each one is carefully
thought out and, in its own way, beautiful. But would they work if you
swapped the hair around but kept the
same clothes and make-up? Would
Miss French Chic look so pared-down

with curls tumbling down her back?
Would the punk appear so anti-estab-
lishment with a neat blonde halo?

Hair is a statement, just like our
clothes, make-up and the rest of our
style. The power of hair lies partly in
its ability to transform. With the twist

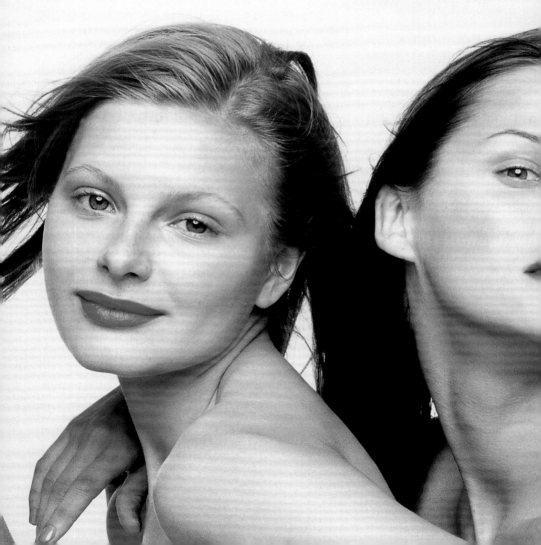

of a chignon, a sharp streak of peroxide blonde or the simple addition of accessories, the look and mood can be changed in an instant. Hair taps right into the psyche and affects us like almost nothing else; its moods and tantrums can knock us sideways. The phrase 'bad-hair day' slipped so neatly and easily into common parlance because it was a phenomenon that we understood all too well – that feeling of utter misery and lack of confidence that comes from hair that will not shine, succumb to our desires or help us look amazingly beautiful. If you know that feeling and want to gain the upper hand, this chapter is for you.

YOU, FASHION & YOUR HAIR

The catwalk is the fashion designer's version of theatre. It exists for show, exhibition and to get publicity. Rarely do the looks shown on the runways translate into real life – and they are not supposed to. The catwalk is about getting a total look, and hairdressers often create extreme hair to re-enforce the designer's statement. Fashion should be secondary, says internationally acclaimed hair expert John Frieda, 'You have to start with a style that suits you, first and foremost. It has to be in proportion with you, suit your face shape, be something that fits into your time frame and says who you are.' Subtle influences from the catwalk filter through to the street. Top London stylist Charles Worthington gives an example: 'If you see a lot of very dishevelled hair on the catwalk, that might translate into wearing a little more product in your hair and ruffling it up a bit. Possibly the catwalk looks are becoming less and less relevant as people are becoming more and more individual. But the key thing about your hairstyle is that it should reflect what you are about. If you are a bold, outgoing character, then experiment with some bold colour or a bold cut. Likewise, if you are a quiet person who likes to melt into the background, then keep your colours muted and your cut classic ... choose a versatile hairstyle that you can change from day to night, weekday to weekend. That way you'll end up with a great total look.'

you & your
hairdresser

No matter how good you are at blow-drying, accessorizing and styling your hair, you need a fantastic stylist. While mastery of technical skills is vital for a hairdresser, it is not the whole story. 'You need chemistry,' says John Frieda. 'Ultimately a woman's relationship with her hairdresser is about trust. People get in such a state about their hair for the same reason they do about their health. They want it to be perfect, but it's out of their control because people can't cut their own hair. Hair is so vital to a person's look, it says so much about them and who they are, but they end up having to put it into someone else's hands. And that can be scary. If you have a great relationship with your hairdresser, it's like a meeting of minds. You must trust him completely, be able to communicate well with him and be able to listen to him.'

Only about one-quarter of British women have a hairdresser they see regularly. Shocked? Surprised? Maybe not. Finding someone with whom you feel a rapport and who makes you and your hair look fantastic is often difficult. But if you do find someone, then stick with them and never let them go – they are priceless. Jo Hansford is one of the world's top colourists and has her own London salon and product range. According to her, the key to finding a fantastic hairdresser is visual. 'If you see a woman with great hair, go ahead and ask her who cut or coloured it. You may be in a restaurant, plane or train, but she will be flattered and it is really the only way to know. Don't just listen to chit-chat and gossip about who is the "hairdresser-of-the-moment". Pick up on visual clues – that's the real test of who is a good hairdresser.'

Find the best hairdresser you can afford. He or she will provide the basis of your look, give you a great cut that you can manage during the day and dress up a little for night, and be an informed sounding board for new ideas, colours and styles. Always look for a hairdresser who keeps updating you and does not

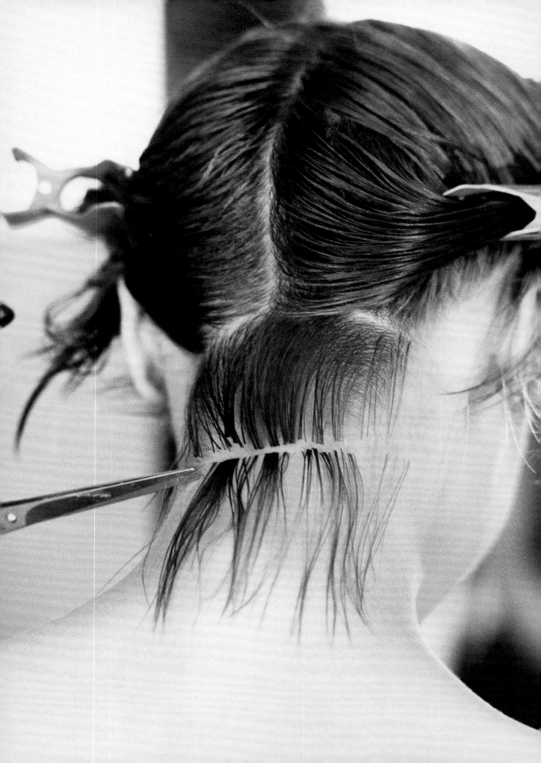

let your look become stagnant. 'You need to build up trust with a hairdresser,' continues Hansford. 'Chopping, changing and going to different stylists every time won't help build up trust. Good communication is also vital between hairdresser and client. If you can communicate effectively what you want and the hairdresser understands and makes you feel confident and comfortable, then you are on the road to success.'

HOW TO FIND A GREAT HAIRDRESSER

1 Look for visual clues. If you see someone with a great cut or colour ask them who did it. 'You'll make their day,' says Charles Worthington.

2 'When trying a new hairdresser for the first time, don't book in for anything radical,' advises John Frieda. 'Test them out with a blow-dry or a trim first, before committing yourself to anything else.'

3 'Pick a good time for yourself and the hairdresser. Don't book an appointment just before a big event when you are under pressure,' continues Frieda. 'Likewise, ask the receptionist when is a good, quiet time for your consultation –

maybe it's the first appointment in the morning, or maybe it's last thing at night. If they are not receptive to you, don't go ahead. You've got your answer already.'

GETTING WHAT YOU WANT

Josh Wood is one of London's top colour specialists and has a coterie of international A-list clients. 'To get the best from your hairdresser you should learn a little bit about what he is doing to your hair. Many people have no idea what they want or what is possible for them to have, and that makes it very easy to be disappointed or frustrated. Find out the name of the colour techniques you are having (for example, "Am I having a semi-permanent that will wash out after six to eight shampoos? Or is it permanent colour that will grow out and leave dark roots?"). Then, when you want to change or update your look, you will be better placed to discuss things with your hairdresser.' Josh continues, 'Also, keep a "look book". It's nothing serious, just a file of hairstyles you like, probably torn from fashion and beauty magazines, pictures of yourself and so on. And keep some pictures of hair that you hate too. It's a great way for your hairdresser to know what kind of look you like.'

If you are starting with a new hairdresser or thinking of changing your colour or style, a consultation is vital. If a hairdresser is not interested in giving a thorough consultation — one that runs through exactly what you want and what they plan to do — then do not go ahead. You are in no way obliged to carry on with an appointment if you suspect that you are not going to get the service and attention you should. Too many women sit through what should be a relaxing and enjoyable experience feeling confused and unconfident. They then pay, go home and weep. No hairdresser wants to give you a style that you hate, but unless you communicate well together (and it is up to you, too!), you will probably have better luck with someone else.

'I HATE MY HAIR' CRISIS

'If you keep repeating the same hairstyle, over and over again, you may begin to hate your hair,' says colour specialist Josh Wood. 'When you reach screaming point, be specific about what you want to change. Never change everything – cut, colour and style – in one go. New hairstyles should evolve and not just appear, just like your own personal style.

'Very subtle seasonal changes are much more modern and flattering than total redesigns. If you are just bored, before you go for a drastic cut, try changing your styling first. For example, if you always wear your hair straight, try styling it curly; if it's always curly, then put some product in it and blow-dry it glossy and straight.

'Condition is critical also. It doesn't matter if your hair is long or short, if it's in bad condition it will look like bad hair. So before colouring, consider if the condition is good enough for colour; you don't want to make your hair look worse. Saying that, changing your hair and make-up is vitally important; colour and form are the two largest factors that make women look dated.'

the cutting edge

All of us want the most flattering haircut for our face — the kind of cut that makes our eyes stand out, our skin seem brighter and makes us feel taller, slimmer and sexier. But is it really possible? Of course it is. The right cut will make an enormous difference to your face shape, to which features dominate and which recede, not to mention to the tone of your overall look. That is why hair is usually the first thing to change when a woman overhauls her image, whether she has just made it in Hollywood, on television, in politics or whether she has just worked it out for herself. If you find the right hairstyle, everything else just seems to fall into place. According to Charles Worthington, there are three points to consider before embarking on any change:

1 Be realistic. How much time do you really want to spend on your hair every day? Is it just five minutes in the morning, after jumping out of the shower? Can you spare 10 to 15 minutes for blow-drying, straightening and taming? Or are you high-maintenance,

never happier than when standing in front of the mirror, fussing and fluffing your crowning glory? In that case, you can probably take on a style that requires maximum effort. If you choose a style that requires time you are not happy to put in, you will never get the look you want.

2 Make the most of what you have got. Whether it is straight, curly, dark or blonde, wavy or wispy, hair always looks best when it is in fabulous condition and has a fantastic cut. Trying to change your natural hair too much may compromise condition and make you a slave to a high-maintenance look.

3 Ammunition. For all hair types, products are essential daily tools for achieving gloss, shine, body and manageability. Experiment a little and learn which products suit your hair best and how to use them (see pages 183–4).

THE KINDEST CUTS

Determining your face shape, and your hair type or texture, will help you find the most flattering cut. Although not a strict guide, it will teach you how to adapt and hone the styles seen on the catwalk or on the beauty pages of magazines into something stunning and individual. According to Charles Worthington, the face shape triggers off the hairstyle. 'Hair is a frame to the face. It's the same with a painting; if the frame is awful, it detracts from the picture. But if you've got the right style for the face shape, then the whole face looks prettier, fresher, the eyes stand out and good features get emphasized.'

HOW DO YOU DETERMINE YOUR FACE SHAPE?

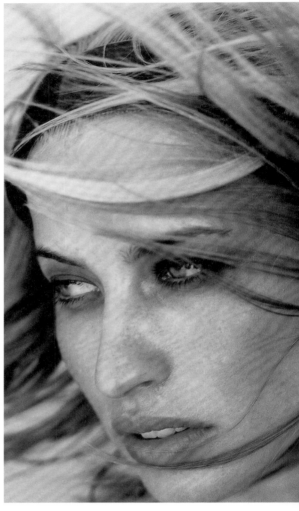

Hold a mirror at arm's length and draw the bold outline of your face with lipstick. What you see will be square, oblong, heart-shaped, round or oval. There, wasn't that fun?

SQUARE: Stay away from angular styles and try layers. A heavy fringe (bangs) is a no-no, but a sweeping fringe adds softness.

OBLONG: A fringe (bangs) is a must. Avoid growing hair too long as it can make the face appear longer; shoulder-length is best. A bit of width in the style can work wonders.

HEART-SHAPED: Avoid very short styles and instead create width at the jaw line or neck, perhaps with flick-ups. Avoid extra height or exaggerated width around the eyes.

ROUND: If the hair comes forward onto the face, then it will not expose the roundness. A soft fringe (bangs) can work well, too.

OVAL: Although traditionally considered the 'perfect' face shape, that does not necessarily make things easier. You lucky girls now have to make choices.

HAIR TYPES

FINE & STRAIGHT: This hair needs guts and strength, but the jury is still out on whether or not to have layers put in fine, straight hair. All hairdressers agree on one thing – don't grow fine hair past shoulder-length. Instead, keep it in great condition with volumizing products and think about a fringe (bangs). London hairdresser Stuart Phillips explains, 'Generally the hair that grows down the sides of our faces is in worse condition than anywhere else; we sleep on it, fiddle with it and style it most often. A fringe gets rid of that hair and leaves only the best-conditioned hair on show. But don't cut a fringe unless you and your hairdresser are really sure it suits. It's too drastic.'

THICK & COARSE: 'Thick hair has the widest choice of styles – anything goes – but it is the hardest to look after,' says Stuart Phillips. 'It's easy to have a strong shape cut into thick hair, and it also looks great with layers or a graduated cut, but you mustn't get it cut too short, or it may stick up and become unmanageable.'

CURLY: There is no rule of thumb with curly hair – it may be fine and fluffy or strong and thick. 'It's really a question of cutting to suit the individual face shape and hair texture,' says Stuart Phillips. 'You can play around with different lengths but, in general, the longer you let your hair grow, the heavier the weight, and that stops it getting too big. If your face is round and your curly hair goes wide, then don't cut it short or add layers around the face – it will only accentuate it.'

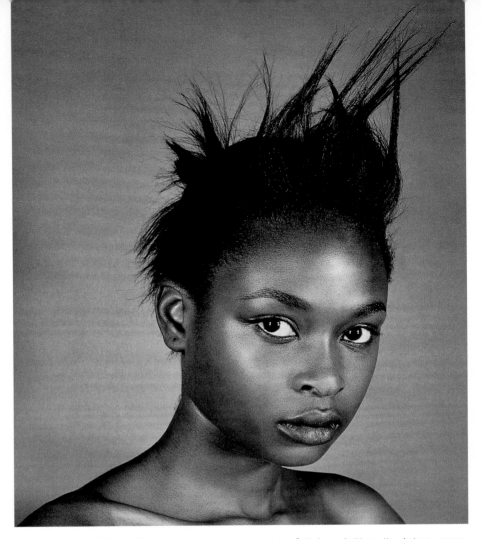

AFRO-CARIBBEAN: 'Black hair is so diverse,' says Lisa Laudat, afro hair specialist and stylist. 'There are so many different textures within that category, but there is really a choice of two things to do with it. Firstly, you can keep it natural, get it in fantastic condition and learn to make the most of it by plaiting it, doing corn-rows or putting it into corkscrews. Or secondly, if you want to straighten it with a chemical process, keep it really straight and shiny. Learn how to blow-dry it, develop a good hair-care routine and learn to use the right products.'

haircare

What is hair? Hair is protein. In fact, it is approximately 97 per cent protein and about 3 per cent water. Each strand is made up of three layers (skin is made up of five layers) and, to all intents and purposes, it is inert, or dead. The condition and health of your hair is a reflection of three factors: your general state of health, your diet, and how well you look after it. Certainly, high-quality, high-tech products can do wonders to repair damaged, lifeless hair, but they can only go so far. If your lifestyle, health and diet are not up to scratch, then neither will your hair be. The hair on your head now is way past the stage of being helped by great nutrition, but every minute of every day, new hair is being made. Any positive changes made now will improve hair sooner than you might imagine. Which leads neatly into the idea that 'beauty comes from within', which is never truer than with hair.

Philip Kingsley is one of the world's foremost trichologists. From his clinics in London and New York he treats many famous names. 'Hair is greatly affected by lifestyle factors – smoking, drinking, drugs and diet, as well as the more obvious factors like pregnancy, menopause, hormone imbalance, ageing and ill health. But you can greatly improve the quality, volume and health of hair through a good, balanced diet. Remember that what is good for the rest of you is also good for your hair. Most women are not eating as much protein as their hair would like and many women of childbearing age are also lacking in iron – another vital nutrient for hair.'

NUTRITION

After four hours without food, the body's vital organs – the heart, kidneys, liver, and so on – begin to draw on nutritional reserves destined for non-vital organs, such as skin and hair. That is why poor nutrition is not only bad for general health, but particularly bad for skin and hair. To redress past misdeeds and improve the quality and condition of new hair, follow Philip Kingsley's advice:

'Three balanced meals a day are important — each containing carbohydrate, protein, fat, minerals and vitamins — and many women are not eating that. Breakfast is the most important meal for hair and it should contain protein, as should lunch, which is the second most important meal for hair. Most people eat enough protein at dinner but that is really the least important meal for hair. For lunch, aim for 120–140 g (4–5 oz) of protein; that is, a piece of fish, chicken or turkey breast, or seafood pasta. There is no quick fix for hair. It will take some months to see a difference, but after 18 months your entire head of hair could be completely transformed and certainly your skin will be glowing.'

Do we need to take special supplements, vitamins and minerals for our hair? Yes and no. Philip Kingsley suggests, 'Remember that what is good for your whole health is also good for your hair, but there is no specific supplement that is good only for your hair. Zinc and iron supplements with vitamin C can be good for hair, but only if you are lacking them. If you have problems with your hair [see pages 207–9], get checked out by your doctor to see what the problem is first, before taking specific supplements.'

THE SUN

The sun damages hair as easily as it does skin. It oxidizes it, dries it out and damages the colour and the cuticle. Unlike skin, which renews cells every 28 days, the average head of hair is 18 months old and may have been burnt over and over again. To keep locks sleek and glossy, treat them with as much care and respect as you do your skin. At the beach and on the slopes, keep hair covered with a scarf or hat. Failing that, slick it with leave-in conditioner, which will be activated into super-duper efficiency with the heat. Blondes have to be extra, extra careful. Why do you think swimming pools are blue? Chlorine is tinged with blue dye, so keep your hair well away — khaki leather looked great when Gucci did it, but you do not want hair to match. Unless you are scrupulously careful, damage incurred during a two-week holiday can take six months to repair. In fact, a fortnight of sun can lift hair colour three or four shades and do more damage than any heated appliance. You have been warned.

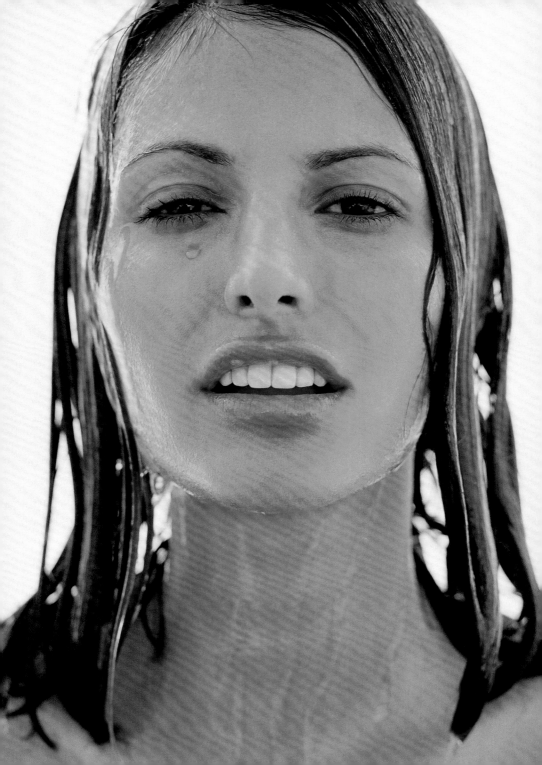

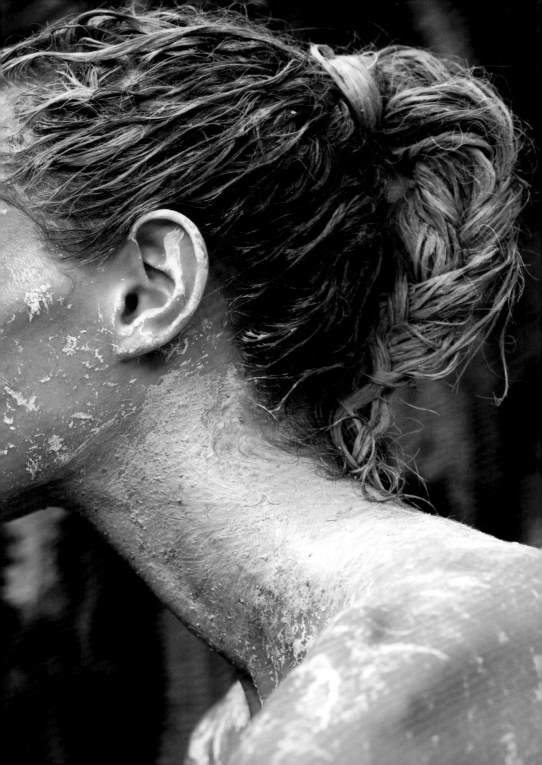

HAIRCARE PRODUCTS

Hair products are not what they used to be; they are much, much better. Like all aspects of the beauty industry in the twenty-first century, they have benefited enormously from advances in technology. Now curls can stay defined and glossy even in humidity, volume can be pumped up on even the finest and fluffiest hair, and shape and style can be kept all day and all night, and still feel sexy and touchable.

Like anything, investing in the best is really worthwhile. If you are paying top dollar for a great cut and colour, there is every reason to carry on the good work when you get home. Many of us are still stuck in that groove of forking out for skincare, but skimping on haircare. That is not to say that you should pay a fortune. When you look further afield than the supermarket aisle for hair products, you will find mid-priced ranges, such as those by L'Oréal Kérastase and Keihls, for example, and hairdressers' brands, such as those by Paul Mitchell, Charles Worthington, John Frieda, Jo Hansford and Trevor Sorbie; they all make excellent, affordable products.

What you will find with top-notch products is that they do not contain the alcohol and resins found in cheaper products, so they work more efficiently and are kinder to hair in the long run. They will also be boosted with extra ingredients, such as sun filters, vitamin-rich antioxidants and deep moisturizing ingredients that are capable of penetrating the hair shaft and strengthening the cuticle day after day.

SHAMPOOS: There are literally hundreds of shampoos out there, so how do you separate the wheat from the chaff? The first rule is to stay clear of the sudsy, detergent shampoos that you could use to wash your dishes. Read the labels carefully and look for formulations that correspond to your hair type exactly. Do you want something deeply moisturizing for dry, coloured hair or something oil-free for fine, limp hair? Whatever you need for your hair, it is out there. Steer clear of two-in-one shampoo/conditioners. Every hairdresser will tell you that one product cannot do two things well at the same time – it is common sense.

CONDITIONERS: Almost every hair type needs conditioning, especially if you colour, blow-dry or heat-style it. Fine, straight, flat hair needs just the ends conditioning, never the roots, and a light, oil-free formula will do. For the curly, porous, dry variety of hair, choose a heavier, more moisturizing formula and use it all over the hair from the roots to the ends, but remember that leaving an everyday conditioner on longer than 30 seconds will not increase the benefit.

DEEP, INTENSIVE CONDITIONERS: Ideally, everyone should use one of these weekly. They pump moisturizing ingredients, such as emollients and vegetable protein, into the hair shaft, repairing damage and weakness head on.

CLEANSING HAIR

'Your hair should be absolutely and completely soaking wet before you shampoo,' says Charles Worthington. 'Don't just flash it under the shower – let it get drenched for 30 seconds to one minute – you'll need much less shampoo and washing will be much easier on your hair.'

According to Philip Kingsley, the more you shampoo your hair, the better. 'Cleanliness is good for your hair, in the same way that it is good for skin,' he says. 'After all, it is going all the same places as your face, so if you wash your face daily because it is dirty, then so should you wash your hair. Washing hair is actively good for it because it is adding water and moisturizers to the hair.' But what about washing away all your hair's natural oils? 'Nonsense,' says Kingsley. 'Hair does not need oil. It needs water and moisture.'

CONDITION, CONDITION, CONDITION, CONDITION

More than anything else, shiny, shiny hair is the Holy Grail of haircare now. No matter if the colour is brown, bronze or blonde, if it shines, it must be good. The craze for lustrous, shiny locks is partly fuelled by the belief that shiny hair is healthy, natural hair (even though we know the prettiest things are not always really, really natural) and partly because product technology is now able to give us shine straight from the bottle. Admittedly, if you have been a nut and damaged your hair, either through sun exposure, overprocessing or some horrible kitchen-sink drama with a dye bottle, it will take more than a slug of serum to get over the worst. But dramas aside, most hair responds well to a few basic strategies to keep it clean, healthy, well nourished and looking good.

1 Let us start at the very beginning. 'Never, never neglect your hair so much that it gets into bad condition in the first place,' says Trevor Sorbie. 'Keep your hair out of the sun, especially if it is coloured. It's the worst thing for it.'

2 Strong detergent shampoos can cause havoc. They do not clean particularly well and they strip hair of its moisture. Baby shampoos are the worst culprits. Look for good-quality shampoos that are appropriate for your hair type.

3 The aggressive friction created when you towel-dry your hair drives curls into frizziness and damages fine hair. Blot, blot and blot again, instead.

4 Almost all hair types need conditioning after washing. If your hair is very fine, use a light, oil-free conditioner from the middle to the ends only. Stronger, coarser, drier hair needs a heavier conditioner and perhaps a leave-in conditioner, too. Blot the hair dry first, apply conditioner, leave it on for 30 seconds and then rinse it off thoroughly. Remember that all standard conditioners stop working after 30 seconds.

5 An intensive conditioner is the secret weapon of every glossy-haired girl. They are not made of the same ingredients as ordinary conditioners, but contain a high proportion of moisturizers, emollients and vegetable protein, which are all able to penetrate the hair shaft deeply and repair any damage and weakness.

HAIR TYPES

When it comes to hair type, you can run but you cannot hide. Do what you will, but try, please try, to like your natural hair just a little bit. Try to appreciate its idiosyncrasies and learn to make the most of them (see also The Kindest Cuts, pages 175–7). Remember, also, that using the right products – those specially formulated for your hair type and lifestyle — will help to heal, tame and coerce your hair. Here are some tips to help you work with the hair that nature gave you.

FINE HAIR: According to Charles Worthington, 'Don't be afraid of washing and conditioning your hair every day, if necessary. If you are using the correct products, you are adding moisture, strength and protection to your hair. Hair is like skin: keep it clean, well moisturized and protect it from heated styling and the sun. Use a volumizer on the roots, not all the way through. Also, do not go too blonde. Blonde can look a little see-through. You would be better with a deeper, richer colour to make hair look lustrous.'

THICK HAIR: Thick, dark hair can be fantastically shiny. However, because it is so strong, it can be resistant to styling, so it needs firm-hold products. Serum is a great way to tame unruly hair into submission, and it makes the hair easier to handle while imparting great shine.

CURLY HAIR: About 60 per cent of the world's population have curly, frizzy hair.

Generally, curly hair is dry hair and needs to be well moisturized. Use a moisturizing shampoo and intensive conditioner. To get control and smooth down the hair cuticle, apply serum to wet hair.

'Be liberal with products,' says Charles Worthington. 'If you don't use enough, you won't get enough effect in curly hair. You'll probably need serum and mousse to define the curls or to blow-dry the curl out. Leave-in conditioner is also a great idea as it moisturizes and protects.' Other hair professionals recommend brushing curly hair straight while you are still in the shower, applying some gel and then leaving it alone for a natural but sleek style.

AFRO-CARIBBEAN OR FRIZZY HAIR: The individual hairs can be quite fine and brittle, so strengthening and moisturizing is very important for this hair type. Often the hair is dehydrated, so leave-in and intensive conditioners are both useful products, especially if the hair has been chemically straightened. To add a little gloss and protection, use a serum.

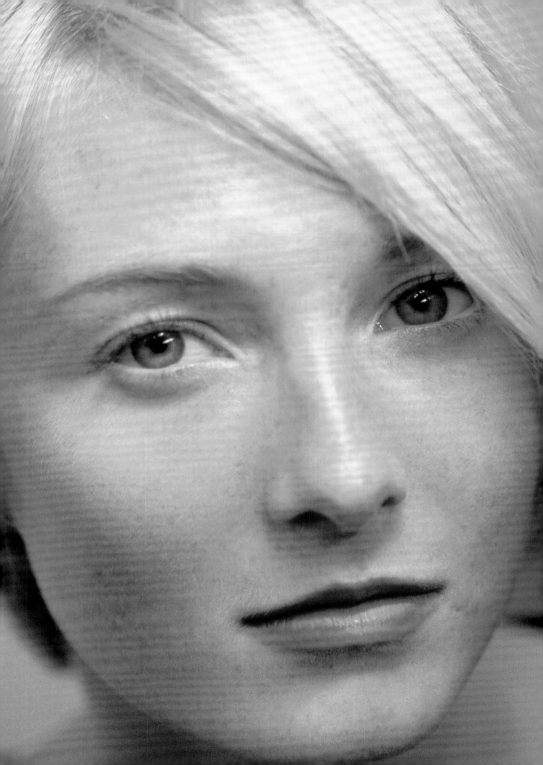

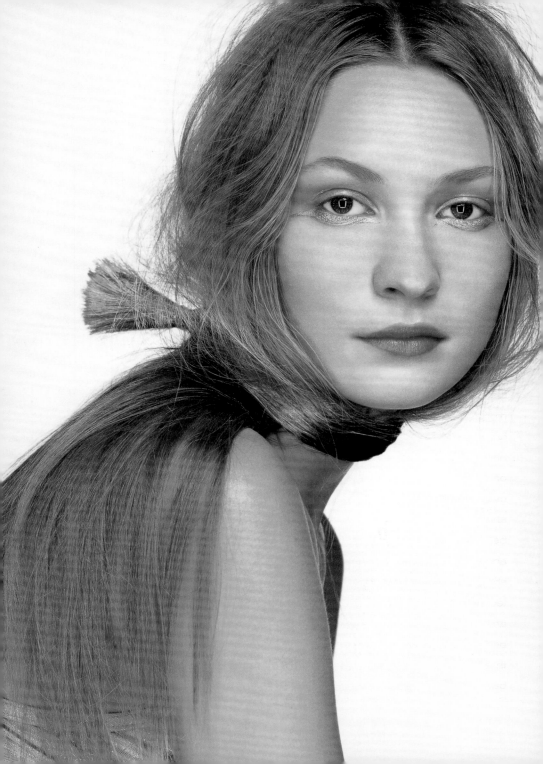

colour

Almost every head of hair looks better for a touch of colour. Whether it is hyper-natural honey highlights that gently frame the face or bold slices of super-shiny bronze in long, dark hair, the effects can be stunning. Do not think that the only choices are blonde, brunette or redhead; the technology behind hair colouring is now so sophisticated that almost anything is possible. If you want to be blonde, you can choose anything from pale cream and liquid honey hues to golden, buttery highlights. Or imagine the luscious myriad colours of chocolate, chestnut, amber, cinnamon and copper – perhaps used as touches here and there, or woven seamlessly into the hair all over, making it seem light-reflective, alive and glorious. Jo Hansford has been colouring hair for film, television and supermodels for over 30 years and she is enthusiastic about the latest technology. 'The new products today are absolutely amazing, incredible, because they are so translucent. I do think that hair colour is important because it's the one accessory that you

never take off. It's not like a dress, which you may spend a fortune on and wear only once or twice. Hair colour has as much of an impact on a woman's look – eyes and skin tone – as cosmetic surgery and you wouldn't have cosmetic surgery unless you'd had a serious consultation, maybe two or three. Now we can get the results that previously we only dreamed of. We've reached a point in hair colouring technology where the fear element has been eliminated. The products are very flexible now so you don't have to play safe any longer. If you've found the right hairdresser/colour technician [see pages 171–4] then feel free to go ahead, experiment and have fun.'

DAMAGE FROM COLOURING PROCESSES

The number one reason people do not have their hair coloured is the fear that it will damage the hair and leave it looking dry, frizzy and dull. Fear not. If done properly, dyeing will not damage the hair; in fact, several colouring techniques actually improve hair condition and increase shine. For example, tone-on-tone colours, such as L'Oréal Diacolor and Wella Color Touch, blend away grey hair and gradually fade or wash out after about 28 washes. The level of peroxide is so low, at 3 per cent, that it just gently swells the hair shaft, leaving the hair glossy and shiny. Likewise, vegetable colours and colour-enhancing shampoos can leave a subtle hint of colour, but mostly they give great shine. There is little doubt that going blonde is still the most damaging colour process. Bleach is used to open up and penetrate the hair shaft and must be handled extremely carefully, so never try it at home. But there are fabulous technicians out there who can lighten hair extremely well and minimize the damage.

The key to keeping coloured hair in super-shiny condition is using the right products. Always look for those specially formulated for coloured hair as they will maintain the pH balance and will not contain alcohol or resins that dry hair. If you are dubious about using special products for coloured hair, then think about this: you would not use the same face cream for dry skin as you would for oily, would you? Also, be religious about using an intensive, deep-conditioning mask every week – they make a huge difference.

COLOURING TECHNIQUES

There is enormous confusion when it comes to colouring techniques. The whole business seems to be shrouded in mystery and muddle, but no longer. Read on and remember.

SALON COLOUR

TEMPORARY COLOURS: These are super-safe and sometimes known as 'water rinses'. The colour does not penetrate the hair and washes away easily, but they are less and less popular now because they do not impart much shine.

SEMI-PERMANENT COLOURS: These will last from six to eight shampoos. The colour stains the cuticle by just sitting on top of it. As they do not penetrate the hair shaft, they are not colouring, in essence, but blending. They will blend away some grey.

TONE-ON-TONE COLOURS: These dyes are mixed with a catalyst and contain 3 per cent peroxide, which gently opens the cuticle for the colour to enter.

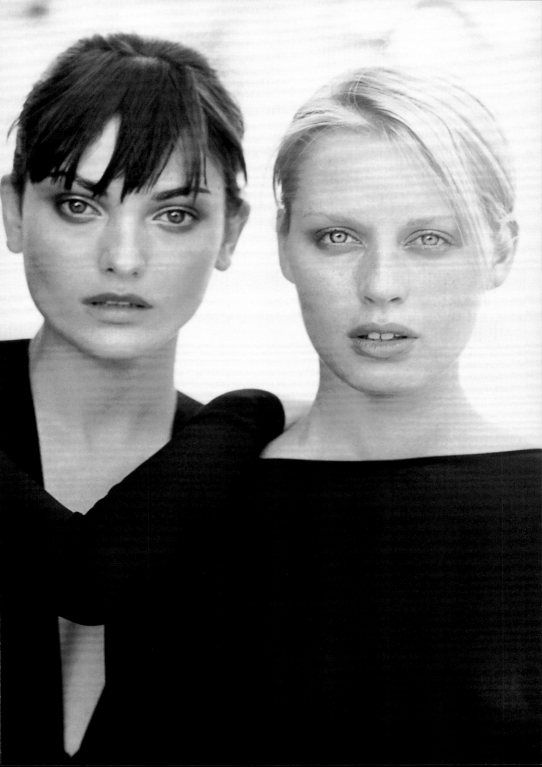

They will last for approximately 24 shampoos, but they do not really wash out. There is slight regrowth, but many more advantages: they do not damage hair; the colours can be bold; they cover grey; they are not permanent; and they give great shine.

PERMANENT COLOURS: If done correctly, these colours do not damage hair, but they do use between 20 per cent and 40 per cent peroxide. Peroxide is acidic and should always be balanced by an alkaline substance, usually called 'high lift tint'. High lift tint does not damage hair because it lifts the cuticle, deposits the colour and then puts the cuticle back. Although knowing the entire technique involved is not necessary, you do need to go to a very reputable technician.

HIGHLIGHTS: These are usually a combination of bleach and high lift tint applied to strands of hair.

LOWLIGHTS: This technique is never damaging because the hair is not being stripped. Instead colour, slivers of browns and reds, is deposited into the hair. Lowlights are generally permanent, but the tint imparts shine.

VEGETABLE COLOURS: The term is a misnomer because these dyes are not made from vegetables at all. They are safe, water-based and contain no harsh chemicals.

AT-HOME COLOUR

LEVEL 1 – TEMPORARY COLOURS: Temporary colours are available as simple sachets, 'colour enhancing' shampoos and boxes of colour that claim to last between six and eight shampoos. They gradually wash away, so no commitment to a colour is required. They are non-damaging, but do not cover grey.

LEVEL 2 – SEMI-PERMANENT COLOURS: These contain two formulas that need to be mixed together. They blend into the hair rather than cover it. They work best in warm, dark and red colours and, although they do not lighten, they do blend in the grey a little.

LEVEL 3 – PERMANENT COLOURS: These dyes cover grey and the colour grows out gradually. Never apply permanent colour on top of permanent colour if only the roots need colouring. Touch up the roots first, then run the rest of the dye through to the ends of the hair for the last few minutes of the required time only.

YOUR COLOUR, YOUR HAIR'S COLOUR

According to Josh Wood, 'Traditionally, most hairdressers have been trained to put their clients into categories, such as autumn/winter or spring/summer. It is probably better to stay within your colour range, but these days that shouldn't be restrictive, as whatever colour you want, you can find it in every tone. For example, there are cool, beige, ash blondes and warm, buttery, golden blondes now. The same goes for browns and reds.' Jo Hansford agrees: 'It is essential to be absolutely sure of what your own skin tone is now – not what it was a few years ago, as we all change as we age. Your hair colour should be in the same family (warm or cool) as your skin colour. If it is not, it may have the opposite effect and not flatter your skin colour. For example, if you have pinky skin and you have cool colours in your hair it will make you look very pink indeed.'

PRODUCTS FOR COLOUR-TREATED HAIR

When choosing haircare products for colour-treated hair, remember that your hair may have been under quite a lot of stress already, so look for products that are moisturizing, hydrating, soothing and calming. If you cannot buy those formulated specifically for colour-treated hair, then choose products for dry, dehydrated or chemically treated hair. 'Don't mix products from different ranges,' warns Jo Hansford. 'Products are formulated very specifically these days and you won't get the best from them if you are using from different ranges.'

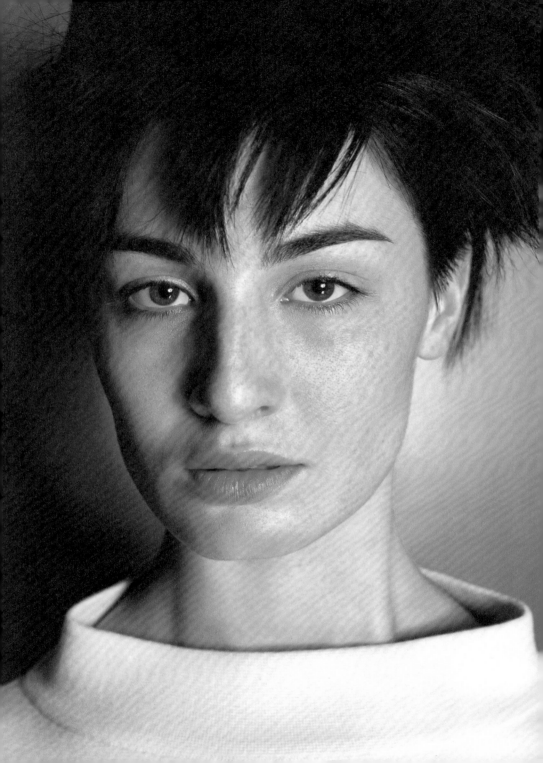

hairstyling

While cutting and colouring are best left in the skilled hands of a hair-dresser, hairstyling is where you have to become your own expert. Of course, the best person to learn from, when it comes to looking after, adapting and playing with your own style, is your hairdresser. So the next time you have an appointment booked, ask for an extra few minutes so your stylist can run through your styling options. The best hairstyles have built-in flexibility, so you can vary your look from night to day, elegant to casual and summer to winter.

The key to unlocking your potential is twofold: learn to have fun with your hair and experiment at home before venturing out; and get to know your products and the new breed of electrical appliances. No matter how well you think you know your hair, or how bored you may have grown, know that your style can be transformed by a simple slick of gel, a pump of volumizer or a headful of heated rollers. It is never too late to learn.

STYLING PRODUCTS

John Frieda is the founding father of modern hair products. He invented serum, the whole haircare-as-skincare concept, and his Frizz Ease range for curly, frizzy and dehydrated hair stands in the beauty hall of fame. 'There are two stages when you're buying hair products. First, "What is my hair type?" and second, "What effect do I want the product to achieve?". Modern products are entirely different from what went before. They do their job incredibly well and still leave hair in great condition. You can get shine and body in one product now, where before you had to buy two. Today there is no trade-off.'

SERUM: Also called glossing spray and available in spray form, serum sits on top of the hair shaft without penetrating it. It coats the hair with smooth, slick silicone, protecting it from outside damage and imparting shine and manageability. Spread only a few drops on the palm of your hand and smooth down the shaft of the hair. For curly, frizzy hair, apply the serum to damp hair before drying it, and also afterwards to leave a little gloss.

VOLUMIZER: This adds volume and guts to the flattest heads, making it a gift to fine-haired women. To apply, part the hair into smallish sections and spray the volumizer at the roots, then blow-dry as usual. The product should not be sticky or heavy, so you can easily get the accuracy you need.

MOUSSE: Probably the first mass-market styling product, mousse is still giving the others a run for their money. For volume and lift, use it only on the roots. Use it all over for curly hair to add volume, define curl and aid styling. Spray a little into the palm of your hand, then distribute it evenly throughout the hair.

WAX: Also called pomade, wax adds texture and 'separates' short hair (think Meg Ryan), making it 'piece-y' (hairdressers' lingo). Wax can also keep hair looking as if you have just stepped out of the shower. Today's versions are not greasy or oily-looking, but a small dollop goes a long way.

GEL: This product gives the strongest hold and is best used on short to mid-length styles that need firmness and structure. All but the best gels can flake and look suspiciously like dandruff, so go for quality and check that the list of ingredients does not contain alcohol.

BLOW-DRY SPRAY: The best sprays can now penetrate the hair shaft, adding moisture and protection while taming hair into a style. It can be used as a pick-up to revitalize flat hair by simply spraying and then blow-drying on a cool setting to restyle.

STYLING CREAM: Basically, this is moisturizer for hair. Blow-drying takes moisture out of hair and styling cream offers leave-in conditioner, protection and some control over frizziness.

STYLING TOOLS

If it is a serious style you are after, you can't do it with just serum and a comb. That is fine for every day, but for sleek, polished locks or head-turning glamour, invest in hardcore hair appliances. Heated rollers, curling tongs (irons), straighteners and hairdryers are what you need. We have all seen the smoke

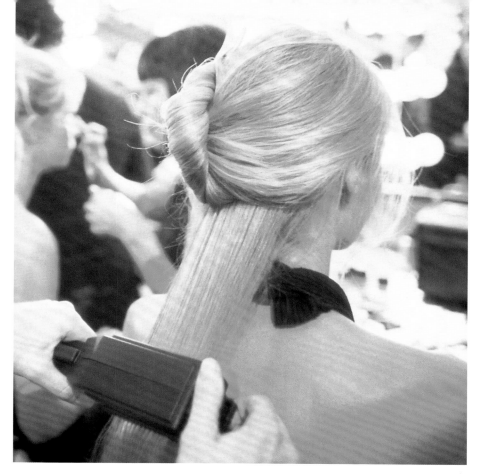

and smelt the singe, and perhaps thought that they were more trouble than they were worth, but today's new crop are proving essential.

HAIR STRAIGHTENERS: At Babyliss, sales of hair straighteners are growing faster than any other electrical hair appliance today. And that is probably because straighteners do more than just straighten; they smooth away frizz, tame or curl the ends of hair and, if done properly, leave the hair cuticle smooth and shiny.

CURLING TONGS (IRONS) & HEATED ROLLERS: Curling tongs, curling brushes and heated rollers are all multi-functional. They add movement to stick-straight hair but can also tame and smooth curly, frizzy hair. But, according to Trevor Sorbie, only the best, salon-quality tools are good enough, 'If you buy the real thing, it will have a longer life by far and you will have more power to achieve whatever style you want. If you don't want to pay up, then just stick your head out of the window.'

DIFFUSERS: These come with almost all new hairdryers, but often get thrown away. Don't do it. They are designed to deliver gentle, diffused heat, which is great for curly hair and gives all hair more volume. The plastic prongs can also be used for lifting the roots of straight, flat hair. A flat concentrator nozzle head also comes with most dryers. It is the opposite of the diffuser; it directs heat at a small, specific area and is great for quick blow-drying.

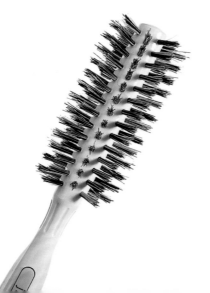

BRUSHES

Trevor Sorbie is a man who knows his brushes. 'Mason Pearson make the best brushes in the world – especially if you have long hair. They may be expensive, but I think they are worth every penny. After all, your hair should be your crowning glory.' Choose a round, boar-bristle brush for blow-drying curly hair. The natural bristles really grip the hair with each stroke, so you do get your money's worth. The longer the hair, the bigger the circumference should be. If you were born with straight, flat and wispy hair, then a brush with natural and stiff nylon bristles helps reduce static.

THE RULES OF BLOW-DRYING

1 'Never start blow-drying until your hair is semi-dry,' says Trevor Sorbie. 'If you begin with wet hair, it will take ages. Blot hair dry first, use the hairdryer to take out the rest of the moisture and then you are ready to begin.' Divide and clip the hair into manageable sections. Dry the underside first, then move on to the upper crown sections.

2 To get smooth, sleek hair, point the concentrator nozzle of the hairdryer

CAN HEAT-STYLING DAMAGE YOUR HAIR?

According to Trevor Sorbie, all good electrical appliances are thermostatically controlled, so they never get too hot to damage hair. 'Perhaps over a long period of time you could do damage,' he says, 'but you would have to be excessive and using them all the time. No matter how bad appliances are, they are never as bad as the sun. In two weeks the sun can do more damage than a hair straightener can do in a year.'

down the hair shaft in the direction of the cuticle, from crown to ends.

3 Heat makes styles drop out, so 'set' with a blast of cold air.

BLOW-DRYING CURLY OR FRIZZY HAIR

1 Apply serum and mousse to gently towel-dried hair, then comb it through with a wide-tooth comb. Dry the hair upside down in the bowl of a diffuser, using a medium heat setting. Touch the hair as little as possible to prevent it from frizzing.

2 If the hair is very unruly, set it in large Velcro rollers and then dry it gently with the hairdryer. Remove

the rollers when they are completely cool. For a sleeker, straighter look, finish by blow-drying the hair further to reduce some of the curl.

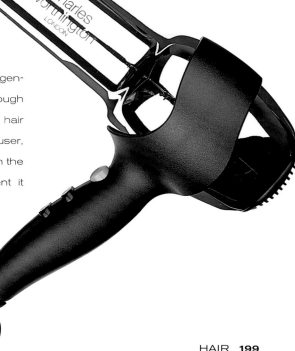

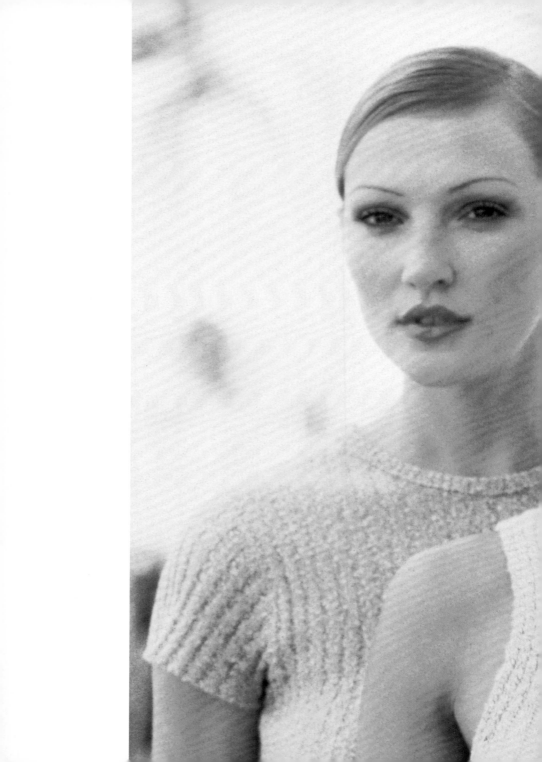

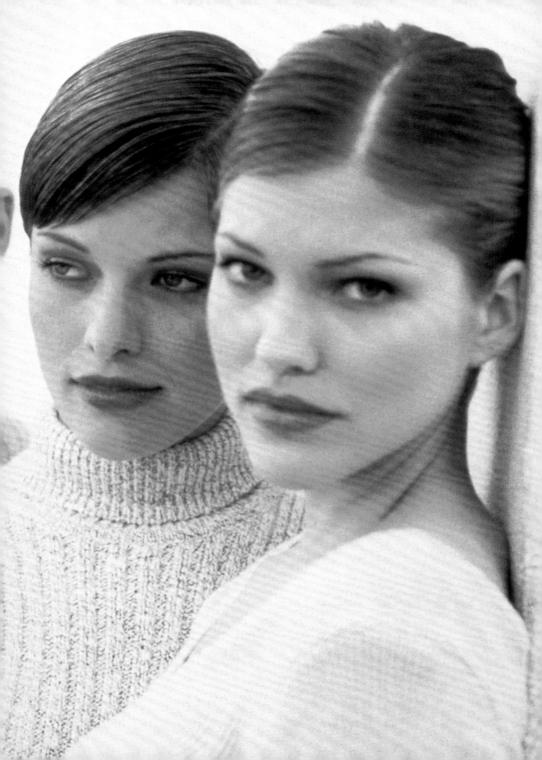

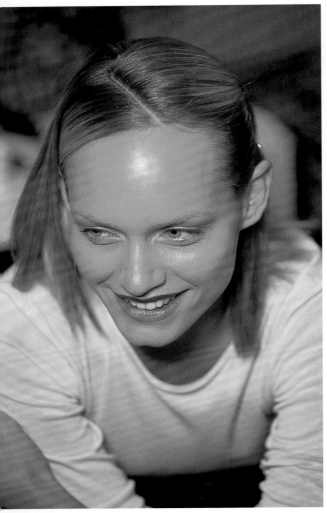

STEP-BY-STEP STYLES

Although it is a well-worn phrase, a 'classic hairstyle' does not really exist. Subtle details change over the seasons and something that seemed quite classic a few years ago probably would not look so now. However, below are four pretty and timeless looks: the ponytail, the chignon, volume for fine hair and perfect curls. They have all had their moment, but they just keep comin' on back and back. Feel free to tweak here and there.

PONYTAILS

1 The style will not work well if the hair is too slippery, so add some mousse or styling spray to give the hair more 'guts'.

PARTINGS

Try different partings to see what suits you. Generally, a middle parting is the least forgiving, as it accentuates any asymmetry on the face. A simple side parting is usually more flattering.

2 Choose the parting and make sure it is straight. Then decide on the height: ponytails should be either high and slicked back (think 1950s) or low-slung and neatly gathered at the nape of the neck.

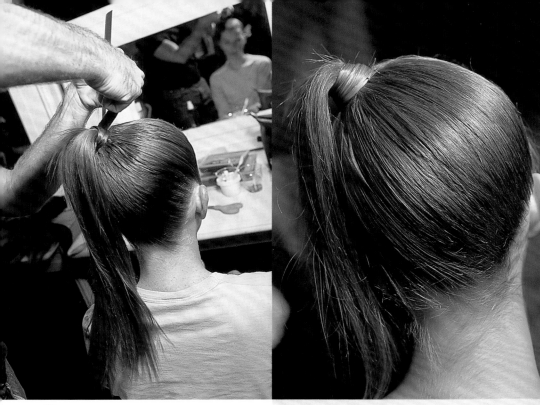

3 Grab the hair in one hand and brush it back with a bristle brush. Keep brushing while holding the ponytail to get good tension between the finger and thumb.

4 Secure the hair with a band. Invisible bands are snag-free and will not tear hair, but bungee bands with two hooks are really the best because they are tidier and grip the ponytail tighter. To use a bungee, wrap it around and around the ponytail, as tight as you like, until the two ends clip together.

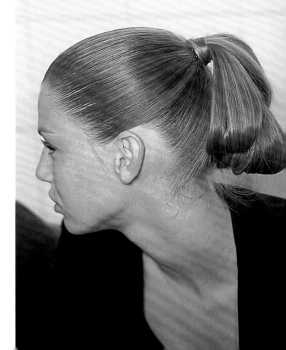

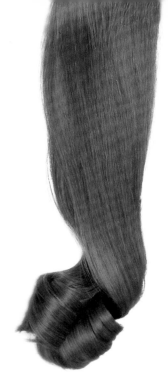

FAKING IT

'Try a false ponytail,' says Charles Worthington. 'Your hair must be long enough to put back and the falsie just clips on the top. But definitely wind a piece of your own hair over the join [see Ponytails, pages 202–3] to make it look natural.'

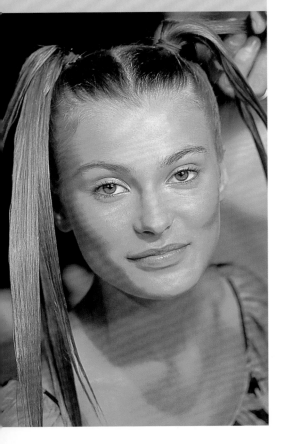

5 For a finishing touch that comes straight from the session stylists, cover the band with your own hair. Take a small section of hair from underneath the ponytail, twist it around the band, spraying it in place as you go, and secure it with a kirby grip (bobby pin) under the ponytail.

CHIGNONS

According to Charles Worthington, 'The most effective "hair ups" or chignons have a bit of volume – whether it's neat at the nape, or soft and dishevelled at the top. It's often difficult to get that much-needed volume naturally, so the best accessory is a "bun ring" [a doughnut-like accessory]. It looks professional and it's easy.'

1 For a clean, neat chignon at the nape of the neck, begin by securing the hair into a low ponytail.

2 Pull the ponytail through the hole in the middle of the bun ring.

3 Dress the hair around the bun ring, securing it with kirby grips (bobby pins).

4 For a softer, spikier up-do, just pull bits out. Cover with an invisible net for a sleek, neat look.

PUMP UP THE VOLUME

There are many ways to achieve volume, but remember that the larger the curler, the less curl and more wave and volume you will get. Big tongs, heated rollers, Velcro rollers, barrel curlers or a heated styling brush can all be used to give hair movement, tame ends and leave the hair shiny, if done properly. The technique is basically the same, no matter which tool you choose, so here is how to achieve volume with rollers.

1 First wash the hair with a volumizing shampoo and lightly condition the ends. Then blot the hair dry with a towel.

2 Divide and clip the hair into rough sections, spraying volumizer only at the roots.

3 Partly dry each section of hair with a hairdryer, brush it gently and then roll it up onto a large-size roller, making sure the ends are nicely smoothed and tucked in. The more rollers, the bigger the hair.

4 For a longer-lasting set, spritz a hairspray or heat-setting spray over the rollers and then blow-dry until the hair is completely dry.

5 Leave the rollers for as long as possible. Remember that heat makes hair pliable, but cold air sets it, so do not take the rollers out until the hair has cooled – or use the cold setting on the hairdryer.

6 Gently take out the rollers and run your fingers through the hair. Mist a little hairspray all over to help keep the curl. Now, don't go out in the rain.

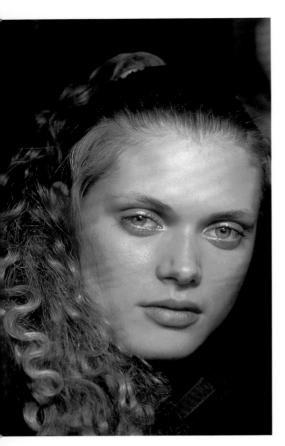

3   Gently dry the hair, putting the curls into the diffuser of the hairdryer and then pushing it up to the scalp.

4   Finish with a blast of cool air. Do not brush out.

VARIATION: To loosen up really tight, Afro curls, roller-set the hair when it is wet. Use proper hair-setting rollers with teeth, which brush the hair smooth. You need the little teeth on the barrel to grip the hair; Velcro rollers will not work. Dry on a low heat, then remove the rollers and smooth serum very gently through the hair to soften the curls.

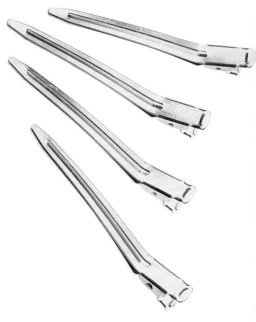

FRIZZ-FREE CURLS

1   The secret to perfect curls is to put product into the hair when it is wet. First apply serum to soften the hair and give it gloss, and then apply a firm-hold mousse.

2   Rake your fingers through the hair to loosen up the curls, but handle it as little as possible to reduce frizz.

hair health

The condition of our hair is a clear indication of the state of our health. Nothing we can do externally can alter the quality of hair that has already grown – we can only tend and improve its external condition. That is why it is vitally important, sooner rather than later, to address the underlying problems of any hair complaints you may have. If you get to the root of things, so to speak, your hair problems may not be solved overnight, but you will be on the way to improving your overall health and growing the strong, healthy hair that you deserve. Whatever you do, do not neglect any hair problems. Like most things, they can probably be solved if they are seen to quickly, but if you delay you may be exacerbating the problem and sapping your confidence at the same time.

DANDRUFF

'There is really no reason to suffer dandruff these days,' says Philip Kingsley. 'Although dandruff is definitely associated with stress, it can be controlled quite easily. Most of the shampoos on the market are effective. You may not like the way they make your hair look at first, but when you get the dandruff under control you will need to use them only occasionally.'

ECZEMA & PSORIASIS

These are recognized medical conditions that can affect the health of the scalp and, in turn, the hair. Both can involve redness, itching, inflammation and flaking on the scalp, as well as on the rest of the skin. Do not think of this as a cosmetic problem. Causes can range from stress, allergies and infections to genetic tendencies. See your doctor and possibly a dermatologist and trichologist.

MENOPAUSE

As we get older, particularly after 40, the diameter of each hair begins to decrease, giving us the feeling that our hair is thinner than it used to be. As with skin, the growth rate of hair slows down, so less new hairs are being formed. To cap it all, streaks of grey may become more persistent, forcing you to colour your hair more often. The only course

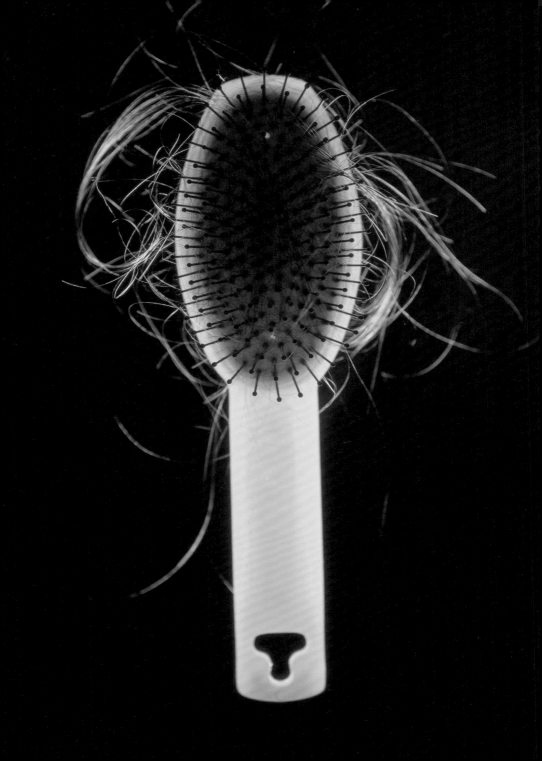

of action is to look after your hair as best you can. Philip Kingsley advises shampooing and conditioning daily to feed moisture back into the hair. 'Scalp massage can also be very good for encouraging faster and healthier hair growth as it "exercises" the scalp. Once a week is enough.'

PREGNANCY

Pregnancy is generally a good time for hair: oestrogen levels are up, androgen levels are down and hair is falling out less. Do not go for more than four hours without food, as the body will start to drain hair-nutrition reserves. As sebum levels are down, hair will become drier, so keep it moisturized, conditioned and protected.

THINNING HAIR

'About 65 per cent of my patients come because of thinning hair, or "loss of hair volume" as I prefer to call it,' says Philip Kingsley. 'They may not be losing actual hair, but each diameter of their hair may be getting thinner and it may stop growing as quickly. Firstly, it is important to find the cause of the problem. Many women, especially those of childbearing age, are anaemic and particularly low in

ferritin and zinc. Get your doctor to test you and get the appropriate supplement if you are lacking. Secondly, improve your diet to include adequate protein, carbohydrate, minerals, fat and vitamins [see pages 43–54]. Thirdly, there may be an underlying hormonal imbalance. It is becoming increasingly clear that polycystic ovaries (PCOS) can cause hair loss and sometimes hair loss is the only symptom ... it is estimated that this might affect at least 30 per cent of young women. If it is found to be true in your case, it is easily treated, either with a birth-control pill or a drug that suppresses androgen levels in the body.'

GREY HAIR

The decision to dye grey hair or not is really one of aesthetics and confidence. 'Grey hair can be flattering if you have pale eyes,' says Frede Geiylly at Michaeljohn in London. 'But it's not really for women with dark eyes. If you are turning platinum, keep your hair well cut, conditioned and groomed, and use a colour-correcting shampoo once a week. Do not forget products: serum could become your best friend as silvery hair can change its texture.'

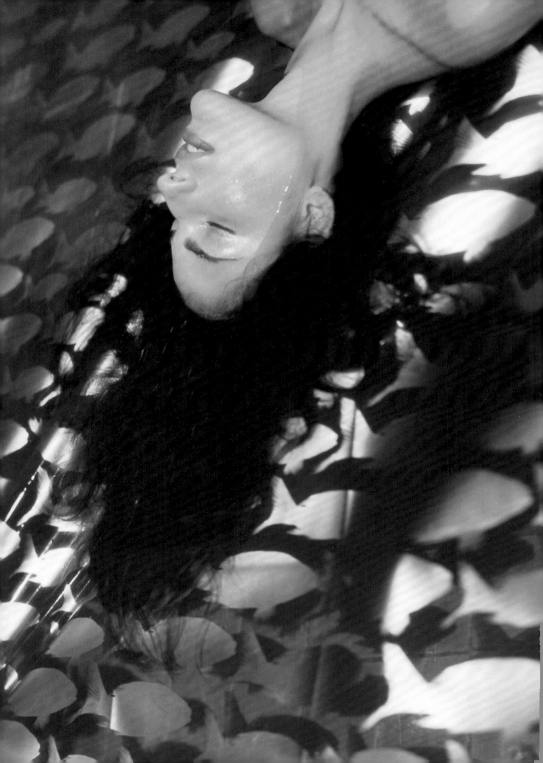

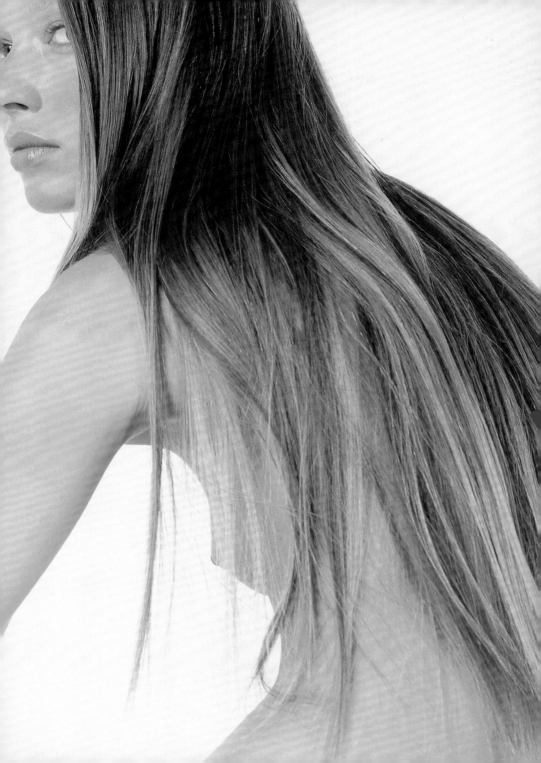

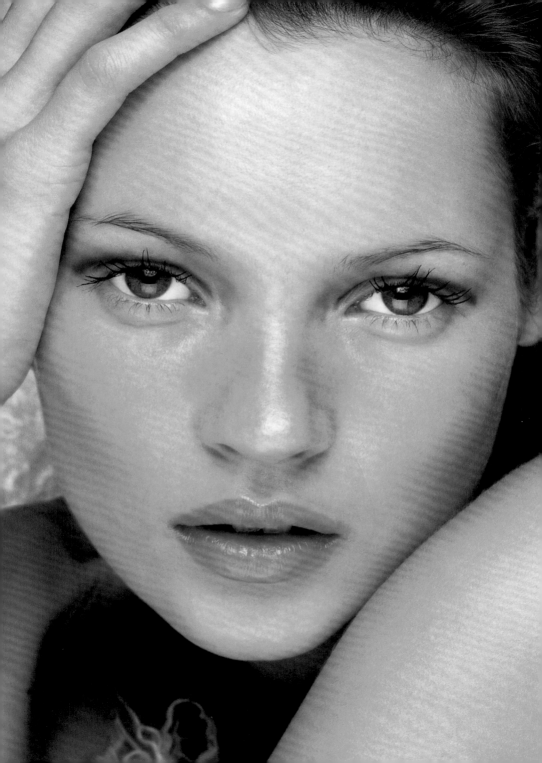

MAKE-UP

Once upon a time painting your face meant painting a questionable moral picture of yourself — wearing make-up usually indicated that you were a stripper, a chorus girl or a whore, and was synonymous with poor values and a poor upbringing. In today's society, where external beauty is (often wrongly) equated with internal good, everyone wants to paint as pretty a picture of themselves as possible. Historically, it is the movie's 'bad' guy who is pictured with a face full of scars, and the wistfully beautiful hero or heroine who dances blissfully off into the sunset. Any way we can cosmetically enhance the canvas nature gave us, makes us look and feel a whole lot better. Bit by bit and decade by decade, make-up has contributed to our idea of ourselves. In the twentieth century alone, the 1920s vamp dabbled with beauty spots, the 1950s starlet sported a painted pout and the 1970s disco queen sparkled as much as a disco ball. By the 1980s and 1990s make-up offered women choice — both 'nude' shades to enhance natural skin tones, and Technicolor products to play with like children let loose in a sweet shop. Happily 'beauty' is no longer a credential given solely to those in possession of a perfect set of classic features. Many of today's icons, such as Chloë Sevigney, Maggie Gyllenhaal, Gwyneth Paltrow and Liz Hurley, to name but a few, have interesting or unusual features which combine with an inner confidence to make them stand out from the crowd. They should be a lesson to all of us: make-up is best used, and often used best, not to change us, but to enhance who we already are.

foundation

Long gone are the days when Esther Williams nose-dived into a swimming pool clad in little but her panstick foundation. Today's bases have more to do with enhancing natural skin tone than hiding it. So fundamental is the change in the approach to foundation that we have even built up a whole new language around it. There is not a woman worth her tinted moisturizer who has not heard of the paradoxical 'no make-up make-up' or 'light-reflecting particles', or even 'compact foundation'. Of all the plethora of products available, foundation is the one most vital to get right. Think of the face as an artist's canvas: without a proper base coat, the rest of the paint will chip and flake – a good foundation ensures the final varnish glides on smoothly and, hopefully, stays put.

CHOOSING A FOUNDATION

Although a good foundation can be expensive, consider the outlay as an investment. As make-up artist Dick Page says, 'When it comes to foundations, buying a cheap and cheerful product is often a false economy. You will get more for your money if you stick to a top-end product from, say, Lancôme or Lauder.' Pretty much all modern foundations are multipurpose, supplying a turbo-boost of sun protection, moisturizers and anti-ageing ingredients, as well as colour and coverage. Far from inhibiting the skin's condition, foundations improve it. Most importantly, they contain ingredients that let the skin breathe, while also protecting it from everyday pollution. Years of research and technological developments have given us the cosmetic wash-off equivalent of new skin. These modern bases often contain a lower pigment concentration than previous foundations, which allows the colour to glide on without creating a solid look. However, actually choosing the right foundation still seems to be the most difficult part of the equation, and the endless choice of texture and colour can confuse even a make-up maven. To make the decision easier, it is vital to understand your skin type. Colour choice is the number one decider on whether you end up with a faultless complexion,

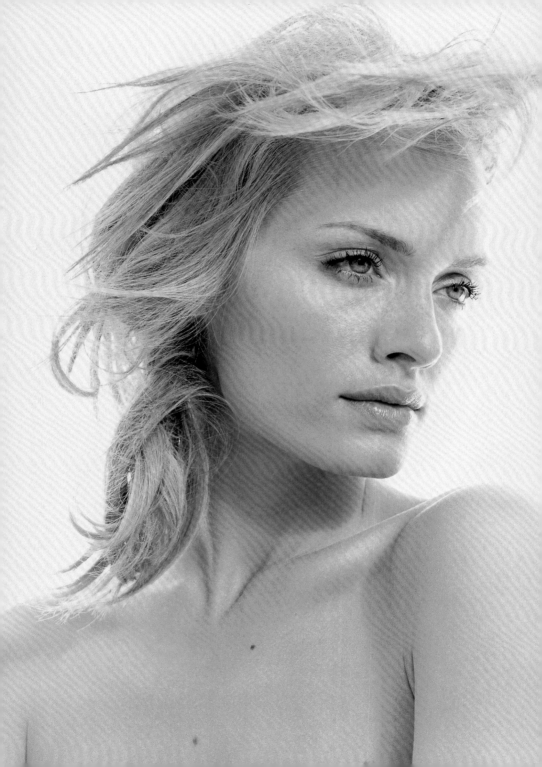

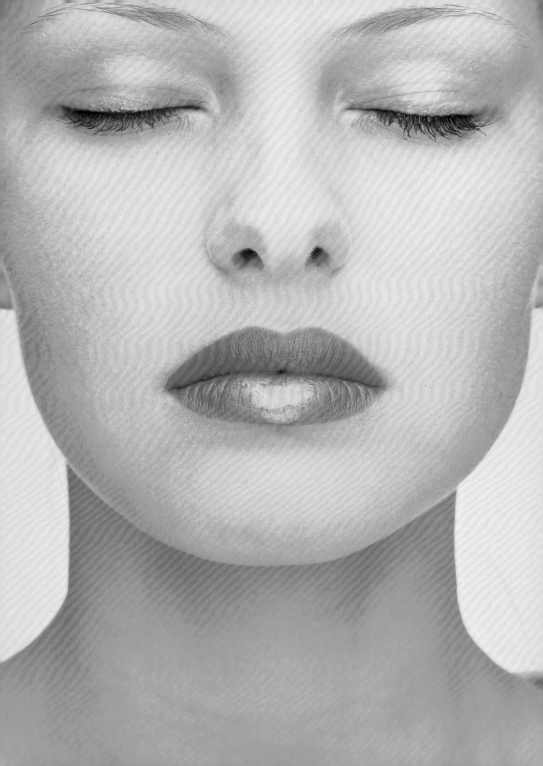

or a less-than-convincing mask effect. Make it a rule of thumb to match foundation as exactly as possible to the skin colour around the neck area. After all, this is where you will be blending the foundation and the skin here is usually fractionally darker than on the face. With many major cosmetic houses incorporating colours for blacks and Asians into their range, the colour choice is endless, which means that the list of 'don'ts' in foundation selection is as long as the list of 'dos'. Memorizing a few of the rules should reduce your chances of ending up looking like an extra from *Cabaret*.

1 Never make a colour decision in artificial light, which is often very deceptive – the foundation can look totally wrong in daylight.

2 Avoid choosing a foundation that is dark enough to look like a suntan.

3 Never try and make yellow-toned skin look pinker by using a pink-based foundation, or vice versa.

4 Choose a foundation that matches the skin tone and then let colour cosmetics do the work afterwards.

5 Allow a test colour to sit on your skin for a few minutes before purchasing it. The acid balance of your skin may affect the colour.

6 The best way to apply foundation is the most basic – use your fingertips. This way you can reach the parts that other tools cannot reach (unless you are a professional make-up artist), and most importantly, learn to blend, blend, blend.

7 There are no rules about where to apply foundation. Just apply it where you feel it is needed and then blend it in carefully.

8 Always use a moisturizer that is specially formulated for your skin type before application to help prime the skin. Applying foundation directly onto the skin will give you a patchy finish.

TEXTURES & TYPES OF COVERAGE

'Texture' has become the buzz-word of modern make-up, and when it comes to selecting a foundation, the consistency of a product is just as important as its colour. Thanks to the endless leaps in technology, ingredients have been refined and refined to the point where foundation takes on a three-dimensional quality. It thus enhances the quality of natural skin, rather than creating a two-dimensional mask which covers it. Considering we all have a unique canvas to work with, with individual marks and blemishes, it makes sense that we should have an individual make-up tailored to our personal needs. Hence the plethora of products available – watch out for key ingredients like 'silicones' (to help foundation glide on easily), 'light-reflecting particles', which bounce light away from surface lines and wrinkles to create a youthful glow, or 'complete coverage', which offers more heavy-duty maintenance.

SHEER FOUNDATION: Sheer base gives the skin the appearance that most of us would like it to have naturally. It usually contains silicones, which help it glide on easily, and gives a soft appearance without looking oily. It disappears into the skin, giving a natural look.

OIL-BASED FOUNDATION: These are great for drier skins, although they do tend to separate in their bottles. If desired, add a few drops of toner to counteract the oil and to make the foundation more sheer. Be sure to shake it well before every application.

LIGHT-REFLECTING FOUNDATION: Containing specially shaped particles that reflect light off the skin, this base gives a youthful appearance. It is appropriate for young girls who want a 'dewy' complexion and for canny older customers who use it to draw attention away from crow's-feet or other giveaway signs of ageing.

MATT FOUNDATION: This is a great choice for anyone with oily skin. Because it does not contain oils, the base dries out quickly once it touches the skin. To counter this, either apply moisturizer first or be prepared to blend very quickly. Do not apply matt foundation too heavily or else you may end up looking like a waxwork.

COMPACT FOUNDATION: A powder and foundation in one, this 'one-stop shopping' of foundation is easy to apply with a sponge.

CREAM FOUNDATION: A smooth, milky foundation that is kind on surface lines and wrinkles, cream base suits older skins. It gives a natural finish while still offering confidence-boosting coverage.

TINTED MOISTURIZER: A moisturizer with a hint of colour, this gives no coverage at all. It is wonderful if you are one of the lucky few who does not need foundation, or to use to enhance a tan.

HIGHLIGHTING STICKS: Not a foundation as such, but these sticks, which add a glow to selected areas, are great for highlighting the face or body and can be used with other foundation products.

GROUND-BREAKERS

Chantecaille's Real Skin is the closest to real skin that foundation has ever got. Colour is suspended in a gel so it glides on easily as well as giving a brighter, sparkling complexion. Future Skin — the 'Real Skin' alternative for those with greasier skin — is an even lighter formulation which is oil-free. Estée Lauder's Spotlight boasts revolutionary optical technology called 'specular reflection'. As the foundation contains many layered particles, hundreds of reflections occur simultaneously and prevent the eye from focusing on any one layer. This, in layman's terms, creates a sense of depth and a youthful glow. Estée Lauder's Lucidity foundation make-up is not only light-diffusing (that is, it reflects light to divert attention from lines and wrinkles), but light responsive, too. Because of a photochromatic pigment it contains, the foundation changes colour in different lights, meaning it looks just as natural in broad daylight as it does in the candlelit glow of evening.

PRIMERS OR
SKIN PERFECTORS

Many a beauty-circuit cynic has suggested that primers are just another wily marketing ploy. However, anyone with a less than perfect complexion may find them worth a try. Skin primers create a smooth layer which helps foundation glide on without going patchy; it will also boost your skin and make it glow. Unlike moisturizer, it stays put, so if you are going somewhere hot, or just want to make sure your make-up doesn't leave the party before you do, a primer may well be worth the investment.

powder

Powder is the 'magic dust' of make-up. Just a whisper, used in the right place and applied with dexterity, can make the difference between an amateur painting-by-numbers and a great master. Invisible but essential, the most effective powder is the one that is sheerest to the touch and the most translucent in appearance. Loose or pressed, powder works as an invisible fixer that helps colour cosmetics brush on easily over foundation without blotching or creasing. Dusted loosely under the eyes before eye make-up is applied, it acts as a magnet for any falling shadow and can be swept off with a soft brush in seconds without leaving your face streaked with colour.

With powder, the means is just as important as the end. Using the right brush will make a surprising difference to the quality of the finish. The more voluminous the brush and (if you are not an animal-rights activist) the more natural the fibre, the better the result. Satisfyingly chunky to hold, a powder brush by Shu Uemura or the revered British make-up artist Maggie Hunt may well set you back

a meal at Nobu, but think of the calories you will save and the prettier you will look the next time you hit Harry's bar (not to mention the undeniably glamorous sensation of caressing your cheek with something so large and soft, it could well have featured in a dressing-room scene in a black-and-white Bette Davis film).

As always, application is everything. After delving luxuriantly into the container, blow any excess powder off the brush. Subtlety is an art not mastered by many, but if you can bring restraint to bear on your technique, a little loose powder placed carefully under your eyes and down the bridge of your nose right to the tip of your chin is a wonderful form of highlighting. Never, ever be tempted to buy powder to complement your foundation. This will create a mask-like effect, which is very obvious to the eye and also looks incredibly old-fashioned. More to the point, most men still associate foundation with panstick, so if you apply your base carefully and finish off with the sheerest whisper of translucent powder, he will never know you are wearing any.

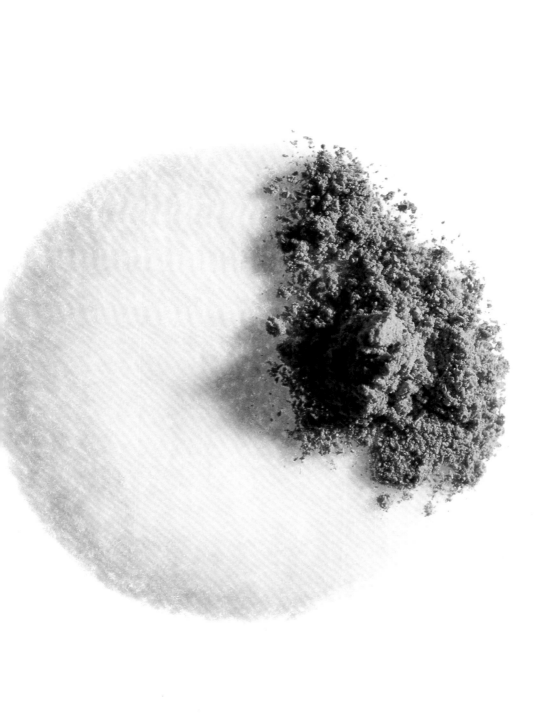

concealer

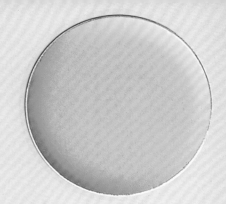

Concealer is meant to look as invisible as the blemish it is intended to disguise. If it is just a shade too dark or a tad too thick, this will not be the case. Nowadays concealer comes in a variety of textures: the cream in a tube; the liquid with a sponge-tip applicator; the simple stick; and the 'hard' product in a compact. For speed and convenience, there are even foolproof dispensers which work similarly to a felt-tip pen: just squeeze the end and the concealer journeys to the tip for easily controlled application. Different areas of the face require different types of concealer. Never compromise the desired effect by using the wrong product — you wouldn't treat a headache with a throat lozenge, would you? Make-up artist Maggie Hunt says, 'The secret to applying concealer is not to overdo it, and always use a brush. A good tip is to add a little concealer to your lip colour if you want to tone it down.'

UNDER-EYE SHADOWS

When it comes to disguising under-eye shadows, the best type of concealer to opt for is a liquid. A harder product has a crumbled-cement effect around crow's-feet. Using a fine-tipped brush, apply liquid concealer in dots along the lowest section of the shadow.

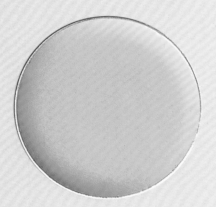

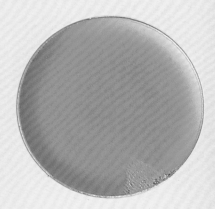

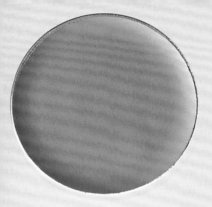

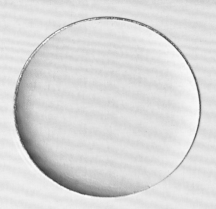

Do not go beneath the shaded area. Pat – don't rub – it in until it disappears. Go easy on concealer – I have heard many a make-up artist groan at the amateur concealer who thinks she has hidden the telltale signs of a heavy night, but has made herself look like a panda.

SPOTS & BLEMISHES

A slightly harder texture of concealer works best to disguise blemishes as it stays put longer than a liquid. Always apply this type of concealer using a brush and avoid the temptation to dis-guise the skin around the blemish itself. A natural-looking finish is achieved by only covering the mark or spot itself.

TOUCHE ÉCLAT

In the world of concealers there is one miracle product so great you will not even want to tell your best friend about it: Yves Saint Laurent's Touche Éclat. Like a magic wand, it knocks years off by radically diminishing shadows in sec-onds. It also works wonders on the creases on either side of the nose, or used as a highlighter on the brow bone.

eyebrows

'Jeepers, creepers, where d'ya get those peepers?' goes the famous song, and it is not surprising that it is the eyes that Louis Armstrong is talking about. The most defining feature of the face, eyebrows can not only be made to look different shapes and suggest a variety of moods, but are also the first place to show your age (if not made up), emotional reactions and state of mind. Much underestimated, the eyebrows are key to defining your look.

Change your eyebrows, and you totally redefine your personality. Just try to imagine Brooke Shields or even Elizabeth Taylor without their trademark eyebrows. While fashions for thicker or thinner brows change quite frequently, if you were born with a strong pair of eyebrows, hold onto them, or at least think twice before plucking them into obscurity. Many a 1960s sex siren now regrets the pencil-thin suggestion of an arc, which remains from years of plucking out a once strongly defined curve. For those who are not blessed with naturally defined eyebrows, there are both permanent and less drastic forms of cosmetic enhancement available. Tattooing is a great option if you are absolutely sure of the shape and colour you want, and it means you can go swimming without worrying that your eyebrow is going to end up drawn around your chin. Pencilling is fine, but use a pencil that is one shade lighter than your natural colour to ensure it blends in without looking obvious.

When shaping the brow, use a really good pair of tweezers (I find that the ones with slanted tips are best but some people prefer pointed). Only ever pluck underneath the natural curve – spiky regrowth on top of the eyebrow looks odd and unsightly. Also avoid leaving a thick bulk of hair near the nose; this 'tadpole' look tends to close the eyes up and draws attention to the nose.

1 Never pluck above the eyebrows. Instead, bleach unruly hairs above the brow until they are no longer noticeable, but be very careful or the eyebrows will become patchy.

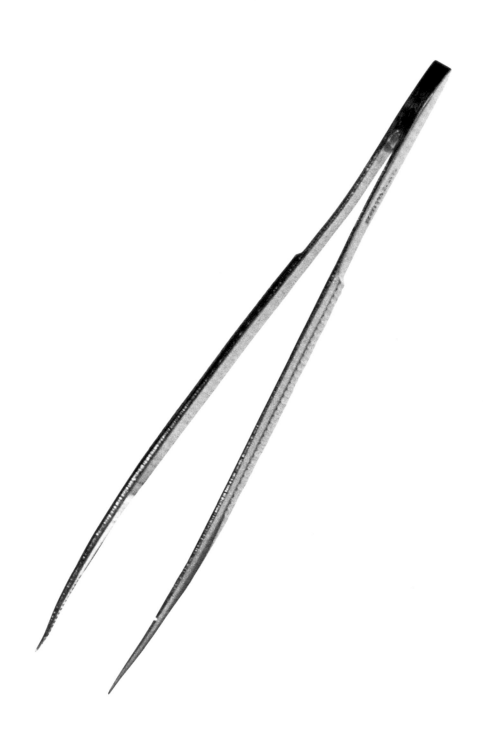

2 Always tweeze one hair at a time. Start at the nose end and work outwards, following the arch and plucking only underneath the brow. To avoid risk of infection, wipe gently with toner and a cotton wool tip afterwards.

3 Get into the habit of using a brow brush to gently sweep the eyebrows upwards. This is a tip adopted by models and actresses to open their eyes up even further and look really groomed.

4 There is one golden rule for using an eyebrow pencil, which seems obvious but is broken remarkably frequently. Use the pencil in gentle, broken movements to create a natural-looking sweep. One continuous motion creates a scary cartoon-rainbow effect.

5 Always pluck hairs in the direction in which they grow. This is the least painful method and ensures that the hairs will grow back flat, as opposed to sticking out.

6 For a gentle, sexy look, bleach the eyebrows about two shades lighter than your hair colour. If you decide to drastically change your hair colour, then make sure your eyebrows match. Facial hair lightener is absolutely fine to use when bleaching eyebrows, but be very careful when washing it off.

7 Avoid the temptation to overpluck the browline. A single line of hair, added or taken away, makes a big difference to the overall look of a brow. Always pluck one hair at a time.

8 If you are fervently anti-plucking, at least brush the brows.

9 If you are pro-plucking, but can't stand the stubbly regrowth suffered by anyone with hair darker than flaxen, electrolysis is a painful but permanent way to get rid of unwanted hair. Only take this route if you are happy for hair today to be gone tomorrow.

QUICK TIPS FOR BROW-SHAPING

Use a white pencil to draw a line along the natural eyebrow. You will be able to see the final desired shape and avoid making a drastic mistake.

eyeshadow

Eyeshadow is an 'ABC of make-up' product, yet it remains one of the most difficult to apply. The best advice is to keep it simple. Once you have mastered the technique for applying just one colour to the eyelid, you are ready to add a second shade. The tools you use are most important. Sponge-tip applicators that come packaged with the shadow are generally useless and far too fiddly to use. Invest in a good-quality eyeshadow brush, which will help the shadow glide on and ensure a more successful result.

A decade ago, the mere thought of applying eyeshadow was enough to kick-start tremors in even the most confident and skilled hands, but with developments in technology, application no longer needs to be such a daunting prospect. Not only is today's colour choice infinite, the skincare benefits and textures have improved enormously. Today, the silicone base ingredients which are used to suspend colour pigments ensure that colour glides on almost effortlessly, grips the lid without a crumbly, crepey effect of yesterday and allows the creation of 'truer' non-streak colours. There is a multitude of textures to choose from – powders, creams, gels and multipurpose sticks all add colour and texture to eyelids while disguising surface lines. Remember that the eyes do not have to be the window to the soul – you can use them to project any picture you like to create.

As the force behind the Body Shop's Colourings range, Barbara Daly has great expertise in getting the best results with the eyes. 'Look at what happens with young eyes – they look dewy and fresh and the skin around the eyes doesn't look dry. To replicate a young-eyes look, use shine or gloss products on the "V" of the inner corner of the eyelid and use as a highlighter on the brow bone and in the middle of the upper eyelid. As a rule, lighter shades of any type of product are far more flattering. Opt for more natural

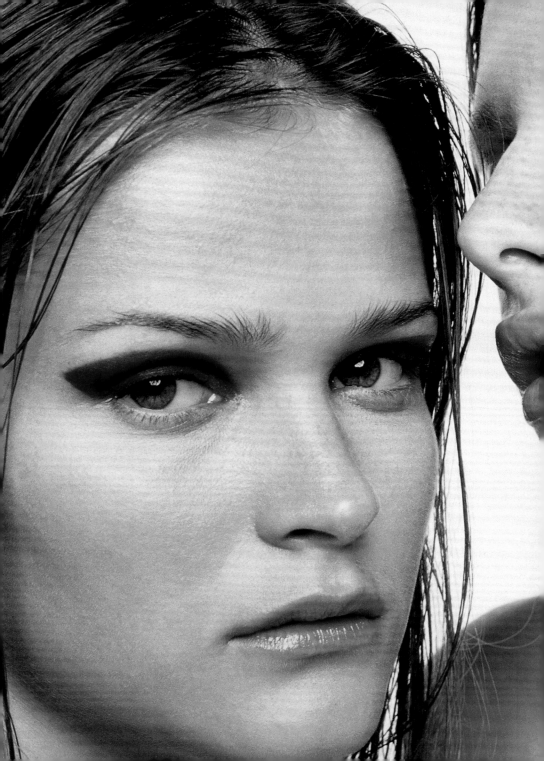

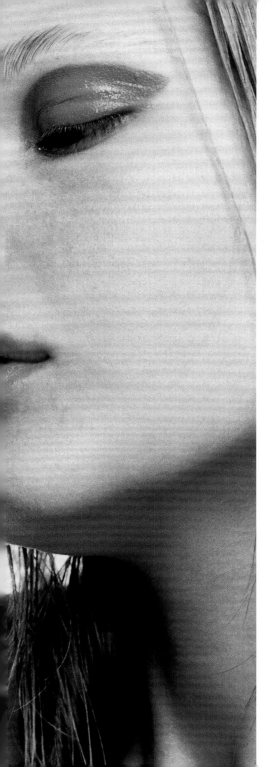

shades like creams, pale peach and tawny shades, and blend and build up colour. Remember that heavy dark shades will make the eyes appear to recede. The more mature woman should steer away from highly pearlized products, as they tend to accentuate the fine lines on the face. A pearlized concealer may look alluring on the back of the hand but it is not good on the eyes. Curling the lashes really does open the eye up. It helps to emphasize the eyes. At the end of the day, I don't think that women should worry too much about the shape of their eyes – I don't think that there is a "perfect shape" for eyes. Make the most of what is naturally yours and remember that smiling eyes are by far the prettiest.'

SHADOW COLOUR

When it comes to colour, anything goes. If you want to add the hint of drama with one shade, or prefer to look like a body double for *Joseph and the Amazing Technicolor Dreamcoat*, let any make-up rules just fly out of the window. After all, the whole point of make-up is to play and experiment. There are so many writers, models and

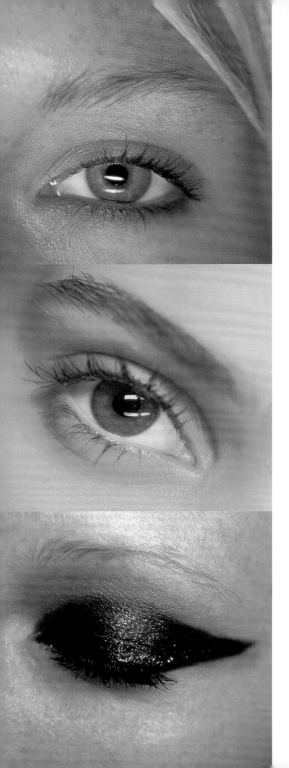

make-up artists espousing rules like the eleventh commandment that sometimes it is easy to forget that the whole point about wearing make-up is that it should be fun.

The eye is a great area to experiment with colour — anything from darker, depth-giving shadows to glittery, light-reflecting options. Although there are no rules, here are a few suggestions to make colour experiments more fruitful:

1 When applying eyeshadow to the crease of the eye, keep your eyes open. This way you can see exactly what shape you are creating, and the colour will go into and slightly above the crease.

2 Do not be afraid of bright colours. Often a pink that looks a bold fuchsia in the box will be a pretty pastel shade once it is on.

3 Try it anyway, even if it is fuchsia.

4 Liquid shadows create a more 'skin-like' effect. Matt shadows look more understated and are much easier to apply than pearlized versions.

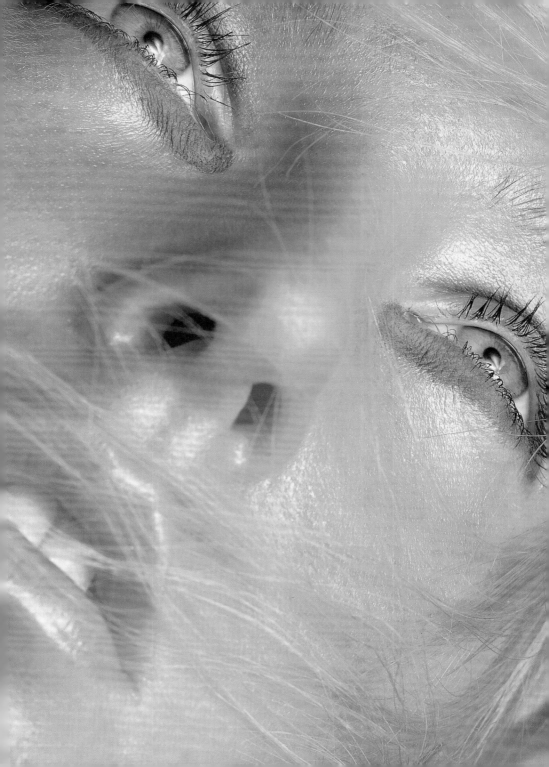

THE DAYTIME EYE

1 Cover the eyelid in foundation or concealer to create a smooth base and help the colour adhere.

2 Brush the lid very gently with a translucent powder.

3 Choose a natural-toned eye-shadow. Using a good brush, start at the lash line and cover the lid right up to the brow bone.

4 Curl the eyelashes. This is a step most women omit, but one a make-up artist would never sacrifice. Curled lashes open the eye up and create a deliciously sexy, fan effect.

5 Apply mascara to the top lashes, concentrating on the tips. Never apply mascara directly to the roots of the lashes, as it looks unnatural and causes the lashes to separate into scary 'spiders' legs'.

6 If desired, apply mascara to the lower lashes, as above.

7 Using an eyeshadow brush, add the same neutral colour used on the top lid under the line of the bottom lashes.

THE EVENING EYE

1 Smoky eyes look really sultry and they work best in softer evening light. First, apply foundation and translucent powder to the eyelid.

2 Next, take a black eyeliner pencil with a rubber hoof end. Apply along the upper and lower lash line, smudging in with the rubber tip.

3 Using either a dark grey or brown eyeshadow, brush colour into the crease of the eyelid, but do not go above the crease line you see when the eye is open.

4 Finish with a natural colour of shadow, applied above the crease and right up to the eyebrow.

5 Curl lashes and apply mascara, as for the Daytime Eye.

THE PARTY EYE

1 First used in black-and-white Hollywood films, the glossy eye has been firmly reinstated at the forefront of fashion. It looks great, but requires major upkeep, so it is a definite 'no no' for everyday. Choose a favourite eyeshadow

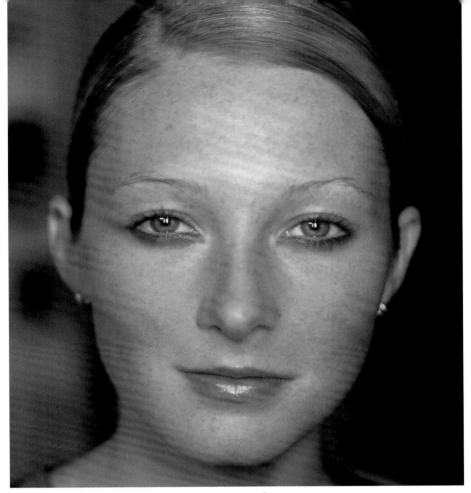

colour – anything from a neutral beige to a citrus orange.

2 Apply mascara at this point. Once the gloss is applied, you will risk smudging the lashes.

3 Blend the eyeshadow well up to the brow. Then simply cover the coloured lid with Vaseline, using your fingertips.

4 If you want a glossy effect, but are prepared to compromise on 'wet look' sheen in return for a longer-lasting effect, substitute a shimmer shadow for the Vaseline.

5 If you are tanned, drop the shadow altogether and just use Vaseline on the bare eyelid. Apply mascara first to avoid smudging.

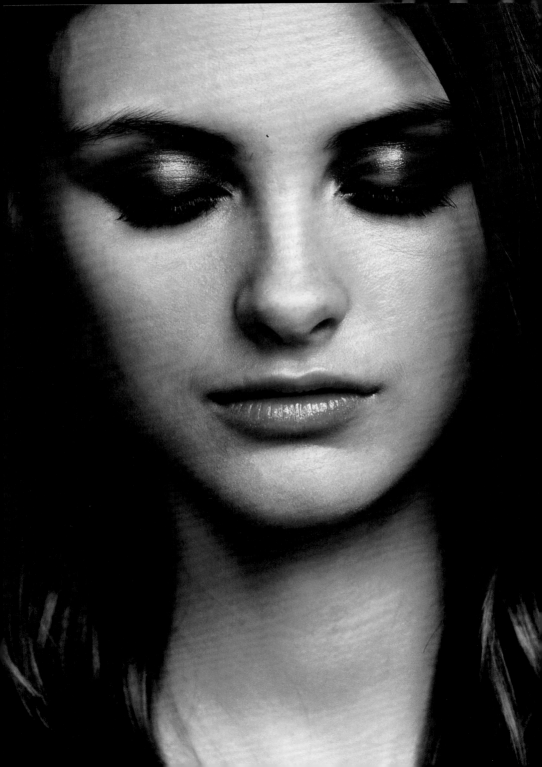

TOP TIPS FOR EYESHADOW APPLICATION

Always pat foundation into the eyelid first as a primer. This helps powder shadow sit smoothly without going patchy and will also help prevent cream shadow from creasing.

The best way to catch any falling powder shadow is to apply loose powder generously beneath the lower lashes before applying the colour. The powder sweeps off easily, taking any unwanted colour pigments with it.

Less is often more. Using a light colour over the whole lid, swept right up to the eyebrow itself, will open up the whole eye area. To avoid closing the eye area in, never use darker shades near the nose; instead, keep them exclusively for the outer edges.

Remember that cream eyeshadow will crack less and lends a more youthful look to the complexion.

Eyeliner pencils are softer than liquids, but best of all is a dark powder shadow line, created by using the tiniest, most pointed brush. The shadow is much subtler and gives you a far sexier 'Bambi' look. Liquid liners are best left to the professionals, but if you insist, use a magnifying mirror, pull the eyelid taut and apply the liner in one continuous movement as close to the lashes as possible.

If you are too busy, or too lazy, to apply eyeliner on a daily basis, a simple alternative is to have a line permanently tattooed around the lash line. Obviously the eye area is very delicate, so finding a very experienced beauty therapist is essential. Do not let associations of other types of tattooing put you off – under-eye (and indeed around the lip) tattooing can look very natural. Be warned, though, it is usually an extremely painful process.

eyelashes

Even the most outspoken make-up minimalist wants a great set of eye-lashes. After all, without them you risk looking like an albino rabbit. Tinting and perming are great wash-proof ways of attaining a perfect pair of flutterers, but for those who are happy to settle down with what nature gave them, mascara, eyelash curlers and even nylon falsies and some rubber gum are enough to create the perfect fringing for your peepers.

Of primary importance are eyelash curlers and most pharmacies sell them. Go gently at first as it is easy to catch the eyelid if you clamp down too hard, which can be extremely painful. The curlers give an instant, wide-eyed effect, but remember to start at the root and squeeze outwards bit by bit along the length. Squeeze down too hard in one place and instead of a gentle curve, you could end up with a right angle.

When selecting mascara, there is a plethora of products that are specifically tailored for your needs, whether you want lash lengthening, thickening, conditioning, transparent colour or waterproof. To apply mascara, sweep upwards in a generous curve. This will make the lashes appear thicker and longer. To keep it looking natural, avoid the roots.

FALSE LASHES

Gone are the days when falsies were the sole domain of cabaret artists, Gypsy Rose Lee and the cast at *La Cage aux Folles*. Now false lashes are not immediately detectable by that unnaturally solid 'rainbow' curve. Falsies are sold individually and in different lengths, which gives a far more natural look. They can be dispersed flirtatiously among your own lashes. When applying falsies, curl them slightly along with your own lashes to keep them in place and stop them falling out. Mix small, medium and long together, with the longest ones in the middle. Always allow the glue to set for a moment and become sticky before applying the lashes.

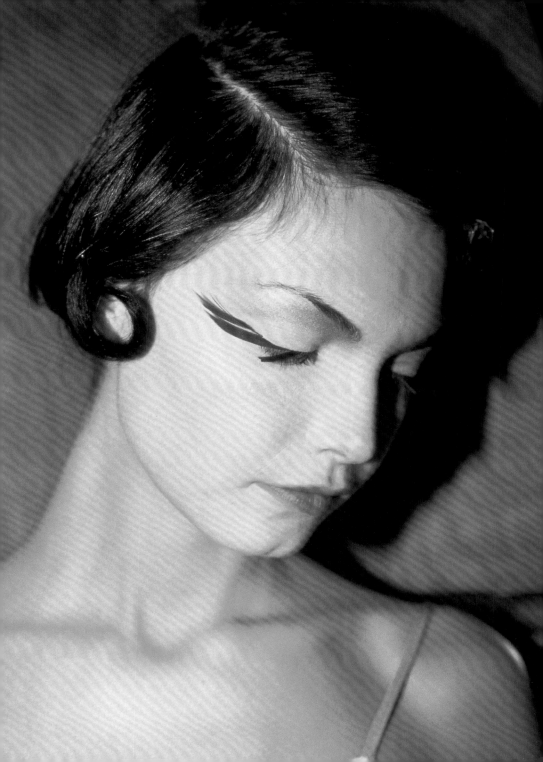

MASCARA FUDGES

1 If the thinnest thing about you is your eyelashes, a thickening mascara with silicones will help create the illusion of a Hollywood sweep. Falsies can also be applied sparingly (the thickest ones towards the centre) before you apply the wand.

2 For those whose lashes are so short they look more like five o'clock stubble, there are plenty of lengthening mascaras available. These contain tiny fibres which attach themselves to the lashes and make them look longer, but avoid if you have sensitive eyes.

3 Waterproof mascara is a cry baby's dream product. This will see you happily through a Sunday night weepy without leaving you looking like Dirk Bogarde in the final scene of *Death in Venice*.

MASCARA TIPS

Avoid the temptation to pump the wand up and down to get an even coverage of mascara on it. This pumping action traps air inside the tube and the mascara will dry out more quickly.

Remember that clear mascara is natural-looking, gives a slightly dewy look, works well with minimal make-up and can double up as a styling agent to shape the brows.

Apply mascara to false lashes in the same way as you would to your own lashes.

lips

Lips are unquestionably the sexiest area of the face, partly because of their subliminal reflection of the lips located elsewhere. Fashion pundits have spent the last few years encouraging anyone with less pout than the flower in the *Rocky Horror Picture Show* to rush for collagen and elastin, and the trend for bee-stung lips looks set to stay. While the phrase 'come to bed' is often associated with the eyes, experience proves it is often the lips that do the talking.

An area where technology knows no bounds, lip moisturizers, plumpers, anti-run agents and sun protection factors are all included in those little sticks of colour, which means that it will not be long before the Paris pout is available in a pot. Gone are the days when a lipstick was just wax and pigment, which stuck to a coffee cup (or someone's shirt collar). If you don't want to leave a giveaway signature, you can even buy non-budge, non-fade lipsticks, which have probably got more staying power than you have.

As you generally have to suffer to be beautiful, this is the one area where you really should put your money where your mouth is. There isn't an icon in every decade who hasn't had a memorable mouth – Brigitte Bardot, Marilyn Monroe, Madonna, Emanuelle Béart and Angelina Jolie all have blissful lips. So for those who want to achieve irresistibly kissy lips without an intrusive procedure, here are some key ways to go about it.

KNOW YOUR LIPSTICK

Know your stain from your gloss: lipstick is available in a variety of textures, so familiarize yourself with what is available. Stains do just that – leave the merest hint of colour, rather like your mouth looks when you have been eating berries. Glosses are slick

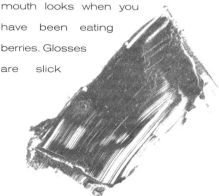

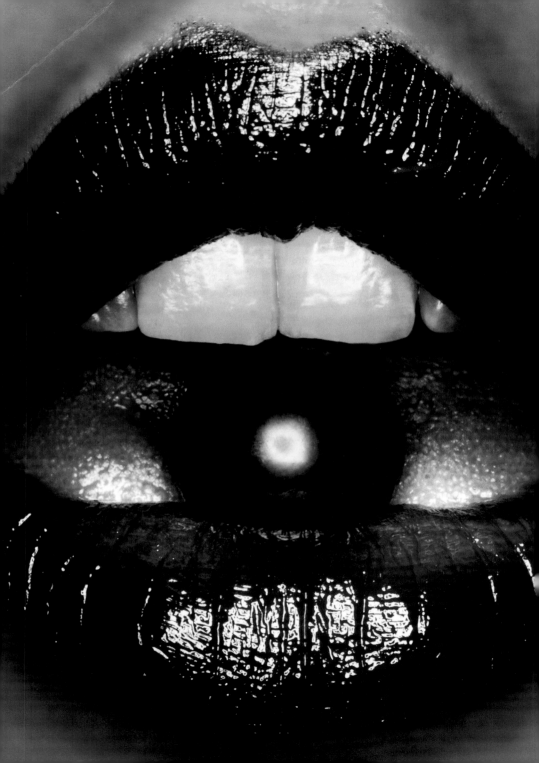

and sexy, and are available in a whole spectrum of colours, but unfortunately they do not have great staying power.

Creamy lipsticks are youthful and suit all age groups. Lipsticks usually contain silicones to help them glide on more easily. Matt versions are great for those who do not like the jammy effect, but they can be somewhat drying and accentuate lines in older mouths. Long-lasting lipsticks stay the course, but they will have to be removed with the cosmetic equivalent of a paint stripper.

LIP COLOUR

Although lip colours come and go, red is here to stay. Red is a timeless classic that bridges the gap of age and culture. The top traditional reds are those by Yves Saint Laurent, Chanel, Revlon, Nars, Christian Dior, Estée Lauder and Lancôme, and if matt versions don't suit you, try a sheer or a stain.

What is the top-selling lip colour? Not red, as you might expect, but shimmering coral – the type of shade usually reserved (at least mentally by myself) for catwalk frippery or one's grandmother. According to a spokesperson for Estée Lauder, 'Our greatest selling lipstick is Frosted Apricot.' And if it's good enough for Elizabeth Hurley ...

Skin tone is and isn't important when it comes to choosing your lipstick. For those who want a classic look, it is safest to stay within the colour chart traditionally associated with your skin tone. Those with pink-based skin (or 'cooler' looks) look great in 'blue' tones, while olive-skinned babes look best in 'yellows'. In layman's terms, while a pinky red would enhance the features of an English rose, a Mediterranean chick would do better with a more orange-based alternative. Blacks and Asians look wonderful in all the deeper, more vibrant colours, but are able to carry off paler colours too.

Remember that for a classic look, your hair colour is irrelevant – Snow White and Pocahontas might both have jet black hair, but their skin tone (and hence their lipstick choices) would be totally different. For the more adventurous, rules are made to be broken. You are free to choose from an entire spectrum of lip colour after all. As with everything in life, if something feels right, it usually looks it.

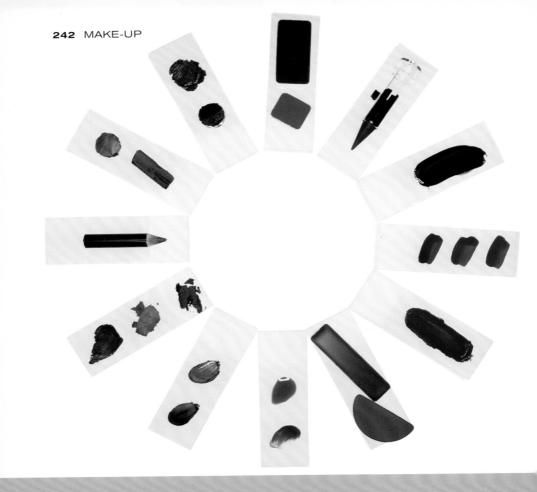

CREATING GREAT LIPS

Make-up artist François Nars offers his own technique for creating luscious lips:

'How do you create the perfect lips? Use a pencil all over the lips, and then apply face powder on top to set the pencil. Then apply your gloss or lipstick on top. In selecting the lip pencil, don't be afraid to select a colour that is different to the lipstick. Provided the pencil is used all over the lip, applying different pencil and lipstick/gloss can create winning combinations. The notion of having to use a lip pencil that matches the lipstick colour is old-fashioned. Try Borneo lip pencil with Tanganyka lipstick.'

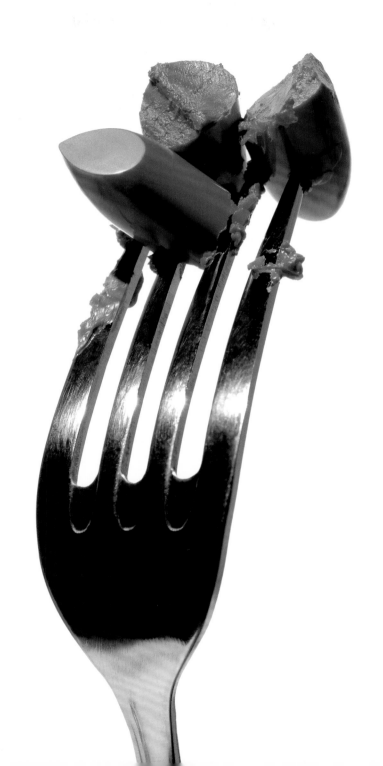

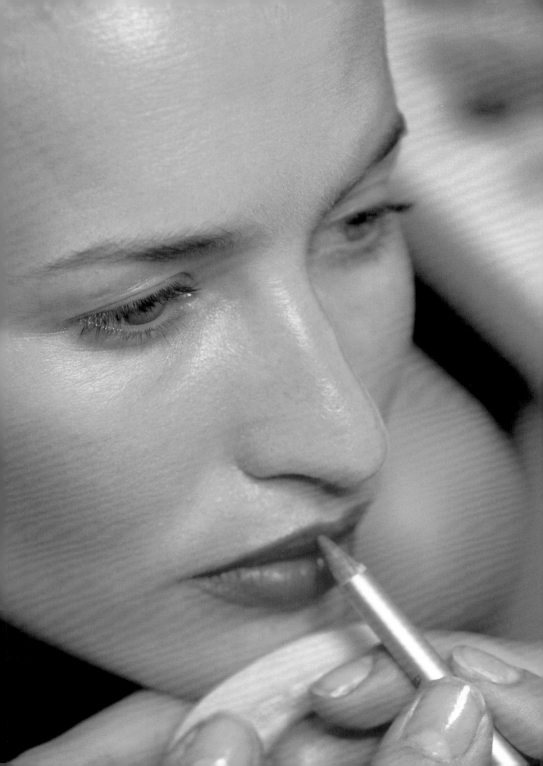

THE PERFECT POUT

1 To disguise imperfections and give a good base, cover the mouth in thin application of foundation and then blot. This also helps to prevent matt lipsticks from cracking and is especially useful when altering a natural lip shape.

2 With a sharpened pencil, follow the outline of the mouth, keeping the lips in a relaxed position.

3 Apply one coat of lip colour with a brush. Powder the lips, then reapply a second coat to achieve a long-lasting look.

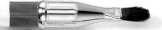

92200 - FRANCE

4 Add gloss only at the end. When it eventually wears off, you will still be left with a coloured 'stain' which will carry you through the evening, or at least until you can reach the cloakroom.

THE PARIS POUT

1 First, blot the lips with foundation. Then, taking a sharpened lip pencil, draw a new outline.

2 Start slightly further in than the corner of your own mouth and draw up towards the peak of the lips to create a rounded shape that ends just above the centre of your own top lip and just below the centre of your bottom lip. Fill in with colour.

LIP TIPS

Blotting with tissue removes excess oil and makes lip colour last longer.

If the lips are dry, apply a dab of Vaseline and buff with a baby's toothbrush.

For an instant evening look, simply add a deeper lip colour to your basic face.

Vaseline is a great conditioner and the best lip gloss around. It also adds life to matt lip shades.

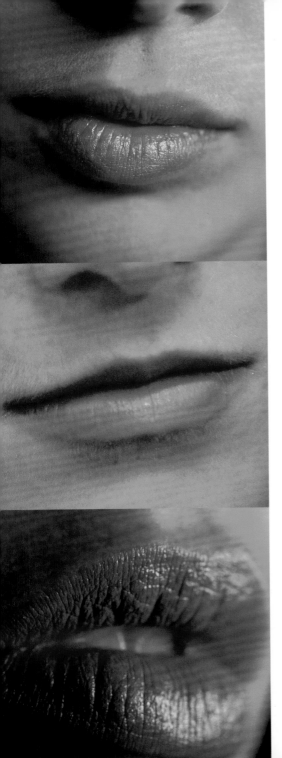

THE NATURAL LIP

1 Take a sharp lip pencil and make sure to relax the lips. Just let the pencil follow the natural lip line without creating any unnatural shapes.

FULLER LIPS

1 Blunt a lip pencil on the back of your wrist and apply foundation to the mouth as usual.

2 With a relaxed mouth, follow the natural shape of the lips, but draw slightly outside your lip line.

3 Fill in with colour and then add a slightly lighter shade in the centre of your top and bottom lips. Always use a pencil in a natural colour and make sure the foundation has been blotted well to prevent the new mouth colour from travelling.

THINNER LIPS

If you are blessed with lips that could be mistaken for life jackets, matt shades are the best choices. Avoid gloss, as this creates an illusion of fullness. Use liner just inside the natural lip line. Stick to lighter shades so that you can divert attention from your mouth by concentrating on deeper eyes.

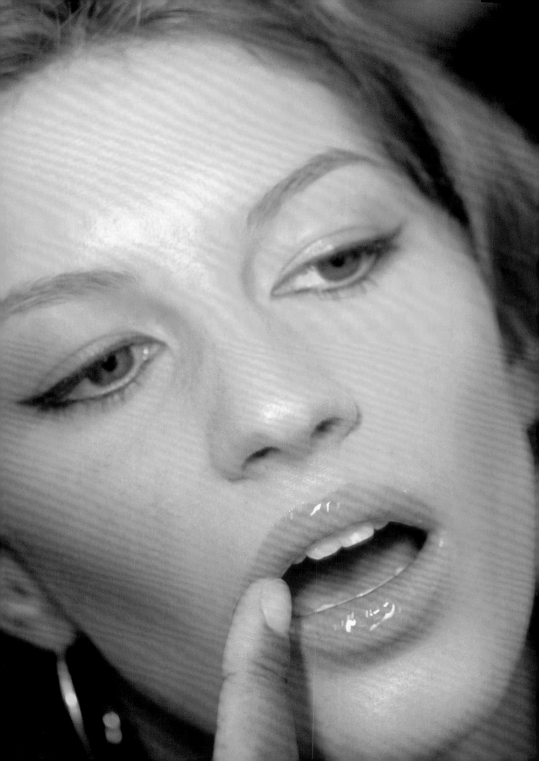

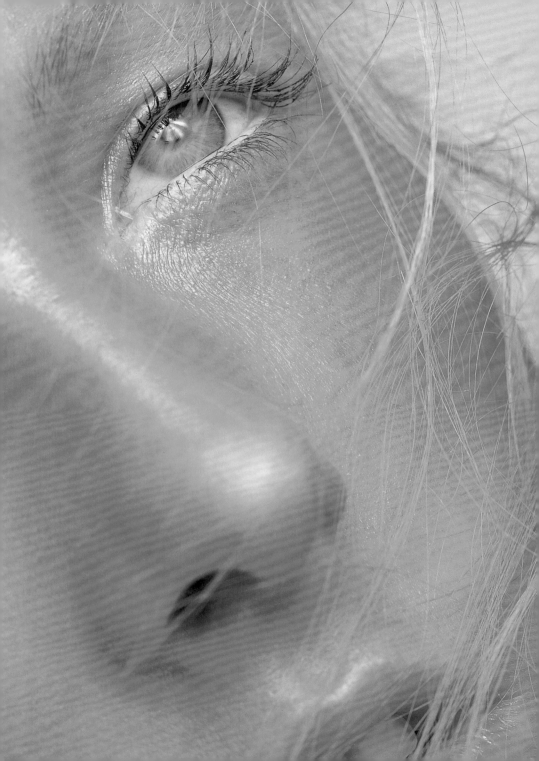

cheeks

A make-up basic, blusher is one of the constant stumbling blocks where women repeatedly get it wrong. The fashion for applying blusher seems to change so rapidly that many get trapped in a 'salad days' application, which may have looked great in the 1960s but does not quite feel right today. Fuchsia rouge accompanied by pearlized highlighter only looks good on a trendy fashion spread, and 'Aunt Sally' circles look simply comic, unless brilliantly applied by a professional make-up artist.

When it comes to colour, you cannot go wrong with a pink or a peach. These hues enhance the natural skin tones and are more forgiving if you aren't a dab hand with your blusher brush. Do not be put off by colours that look vivid in the container. Often a whisper across the cheek results in a fine, subtle finish. While cult brands Nars, MAC and Stila offer a superb array of colours, I personally always stick to the traditional houses of Chanel, Yves Saint Laurent and Christian Dior when it comes to blusher – the purity of colour they offer, combined with the silky texture, is hard to beat.

APPLYING BLUSHER

The key to successful application is knowing your own face. It is vital to flatter the bone structure, or at least create the illusion of having a bone structure. The best way to successfully apply blusher, whatever your age, is to keep it simple. A superlative graduated-bristle brush is worth the investment and Shu Uemura makes the Manolo Blahnik of blusher brushes.

1 Stand in front of the mirror and smile. Touch the rounded 'pillow' area created on each cheek and envision this as the starting point.

2 Whip the colour round in circular motions, remembering to blow excess colour off the brush first.

3 Stop smiling and move the brush up and down.

4 To create the illusion of looking younger, dab the blusher across the forehead, down the nose and on the chin to reflect light.

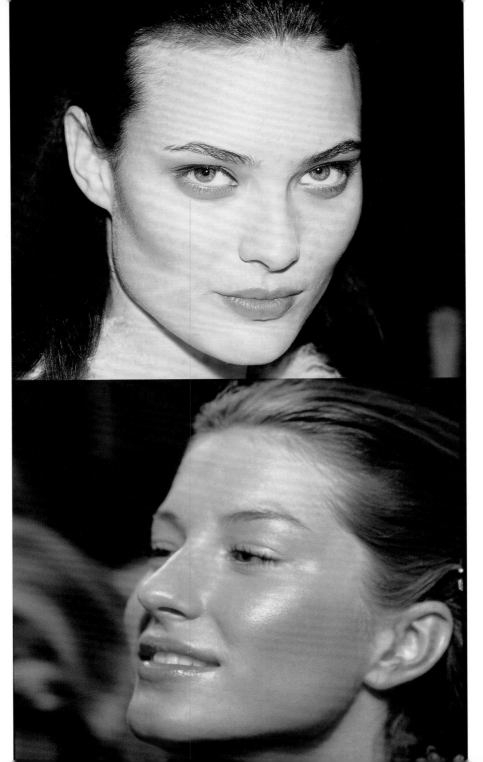

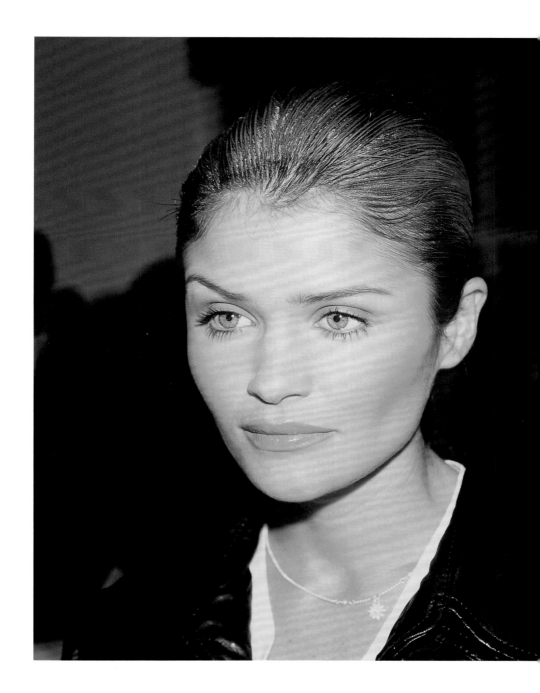

For those who feel that powder blush is something they will never master, product advancement means that cheek colour is now available in cream and fluid textures. One of the great things about these is that they are applied with the fingertips – though it is vital to blend, blend, blend to avoid the zebra effect. Most importantly, after applying a creamy blush, finish off with the sheerest whisper of translucent powder on top to create the illusion that the blush itself is coming from within.

As with any area of make-up, remember that you do not need to be limited by labelling. Multipurpose blush sticks, like those made by François Nars, contain subtle, glittery particles that reflect light and create a youthful glow. These can be used just as successfully on the décolletage or shoulder blades as on the face.

BRONZERS

For those who find the mere thought of blusher in any shape or form a turn-off, bronzing powders are a great way to create a sun-kissed look without risking sun damage. When applying bronzer, never go darker than your natural tan shade or you will look like a 1980s throwback in an ad for Ultraglow.

Choice is once again of the essence, as today bronzers are available in classic powder form (Chanel make my favourite), gel and cream suspensions (Guerlain have an unbeatable range) and wash-off skin tints which work rather like a non-stick fake tan. For those who want to create a sexy, kissed-by-the-sun look, there are wonderful, shimmery sticks which add a bronze glow to cheeks, shoulder blades, décolletage and anywhere else you choose to expose. Companies like Estée Lauder, aware of the craze for 'safe' (non-UV-exposed) tans, have come up with marvellous pots of bronze-in-a-jar gel, which add instant sun-kiss to the sallowest cheeks, and can be applied in seconds with the fingertips.

For a simple, tanned effect, stick to matt, but to create a dewy, remains-of-being-away look, nothing looks better than a slick of a shimmery bronzer across the cheek bones and a pair of lips which are moist with Vaseline.

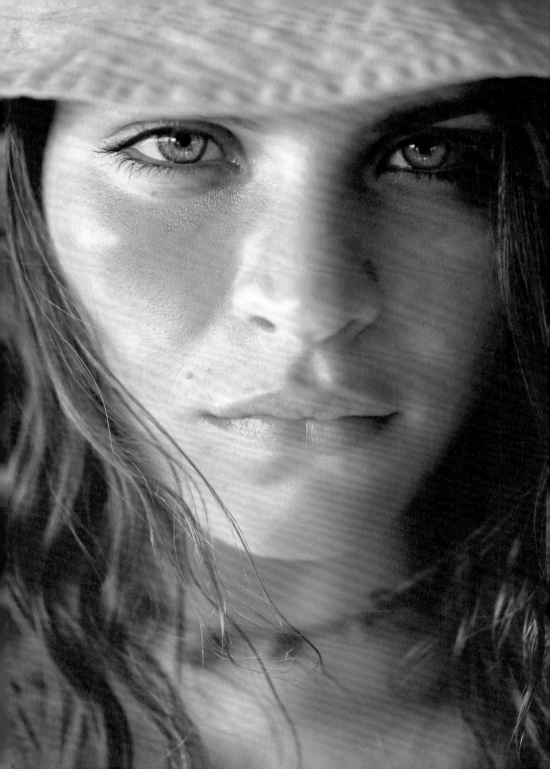

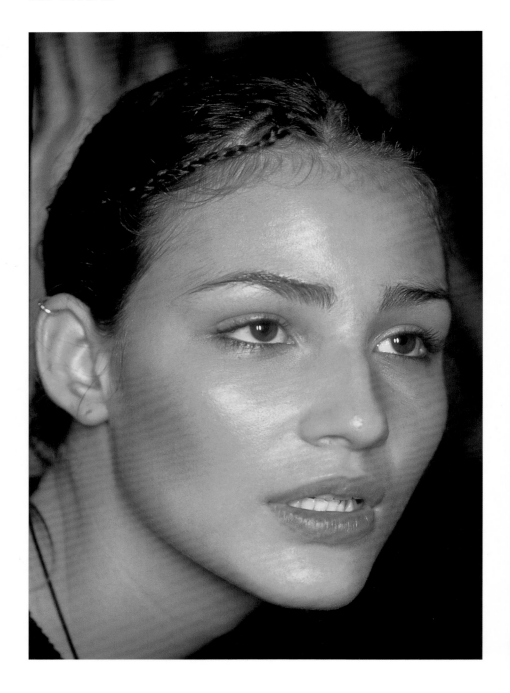

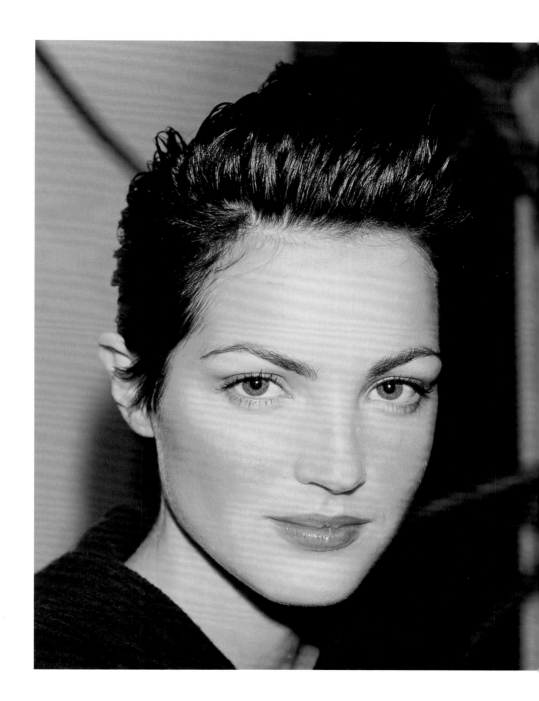

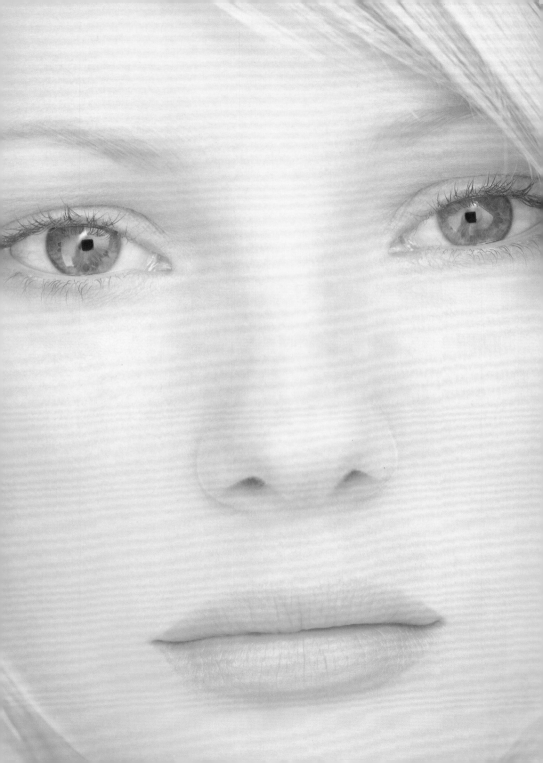

get the look

While fashions come and go, season after season, there are some key looks which, properly mastered, will take you anywhere (without a make-up artist) with confidence ...

NATURALLY BEAUTIFUL

1 Using a liquid concealer several shades lighter than the skin, create a dot-to-dot around under-eye dark circles. Do not apply beneath the shadows. Blend in with your fingertips.

2 Blend foundation into the cheeks, forehead, nose and chin, either using your fingertips or a good make-up sponge. If a certain part of the face does not need foundation, do not apply it. Once the foundation has been applied, use a harder concealer to cover any blemishes.

3 Take a large brush, dip it in loose translucent powder and blow off any excess. Dust the powder all over the face, applying extra underneath the eyes to catch any falling eyeshadow.

4 Using an eyeshadow brush, apply a neutral eyeshadow in any shade from oyster to beige-brown all over the eyelid. Start at the lash line and continue right up to the brow. Brush away any excess loose powder from under the eyes.

5 Curl the lashes with an eyelash curler. Squeeze gently at the roots, then gradually move out to the tips of the lashes.

6 Apply mascara, avoiding the roots of the lashes to prevent a spidery look.

7 Use a natural-coloured lip liner to outline the natural shape of the lips, and then fill them in with the same pencil. With a brush, apply a natural shade of lipstick all over, blot and reapply.

8 Smile into a mirror. Using a good blusher brush, apply an apricot blush to the apples of the cheeks, the bridge of the nose (this will also make a broad bridge appear narrower) and the chin.

THE 'AUDREY'

1 Apply under-eye concealer, foundation and powder, as for Naturally Beautiful (pages 256–7).

2 Use a brown eye pencil to define the eyebrow, drawing above the natural brow line but not below it. Make sure the part of the brow nearest the nose is the thickest, thinning out slightly towards the top of the curve, and then tapering towards the outer corner of the eye.

3 Using an eyeshadow brush, apply a neutral eyeshadow to the eyelids, up to the crease only. Apply a neutral cream shadow from the crease up to the eyebrow.

4 Use clear mascara to sweep the eyebrows upwards.

5 Curl the eyelashes and then apply a dark mascara to the top and bottom lashes.

6 Using the blusher brush in circular motions, apply a pale pink blusher to the apples (or 'pillows') of the cheeks only.

7 Define the lips by lining with a flesh-toned lip pencil. Fill in the whole area with the same pencil. Finish with a coat of gloss or Vaseline on top of the colour.

ALL THAT GLIMMERS IS NOT GOLD

1 Apply under-eye concealer, foundation and powder as for Naturally Beautiful (see pages 256–7).

2 Using an eyeshadow brush, apply a neutral, matt cream eyeshadow as a base colour, taking it from the eyelash line right up to the brow.

3 Next, outline the eyes with a dark eyeliner pencil or a dark shadow applied in a thin line with a tiny brush.

4 Choose a really frosted shadow in any colour, though pale colours look the least retro. Smudge the shadow onto the brow bone, just below the eyebrow and tapering out towards the eyelid crease. This opens up the eye.

5 Curl the eyelashes carefully and then apply mascara, as for Naturally Beautiful.

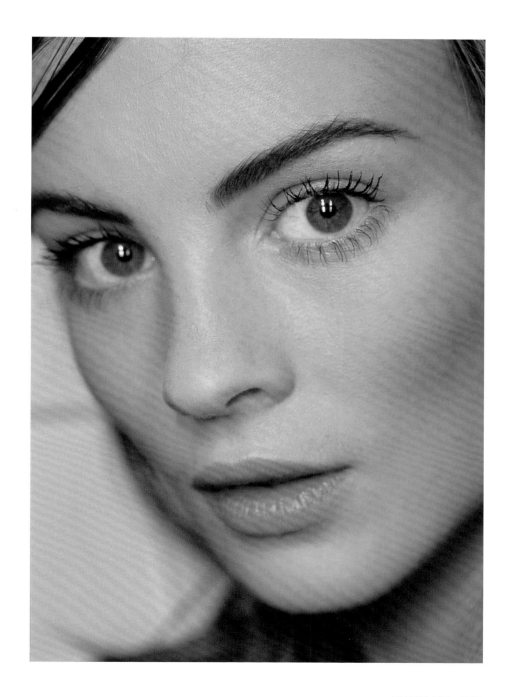

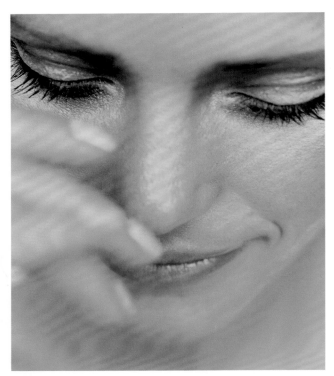

TOO HOT TO TOUCH: THE SEX KITTEN

1 Apply concealer, foundation and powder as for Naturally Beautiful (see pages 256–7).

2 Dust a generous amount of extra loose translucent powder onto the bridge of the nose, under the eyes and on the chin.

3 Use an eyebrow pencil to fill in patchy eyebrows and brush hairs upwards with an eyebrow brush.

6 Choose a lip liner several shades darker than the main lip colour. Outline the lips carefully.

7 Fill in the lip shape with a frosted lipstick. For added shine, sprinkle glitter in the centre of the top and bottom lips. Finish with a coat of gloss or Vaseline.

4 Blend a beige cream shadow into the eyelid up to where the crease forms when the eyes are open.

8 Apply a matt blusher. Using a shimmery highlighter, rub a little glitter into the cheekbone itself and onto the shoulder blades, back or décolletage.

5 With an eyeshadow brush, apply white frosted powder shadow from the lash line up to the eyebrow. Sweep it generously towards the outer corner of the eyes. Do not worry if the shimmer ends up beyond the corners.

6 With a steady hand, apply black kohl pencil to the upper lid. Make sure the pencil is as sharp as possible and use one continuous motion. Slope the line downwards, and then let it flick up slightly at the corners to create a sleepy 'come to bed' look.

7 Curl the lashes gently with an eyelash curler and then apply black mascara to top and bottom lashes.

8 When the mascara has dried, use a very thin eyeshadow brush to draw a line of smoky shadow under the lower lashes, sloping downwards towards the outer corners to match the upper lids.

9 Sweep a pinkish blusher upwards on the cheeks, following the line of the cheekbones.

10 Line lips with a fleshy red pencil, filling in with a pure red lipstick. Blot, reapply the lipstick and add lip gloss or Vaseline to complete the siren look.

THE BRIGHT SPARK

1 Apply the same base as for Naturally Beautiful (pages 256–7).

2 Line inside the top and bottom eyelids with a blue eyeliner. Using an eyeshadow brush, apply a blue eyeshadow (about two shades lighter than the liner) to the top eyelid from the lash line to just above the crease. Add a little colour underneath the eye. Blend well so the colour fades naturally without an obvious line.

3 Apply a beige liquid eyeshadow to the centre of the lids and blend in well so the colour appears graduated rather than a block. Curl the eyelashes and apply mascara, as for Naturally Beautiful.

4 Apply a coloured gloss or lip stain to the lips. Do not outline the mouth or you will look like Coco the Clown.

5 For a 'pinched' look, blend cream blush into the cheekbones.

THE BLONDE BOMBSHELL

1 For a 'wide eyed' effect, apply concealer, at least two shades paler than the foundation) to the under-eye area. Lightly smooth in the base and powder, then highlight the T-zone with extra powder.

2 Blend taupe eyeshadow up to the crease of the lid. Add ivory or white frosted powder shadow from the lash line up to the brow bone, extending past the creases at the outer edge of the eyes.

3 Next (and this requires a very steady hand), follow the line of the lashes with a black liquid eyeliner, keeping as close to where they meet the lid as possible, and flicking up to create a 'cat eye' look at the outer edges. Always do this in one movement.

4 Curl eyelashes and apply black lengthening mascara, paying particular attention to the top and bottom outer lashes.

5 Sweep pale pink blusher under the cheekbones, and across the forehead and chin.

6 Line the lips in a red-based lip liner, then fill in with a bright red lipstick. Blot, reapply and coat generously with lip gloss.

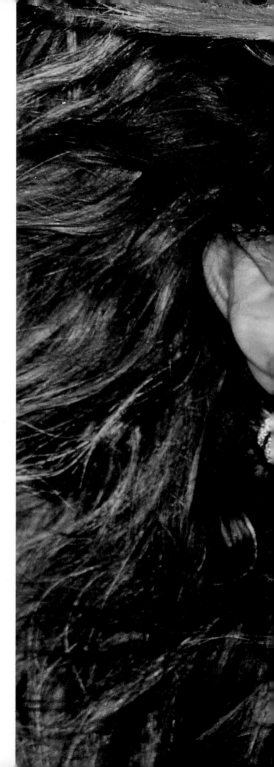

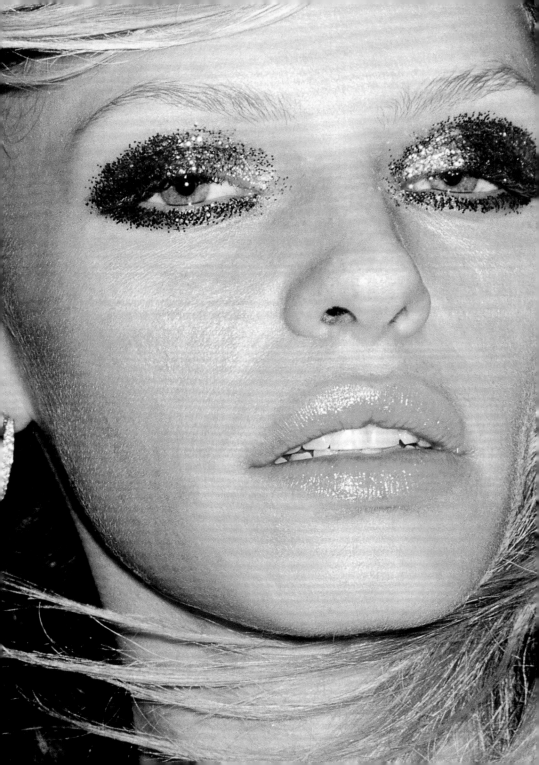

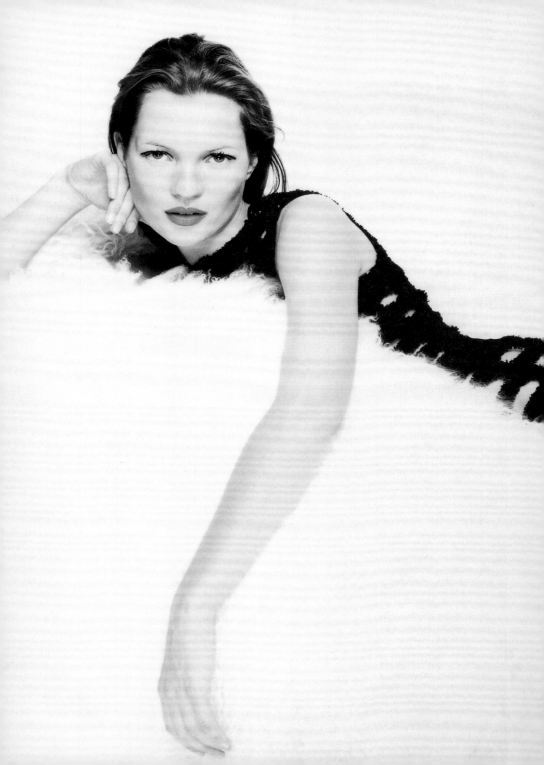

HOW TO LOOK GOOD IN PHOTOGRAPHS

OK, admit it. How many times have you looked wistfully at pictures of movie stars and supermodels and thought, 'why can't I look as good as that?'. What you do not realize is that, more often than not, they look at their glossy maga-zine alter-images and also wish they looked like that. A successful photograph is often as much to do with the skill of the photographer and the make-up artist (not to mention the guy who airbrushes wrinkles and cellulite from the picture afterwards), as it is to good genes. While no team in the world could turn Old Mother Hubbard into a budding Kate Moss, there are some canny tips that can improve a look. If you master the art of optical illusion, you will not be filled with dread the next time somebody threatens to capture you on Kodak. Also, consider British make-up artist Maggie Hunt's advice: 'You may notice that in photographs your face tends to appear a lot whiter than your body. This is because the flash reflects light off the foundation and powder on the face, and the bare skin of your chest or neck absorbs the light. Be sure to apply a bit of powder to your neck and chest too, or wear little or no foundation.'

Use good posture. Standing tall immediately gives you presence and takes away unsightly shadows because your head is properly held up.

Know your best features. Do not flash a cheesy grin with your nicotine-stained teeth. Instead, give a half smile.

Appear relaxed even if you are not and behave as if the camera is not there. 'Natural' shots are more attractive than static, posed pictures, which convey no atmosphere. To appear natural, relax the shoulders and you will find the rest of the body relaxes, too.

Be prepared. Knowing when you are likely to be photographed, such as at a wedding, means you can make up your face with the camera in mind.

tools of the trade

A bad workman is quite right to blame his tools when it comes to applying (or rather not applying) make-up. Having the right equipment is paramount to achieving the desired effect and can make all the difference between looking great or ending up like a 'before' pose in the 'after' picture. While some items are worth a large investment, others can be found very reasonably at your local pharmacy. Remember, all these are essential. No girl worth her Prada make-up pouch would be without them …

SPONGES: Handy for applying foundation (especially around the nose and eye area), they are also good for applying powder. Wash them frequently and dry naturally to maintain their condition.

POWDER BRUSH: The larger the brush, the better. Be sure to blow excess powder off the brush before using it. Wash it in a light shampoo and allow to dry naturally. A mild hair conditioner keeps natural fibres in peak condition.

BLUSHER BRUSH: Although smaller than a powder brush, a blusher brush is far larger than the freebie found in a compact. The quality of the brush makes all the difference to the application and is worth investing in. Wash as above.

LIP BRUSH: This is an essential tool for applying non-budge lipstick. It is also much easier to control: have you ever tried manipulating a whole lipstick into the pointy bits of your mouth? Wash frequently to avoid colours bleeding into one another.

EYESHADOW BRUSH: Ditch the sponge applicator and use a decent eyeshadow brush for a smooth and even application.

EYEBROW BRUSH: This is an underestimated cosmetic tool, but the key to a groomed look. Brush the eyebrows upwards to create a wide-eyed, open-faced look.

EYELASH CURLER: No professional make-up artist would ever be without an eyelash curler.

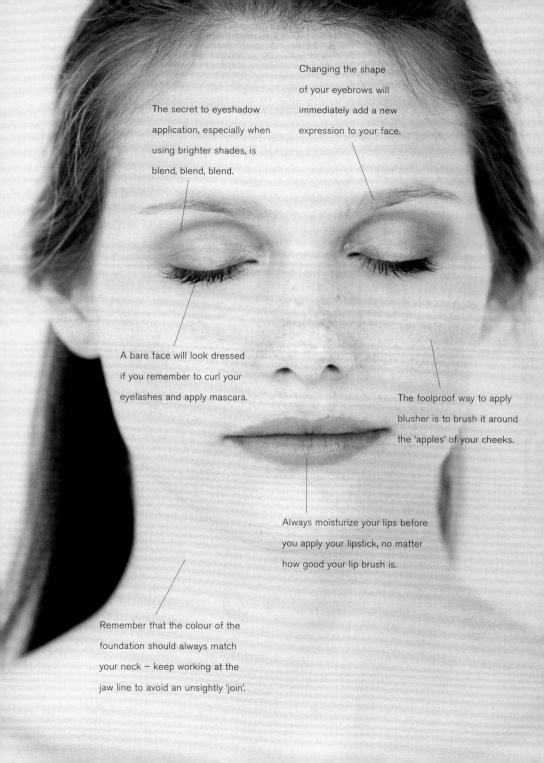

Changing the shape of your eyebrows will immediately add a new expression to your face.

The secret to eyeshadow application, especially when using brighter shades, is blend, blend, blend.

A bare face will look dressed if you remember to curl your eyelashes and apply mascara.

The foolproof way to apply blusher is to brush it around the 'apples' of your cheeks.

Always moisturize your lips before you apply your lipstick, no matter how good your lip brush is.

Remember that the colour of the foundation should always match your neck – keep working at the jaw line to avoid an unsightly 'join'.

SCISSORS: An indispensable tool for anything and everything.

EYELASH BRUSH: Use this tool between each coat of mascara to prevent lashes from clogging.

TWEEZERS: Only the blondest of the blondes never has a stray hair that needs whipping out. When buying tweezers, make sure that the ends meet perfectly, otherwise they will only do a second-rate job. I find that the ones with slightly sloping edges work best.

SHARPENER: Essential for great results with a lip or eye pencil.

ELIZABETH HURLEY'S FIVE-MINUTE MAKE-UP:

Start with a scrupulously clean and a well-moisturized face. I always begin with my eyes first and start by concealing any dark shadows.

Then I use a soft brown eye pencil and draw smudgy lines close to the lashes, top and bottom. I blend these further with a brush, which I have dipped in a gleamy brown powder shadow. This stops the eye pencil from running during the day; powder alone will not last.

I curl my lashes and apply black mascara. After pencilling in my eyebrows, I set them with brow gel so they don't rebel during the day.

Next, I use a light stick foundation, which I blend with my fingers, and then a stick blush in pink, which I also blend very well. I use a very small amount of loose powder just to set the foundation, as I loathe seeing powder on the skin.

For lips, I first use a pencil and then one of the new Estée Lauder Go Pout lipsticks, which make your lips look huge.

body art

You'd have to have kept your eyes wide shut not to have noticed fashion's focus on body decoration. While the torso-tinted models at Alexander McQueen and Julien Macdonald splashed onto the catwalk like droplets of paint on an artist's palette, and Bollywood film stars are graced with intricate designs of henna on their hands, the general public seems to have a never-ending fascination with celebrity tattoos. The trickle-down effect is that every woman these days thinks of her body as she does her face. Whether through body shimmers, fake tan or body art, no modern woman would expose bare skin without treating it cosmetically in some way.

For those who think an artist should bare her soul but not her body, there is, of course, a safer middle ground than head-to-toe body decoration. So if being a 'couture canvas' is more than you can bare, why not opt for a ready-to-wear version?

Where runway fashions lead, cosmetic houses are fast to follow, which means

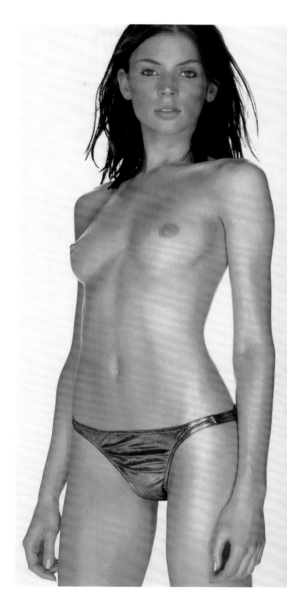

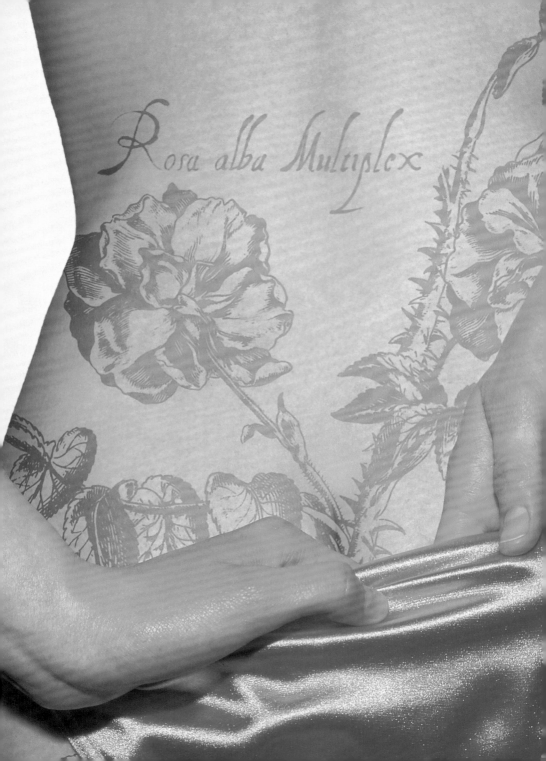

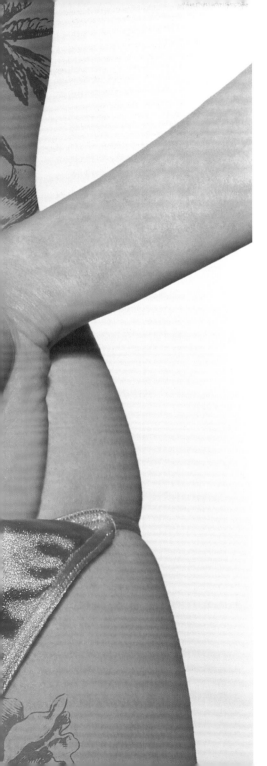

that at any department store today you'll find the cosmetic counters positively groaning under the weight of body make-up. For those who want to test the water with the merest glint of body paint, there are hundreds of glittering gels, iridescent creams, sparkling bronzers and pearlized powders for you to dip into. Smudged across the cheeks, nestling between the shoulder blades, or whispered round the décolletage, these products will ensure your body looks as well kempt as your face. For the more adventurous, temporary tattoos or stencils are bound to liven up your evening — round the upper arm, just peeping out of your boob tube, or hidden right at lowest point of your back work wonders — and, best of all, can clear off when you do. If you really feel like going for it (or have just been looking for an excuse to change the bathroom carpet), then you can even find body paint itself in DIY versions. For the girl who feels naked without jewellery, a diamanté body jewel is an erotic way to embellish your navel. As long as your tummy is more Elizabeth Hurley than Morocan belly dancer, it is certainly one way to make sure you are the brightest spark at the party.

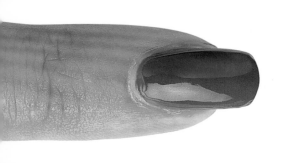

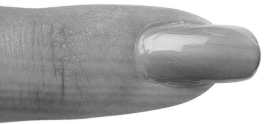

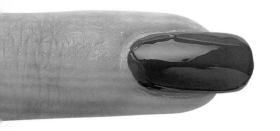

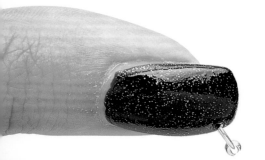

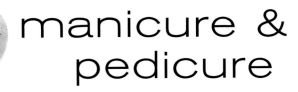

manicure & pedicure

Until recently, most women did not dedicate even a quarter of the time to looking after their hands as they spent cleansing, toning and moisturizing their faces. Suddenly everything has changed as nails have become as much of a fashion statement as wedge heels and a Balenciaga handbag. For years they were coated with transparent varnish, then they were coloured and now they are three-dimensional. With designers sending models down the runway sporting barbed-wire spokes and diamanté fingernails (a statement most of us would never dream of stretching to), a marked change is occurring in British attitudes. Susie Fitouri, manicurist at Alexander McQueen's shows, says, 'English women used to keep quiet about their nails and would traditionally stick to pale colours or a predictable red. These days they enjoy experimenting with streaks and multicoloured effects. Blue, black and yellow are no longer the domain of the outlandish – normal women paint their nails these colours, too.' The greatest aspect of nail technology today is that you do not have to be genetically programmed to have a beautiful set of fingernails. Contrary to popular belief, fibre-glass tips, if properly applied, do no real damage to the nail bed and can create a convincing set of claws for even the most hardened biter.

FEET GLORIOUS FEET

When it comes to sex appeal, shoes have it. Forget see-through, will-o'-the wisp dresses – to be truly provocative, it is time to put your best foot forward. Fashionable shoes necessitate a pair of perfect feet. No girl worth her Manolo slingbacks would set foot outside the house with trotters encased in hard skin. Slapping a layer of the latest nail polish over ten flaky toenails will not disguise unsightly feet.

So what is the best way to achieve soft skin and radically improve their appearance? If a regular pedicure takes up too much time and money, there are still some tricks worth mas-

tering in the comfort of your own home. Walking barefoot as often as possible is very good for the feet, as it stimulates the circulation and frees the bones from the confines of restrictive high-fashion shoes. It also reduces the chances of developing corns and bunions.

HOME CARE

Remember that feet take the full force of the body's weight every time you stand up, so it is essential to occasionally relieve them of the pressure. Set aside ten minutes on a weekly basis and put your feet up. Soak them in a bowl of steaming water, as hot as possible, doctored with a little aromatherapy oil to help soften hard skin. My favourite is Aromatherapy Associate's lavender oil, but other oils worth trying are eucalyptus and tea tree, which both have antiseptic properties, or peppermint, which deodorizes.

The best way to remove hard skin from the balls of the feet is with a pumice stone. Those who suffer from hard skin on their heels should scrape with a foot file on a nightly basis.

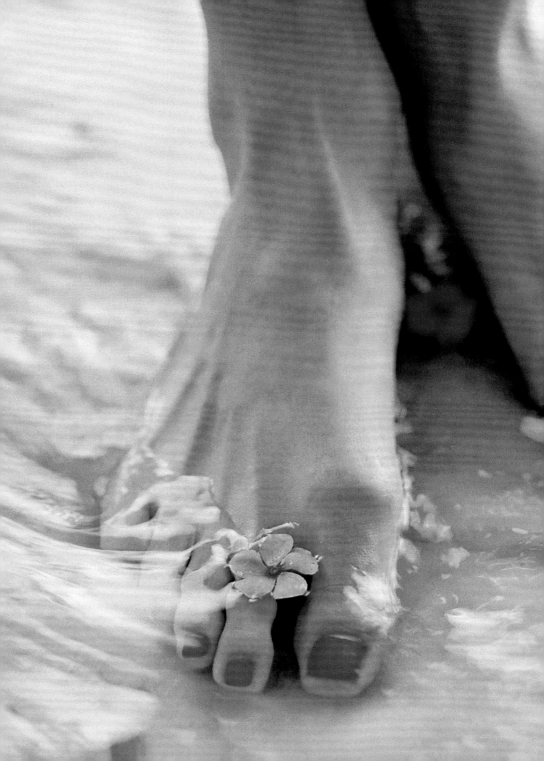

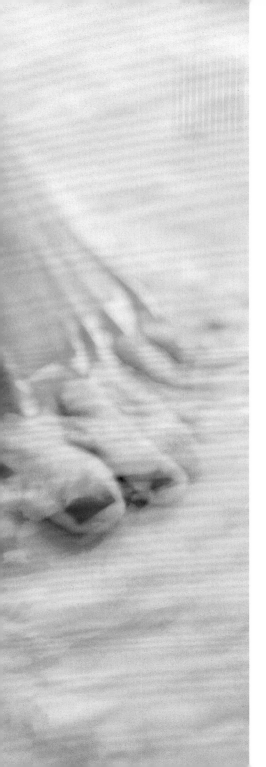

When it comes to cosmetic appeal, remember that toenails should always be cut straight across, and the most effective way to shape them is with a clipper. Use warm almond oil to soften the cuticles and a body moisturizer to keep the skin supple. When applying coloured polish, separate the toes with cotton wool to avoid smudges. As a simple rule, brighter, darker colours look best on toes.

Keeping hands looking good does require a little effort. Moisturizing is essential. Like facial moisturizers, hand creams now contain sun protection filters that prevent premature ageing and keep hands looking young and smooth. Rubbing Vaseline into the cuticles and down the fingers before bed will help to strengthen the nail bed, and only adds a couple of minutes to a nightly beauty regime. On the weekly front, there is nothing that improves nail condition more than a soak in warm almond oil and a little attention from an orange stick.

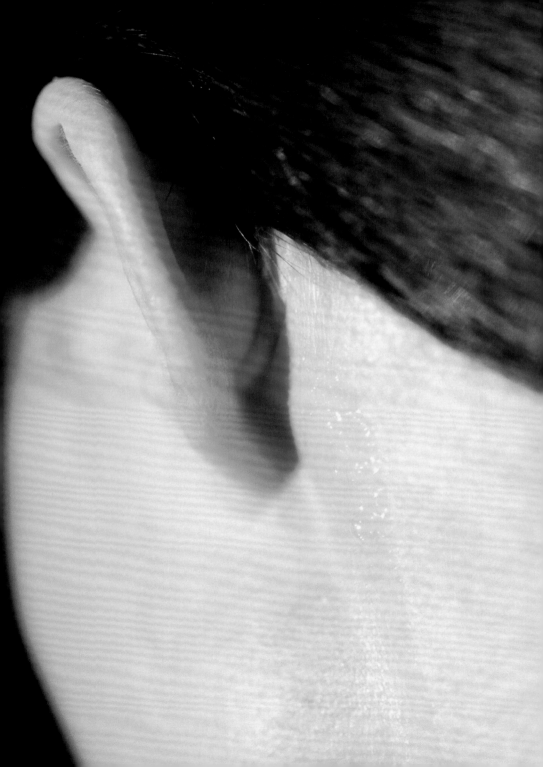

SCENT

The smell of the back of a lover's neck, a new baby's head, the pages of a favourite book; the scent of a Sicilian orange blossom orchard in May, a southern French lavender field in July or a bunch of hand-picked English garden roses in August. All smells are airborne molecules that reach our brains at their most evolutionary regions, bypassing all logic and hitting us where we feel — where we love, where we hurt and where we never, ever forget. Perhaps you fell in love in India one year, while the scents of jasmine blossom and sandalwood mingled in the hot night air with spices like cardamom, cumin and coriander. Maybe it was while skiing at Christmas, with pine trees on the mountains, hot rum punch in the kitchen and tangerine peels thrown on a crackling log fire. Or perhaps your heart always lies at Granny's, where the kitchen was filled with warm vanilla sponge cakes, hot apples and custard, and sweet violet cologne.

When we smell, we smell not just with our nose, but also with our heart. We ignore our rational selves and can be thrown into moments of fantasy, chasms of memory and fits of melancholy. Smell is a fiendishly powerful sense, which can hold us in its grip. We choose and leave lovers because of their smell and can detect love triangles by an unfamiliar waft of perfume. Even those smells associated with our most dreaded demons — death, illness, poison and decay — have the ability to make us recoil, retch, heave and even, quite possibly, pass out.

Smell and its partner-in-crime, perfume, have moved seamlessly through the course of human history. References waft in and out of literature; Horace, Shakespeare, Byron, Goethe, James Joyce, Graham Greene and Erica Jong, to name a few, have all written about the power of smell in human love, lust and power struggles. Scented objects and offerings play a role in almost all religions. In the Bible, the three wise men brought frankincense and myrrh to Jesus and incense is still burned in Christian ceremonies today. Ancient Egyptians and Greeks offered scents daily to their gods. A sixth-century 'perfume laboratory', attached to a synagogue in El Gedi in Israel, has been recently uncovered and in The Koran Mohammed spoke of the effect that perfumes have on the spirit of man. Today the perfume industry is at the cutting edge of research and technology, but far from undermining the magic and mystique, scientists are uncovering even greater intricacies, such as the role that smell has played in human biological development and psychology.

Perhaps the most enticing aspect of the world of perfume is that it allows us to manipulate our own odour and influence our mood and that of those around us. Smells communicate, just as words do. Through the art of the perfumer, we can choose not only how to smell, but also how to be remembered, what impressions we make and what mood we leave lingering behind us. As Jean-Paul Guerlain says, 'Perfume is the most intense form of memory.' But in today's beauty market there is a difficulty when it comes to choosing and buying scent; it is the embarrassment of riches ...

CHOOSING A SCENT

How are we to choose when there are department stores, perfume boutiques and airports crammed full, from floor-to-ceiling, with every different type of scent? Which one is the one for us, the one that will fit us like a glove, fulfil our fantasies and make others fall in love with us, over and over again? 'Choosing a scent is like choosing a lover,' says Roja Dove, international fragrance expert. 'You have to sleep with it first, to know how well suited you are.' And yet very few of us today have one special scent that we can call our own, that we wear day-in and day-out, year-in and year-out, that we identify with and that

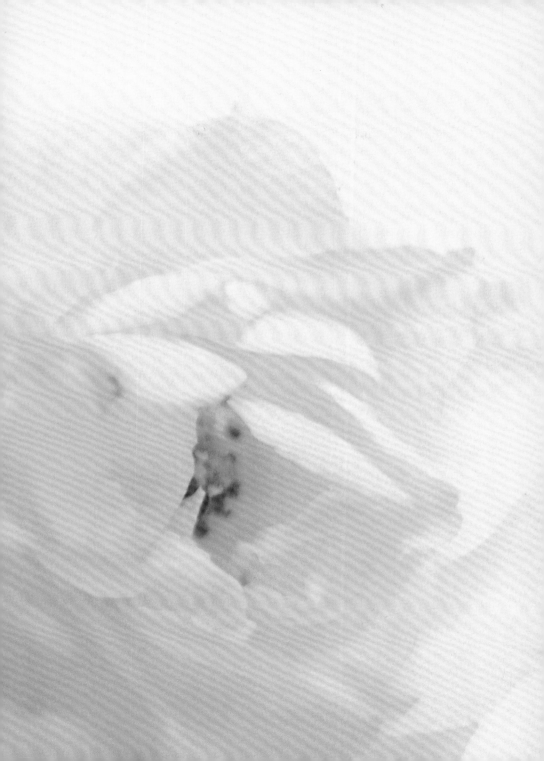

always makes us feel fantastic. And yet, it is probably out there, if only we knew how to find it. Perhaps our vacillating is a pattern of our times, and one that is mirrored in twenty-first century relationships, too. The current trend is to have lots of scents, each a different brand and each expressing a different fashion, mood or moment in time, and to pick and choose between them.

Whether you yearn to find that one special scent to call your own, or to play the field with a whole host of colognes, eaux fraîches, parfums and body spritzes is really a matter of personal choice. But make sure that it is your own decision and not one that is thrust upon you by an advertising campaign, a marketing executive or a piece of clever copy. Scent is a multi-billion dollar industry now and perfume is seen, by some, as just a product. To others, though, a beautifully constructed scent is more like a work of art. Old-world perfumers took years to perfect their perfumes. Like great painters or composers, they would work diligently on a single formula, spurred on by a love story, a particular woman or the memory of a fleeting smell. Working in isolation, without marketing and advertising teams, they had only themselves and a select few to please.

Today most new scents are not created by one person, but belong to companies and the teams that work on their conception, production, marketing, advertising and distribution. Like anything else, some scents are wonderful, while others are terrible. Some will stand the test of time, while others will be no more than flashes-in-the-pan – and all at our expense. When choosing a perfume, trust your sense of smell. Unplug the telephone, close your eyes and spend some time before making your choice. Ask for samples, or spray the tester on a blotter or page of your diary when in the shop, smile sweetly and then go home. Do not be harried, targeted or manipulated. Make up your own mind about what you think. Maybe it will be a *coup de foudre*, a brief affair, or perhaps love will smoulder gradually. But make it your decision and not someone else's. We each smell differently, have our own unique sense of smell, skin type, style and personality. Learn to find the scents that suit you and make you feel wonderful. It may be the most exciting journey of your life.

the world
of perfumery

A perfume is difficult to express with words only. Our rich vocabulary somehow falls short when it comes to revealing the nuances of smell. However abstract smells and perfumes may seem, the evolution of scent and the rise of the commercial industry is anything but abstract. Perfumes are a record of the times, perfectly capturing the changes and evolutions of culture, society, arts and industry. If we take just a little peek at the most beautiful and best-loved scents, we see more than lists of ingredients. We can see some of the milestones of the past hundred years: the impact of urbanization, industrialization and technology; the liberation of women and the unleashing of female sexuality; the rise of the consumer and the power of money. In fact, there is almost no human experience, no matter how intense and personal, that cannot be captured and bottled by a skilled perfumer.

THE PERFUME INDUSTRY

The modern perfume industry is a by-product of the leather industry – in particular, glove manufacturing. In Europe during the sixteenth century, gloves were a fashion statement and status symbol. The tanning process involved the use of urine, so scenting the gloves became a crucial process. Soon the southern French town of Grasse, the home of glove-making, became a tanning and perfume capital. Due to the superb weather conditions, flower fields flourished, and when the vagaries of fashion and new taxes wrought the decline of the glove industry, the rolling fields of rose, lavender and jasmine gave birth to the modern perfume industry.

GUERLAIN

In 1828 in Paris, Guerlain was founded, marking the beginning of a new era. To this day, considered by most to be the world's greatest-ever perfume house, Guerlain broke the hold that the English had on perfumery until then. During the puritanical Victorian era, English perfumery was riding the crest of a wave with simple, single-note, non-sexy flower

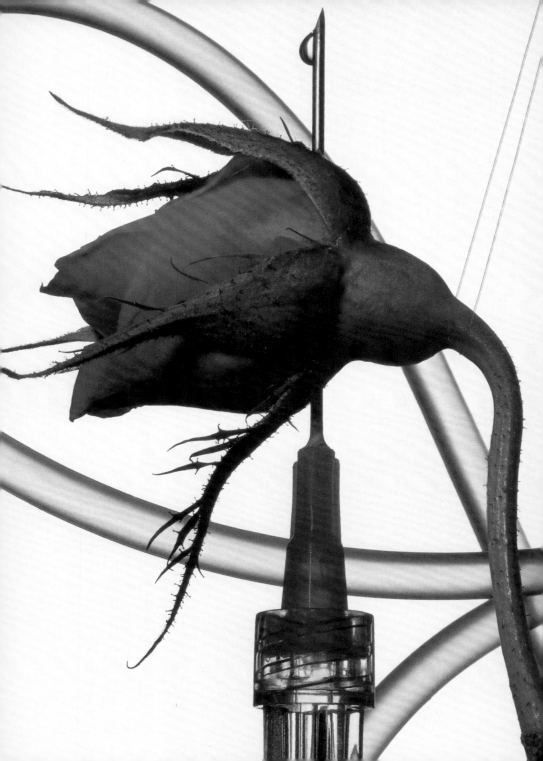

waters, such as rose and lavender, which the ladies dabbed onto their handkerchiefs. Due to its erotic associations, musk was banned and the practice of scenting the skin was deemed too sexual. Guerlain eventually changed all that by making scents, such as Jicky, in 1889, that appeared simple and decorous at first whiff, but revealed a hidden sensuality on the skin a few hours later. The company still use only the highest-quality ingredients, no matter how rare or difficult they are to obtain, and constantly push back the boundaries of what is acceptable and possible. What was so exciting about Jicky was that it was not a perfume that was trying to re-create nature. It used two new aroma chemicals — coumarin and vanillin — and smelled of something other-worldly and intensely modern. The intoxicating L'Heure Bleue, 1912, tapped into the mood of the *belle époque* perfectly. And when Mitsouko came out in 1919, its delicious and daring note of ripe peach skins (a newly discovered ingredient) captured the post-war optimism and Art Nouveau spirit. But Shalimar was another thing altogether. Still one of the most provocative scents around, in 1925 it stopped men dead in their tracks. Created by Jacques Guerlain,

the perfume was inspired by the feverish, intense love of the third Mogul emperor of India for his wife, Mumtaz Mahal. He created the Shalimar gardens for her in Lahore and when she died, amid his sorrow, he built the Taj Mahal in her memory. Romance, exoticism, seduction and a love of the Orient was bottled, and the world of perfumery never looked back.

During this period, perfumers were masters of their own destiny and that of the elite who were able to afford their scents. They could bring out delectable new concoctions whenever they felt inspired or hit upon some new ingredient. Some perfumers worked freelance while others founded their own small-scale perfume houses which reflected their particular style, ethos and talents. One of these was the great François Coty. His aim was to use the new synthetics to make good-quality scents at affordable prices to the emerging bourgeoisie. L'Origan, 1905, Chypre, 1917 and L'Aimant, 1927 became popular classics because each bottle captured the new mood — they were bold, sexual and democratic. More to the point, François Coty began the trend for marketing and advertising by adding a visual element to his scents.

the emergence of fashion

The fashion world revolutionized perfumery and, in fact, has made it what it is today. Now every designer has their own scent, which makes them more money than their clothes ever can, and which radiates more awareness and press coverage than their catwalk shows, no matter how innovative they may be. The successful designer scents have more than their smell to thank; somehow they manage to capture the essence of the designer and encourage customers to share in that style with just a couple of squirts a day. After all, the clothes of Prada, Gucci, Chanel, Stella McCartney, et al, are available to relatively few, but we can all enjoy their perfumes and cosmetics.

The couturier Paul Poiret began the crossover of scent into fashion. A lover of perfumes, he brought out his own in the 1910s. With no precedent before him, he was unconfident and claimed, 'No one will ever wear a perfume with a dressmaker's name.' As a result he branded his scents Les Parfums de Rosine instead of Poiret. How wrong could he be. He lavished enormous care, money and creativity on his scents and was the first designer to truly appreciate the link between the fashion mood and the scent a woman is wearing. He told his clients, 'That dress fits you wonderfully, but one drop of my perfume on its hem, and the dress will make you ravishing.' Paul Poiret was a trail-blazer but he only dipped his toe into the water. It took the indomitable, irrepressible Coco Chanel to change history.

COCO CHANEL & NO. 5

When Gabrielle 'Coco' Chanel brought out No. 5 in 1921, it was not only her avant-garde fashion status that led to its success: the scent itself was extraordinarily new and shocking. It contained the new perfume ingredients, aldehydes, which were extremely powerful synthetics that can have a fatty or waxy smell, but smell sparkling or fizzy when considerably diluted. The perfumer

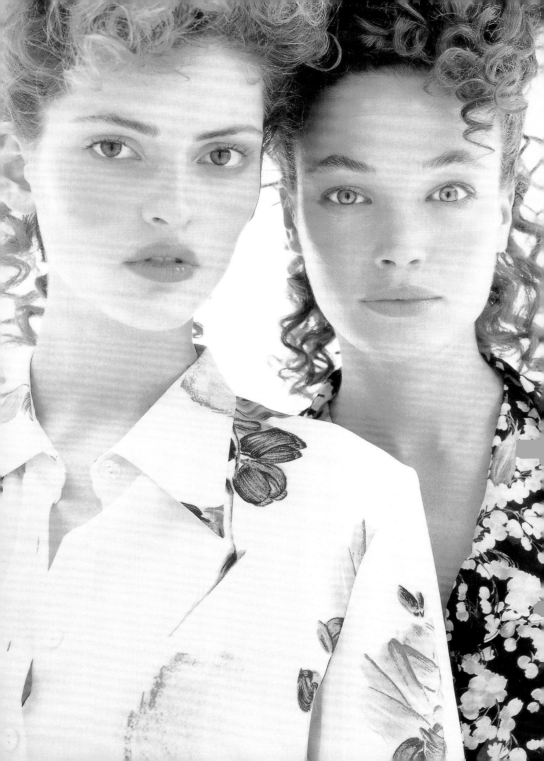

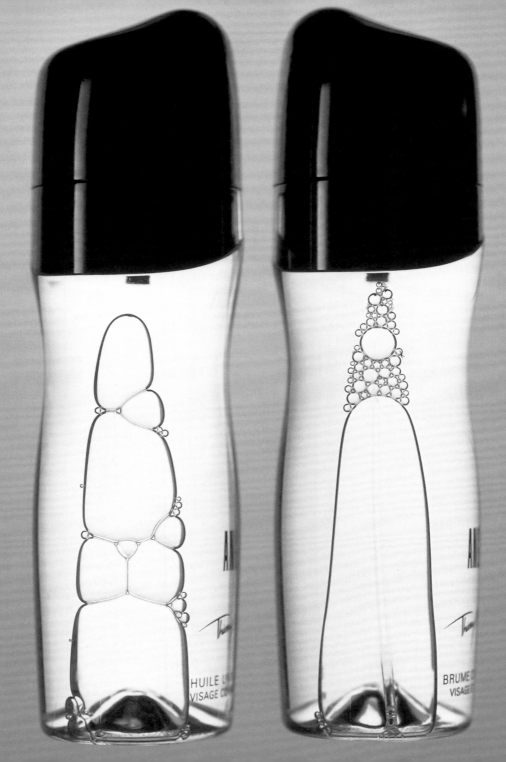

Ernest Beaux added this sparkling top note to a heart of jasmine, orange blossom and May roses from Grasse, ylang ylang from the Commoro Islands, sandalwood from Mysore and Bourbon vetiver. Chanel herself described the scent as 'an armful of abstract flowers' at a time when the abstract art of Picasso, Mondrian and Kandinsky was beginning to take root and Ernest Beaux described it as 'the smell of a snowy landscape'. Whatever. At first Coco Chanel did not sell the scent but began spraying it around herself, surreptitiously and in public places, to watch the reaction. Soon she was scenting her salon with squirts of No. 5. When asked what the smell was she would reply, 'Oh nothing much. A little perfume I thought up myself ... If you insist I'll give you a bottle.' Soon No. 5 spread around Paris like a rumour. When it was finally launched to the public, Coco Chanel acted as if she were reluctant and her hand had been forced. The perfume went on to make a lot of women happy and to make Chanel a fortune, but no one had missed the trick of creating an aura of desirability and exclusivity around a brand and soon everyone was at it.

THE COSTLIEST FRAGRANCE

In 1927 Jeanne Lanvin, now the oldest fashion house in Paris, launched the incredibly sophisticated Arpège to an eager audience. At the time the scent was seen as an attempt to out-do nature and create the smell of a flower that surpassed all the fields of flowers growing in Grasse. The extravagant and indomitable Jean Patou launched Joy to the public in 1930, immediately after the collapse of Wall Street and a worldwide economic depression had set in. Heedless of general cutbacks and economic frugality, he threw caution to the wind and launched what was to become known as 'the costliest fragrance in the world' — an extravagant, audacious bouquet of the most expensive May roses and jasmine. When the perfumer Henri Almeras presented the sample fragrance to Patou, he employed much the same trick as Coco Chanel. History, or myth, tells us he tried to hold back from presenting it, saying that it was far too expensive, far too precious, ever to be made public. Of course, this was joy to the couturier's ears. He loved the idea that nothing was too precious or extravagant for his clients. A perfume legend was born.

FROM SMALL-SCALE
TO MAJOR BUSINESS

Until now, perfumers and couturier-perfumers had existed happily side by side, but vibrant industrialization and the Second World War put an end to that. Artisans in all fields could not keep up, and the small independent perfume houses just could not compete with the richer couturiers, so many fell by the wayside. Furniture-making and textiles went the same way, with mass production being the only way to keep up with demand. It seemed that if the perfume industry was to survive, it needed more financial backing than freelance perfumers could provide. When Elsa Schiaparelli, referred to as 'that Italian' by rival Coco Chanel, launched her scents – including the famously sexy Shocking – in the early 1920s, she was breaking new ground. Not only was she marketing her scents visually, with the help of Salvador Dali, Jean Cocteau and Man Ray, but she also used a compound house to make the 'juice' rather than a traditional perfumer. A 'compound house' was a wholesale fragrance/flavours/chemicals company and Schiaparelli was the first fashion house to employ one, thus changing the entire nature of the perfume industry. No longer was perfumery a small-scale operation, run by perfumers and amateurs, but a post-war commercial industry.

Today, with the exception of a select few, every single perfume available is made by compound houses. Quest, IFF Firmenich and Givaudan-Roure are names that consumers rarely hear, but they are the power behind the throne. Perfumers now work for these multi-billion-dollar empires, dividing their time between concocting new scents for various clients and working on the development of new ingredients in their labs and in the field.

But it is not only designer scents that compound houses make. A large part of their business is to create flavours for food products and fragrances, for everything from soap powder to toilet cleaners. In fact, that is how almost every young, modern perfumer starts in their business: making scents for household products before moving on to the more glamorous area of fine, designer fragrances. Because of their enormous size and huge budgets, these compound houses are at the cutting edge of perfume technology.

PROFILE: CALICE BECKER

Calice Becker is a young, modern perfumer and was the 'nose' behind Christian Dior J'Adore. She is also senior perfumer and vice president of Quest International.

'I love my job because I get to create perfumes that are part of my dreams and I get to indulge my fantasies. In nature there are so many wonderful smells that inspire me and I work hard to combine those amazing ingredients with the needs of my clients and their customers.

'When a designer comes to me with an idea for a perfume, the most important thing is for me to listen to them very, very carefully. After all, I have the job of interpreting their dream and bottling it eventually for their customers. They have certain expectations of how the scent should smell, and I have to draw on my memories and reserves to realize that for them. Maybe they want it to be a sporty fragrance, for women to take to the gym with them, or maybe they want something feminine and fruity.

'First, I draft a very simple set of accords for them and make up a very simple fragrance. It is a bit like being a painter doing a preliminary sketch. I have to harmonize the various different elements and then bring together the technical qualities that are necessary for a perfume. It should have a bright top note, a heart, and then the base notes must linger on the skin and still smell beautiful after several hours.

'Then I play around with the smells and mix and match various ingredients as if I were a painter doing a still-life. When you think of all the perfume ingredients there are in the world, and you think of the millions of different combinations you can make, well, you could make scents into infinity ...'

fragrance families

All scents, from Diorella to Diesel, from Youth Dew to Yohji, belong to five fragrance families: floral, oriental, chypre, fougère and ozonic. Within each category there are many sub-categories, such as floral-orientals, fruity chypres and ozonic florals, but fundamentally every scent corresponds to one main family.

FLORALS

In the beginning, all perfumes were floral. Rose oils and lavender waters were

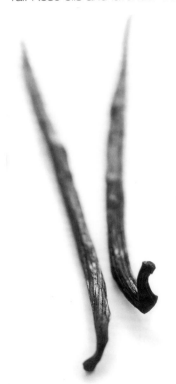

the height of the perfumer's art and exactly how 'ladies' were expected to smell. Today, floral scents are a lot more enticing and exciting, provoking images of dewy summer gardens with their notes of sweet pea, freesia, lilac, lily and carnation or springtime bouquets of freshly gathered paperwhites and hyacinths. Florals are the 'safest' scents of all, being rarely overpowering, demanding or difficult to wear. They can be sweet, subtle and feminine, and as rare and beautiful as the flowers they try to re-create.

Annick Goutal **Gardénia Passion**

Caron **Fleur de Rocaille**

Chloé **Chloé**

Christian Dior **Diorissimo**

Estée Lauder **Pleasures**

Gucci **Envy Me**

Houbigant **Quelques Fleurs**

Jean Patou **Joy**

Jo Malone **Red Roses**

L'Artisan Parfumeur **Mimosa Pour Moi**

Lancôme **Miracle**

Prescriptives **Calyx**

Stella McCartney **Stella**

ORIENTALS

Oriental perfumes are the most sexy of scents, smelling of sultry warmth, night-time and Eastern exoticism. Some can be quite heavy, heady and overpowering but they are also long-lasting. They combine hints of ambergris (which smells warm, velvety and musky) with woody, spicy tones and often include nuances of fresh flowers to counteract the heaviness with a breath of fresh air.

Calvin Klein **Obsession**

Cartier **Must de Cartier**

Chanel **Coco**

Christian Dior **Dioressence**

Estée Lauder **Cinnabar**

Estée Lauder **Youth Dew**

Guerlain **Samsara**

Guerlain **Shalimar**

L'Artisan Parfumeur **L'Eau d'Ambre**

Shiseido **Feminité du Bois**

Serge Lutyens **Ambre de Sultan**

Yves Saint Laurent **Opium**

CHYPRE

These scents tend to smell of autumn forests and mossy woods and often have animalistic notes. A classic chypre scent contains oakmoss, sandalwood and musk, combined with rose and jasmine, and maybe something bright, light and citrussy squeezed on top.

Antonia's Flowers **Tiempe Passate**
Christian Dior **Miss Dior**
Coty **Chypre de Coty**
Clinique **Aromatics Elixir**
Givenchy **Givenchy III**
Hermès **Calèche**
Crown **Marechale 90**
Jo Malone **Fleur de la Forêt**
L'Artisan Parfumeur **Voleus de Roses**
Robert Pignet **Bandit**

FOUGÈRE

Fougère is French for fern, but ferns have no smell. Basically, this is a 'fantasy' fragrance type, which may smell wonderful but is nothing like ferns in nature. It was invented by Houbigant in 1882 to smell aromatic, with notes of lavender and fresh hay. So daring and popular was Houbigant Fougère Royale – because it was not a copy of something in nature, but of something 'imagined' in nature – that it spawned a whole new genre of perfume. Today fougère fragrances are big news because they are often unisex and contain fresh, zesty notes with dry, foresty tones and lavender.

Bronnley **French Fern**
Calvin Klein **CK Be**
Creed **Orange Spice**
Diptyque **Eau d'Elide**
Estée Lauder **Alliage**
Etro **Lemon Sorbet**
Fabergé **Brut**
Guerlain **Jicky**
Penhaligon **Eau Sans Pareil**
Penhaligon **English Fern**
Penhaligon **Esprit de Lavande**

OZONICS

Ozonic scents are relatively recent additions to the perfume world, which have been made possible by the discovery of aroma chemicals that smell of watermelon, but which impart a sense of fresh air and the seaside. They characterize many fragrances of the 1990s, such as L'Eau d'Issey and Calvin Klein Escape, and they are instantly recognizable: you either love them or you hate them.

Aramis **New West for Her**
Calvin Klein **Escape**
Christian Dior **Dune**
Elizabeth Arden **Sunflowers**
Issey Miyake **L'Eau d'Issey**
Ralph Lauren **Polo Sport Women**
Giorgio Armani **Acqua di Gio**

perfume
pyramids

Whether you love or loathe a particular scent, you know that the smell of perfumes change over time. This is because perfumes are constructed in the form of an imaginary 'pyramid' with a top, middle and base.

PERFUME NOTES

The top notes are the short burst of fresh, zesty, green notes that are immediately noticeable when you first spray on a scent, but which fade after about 30 minutes. Lemon, mandarin, peach, orange, lime, bergamot, blackcurrant, grapefruit and aldehydes are all common top notes.

The middle notes develop over time and are usually flowers. This 'heart' of a fragrance is perhaps the most important part because it defines the essence of the scent and will last between two and four hours. This is really what you buy the scent for. Rose, jasmine, gardenia, freesia, tuberose, lilac, ylang ylang,

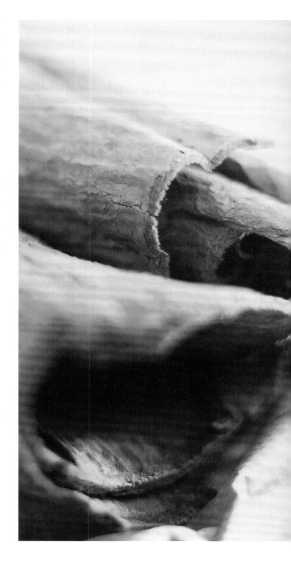

carnation and lily-of-the-valley are popular middle notes.

The base notes are the rich, long-lasting tones that give scents their tenacity and depth. When buying a scent, these are the notes that you will not smell until you get home and go to bed. They may be there from the beginning in oriental scents, but mostly you will have to bide your time to see if you like them. You probably will because they smell fleshy, sexy and human. Amber, musk (both real and synthetic), sandalwood, patchouli, vetiver and some woody oils are all base notes.

TIME CHANGES EVERYTHING

Never, ever buy a scent in a hurry. The scent you spritz on in the shop is not the same scent that you will smell in one, two or five hours' time. Due to their pyramid construction and your own unique skin type, scents will change – so be patient. Get samples to take away, or at least spray the perfume on tester blotters. You will not regret it. Remember that maxim 'Marry in haste, repent at leisure'? Well, something similar to this applies to perfume ...

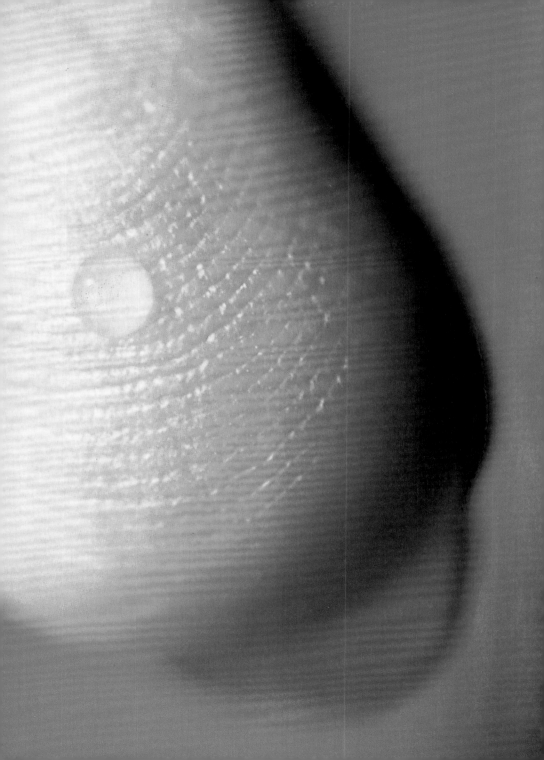

ingredients

When it comes to natural raw ingredients, perfumers draw on the whole planet. The warm climes of Morocco, Sicily, India, Brazil and Australia grow much of the world's production of jasmine, lemon, neroli, bergamot and sandalwood, while Russia, Bulgaria and Turkey provide heady, velvety damask roses. But like any natural commodity, there is a finite supply. It takes 6–7 million jasmine flowers to make a kilogram of jasmine absolute, and some ingredients, such as orris (from iris roots), natural musk, ambergris and tuberose, cost several times their own weight in gold because they yield so little, if any, essential oil.

Weather conditions, wars, political exclusion zones and natural disasters all play a major role in the cost of perfume. Famine in Eastern countries means that they will plant rice instead of patchouli one year, and 'ethnic cleansing' and population migration can mean that labour is not available for flower picking. A magnificent scent is a careful balance of precious essences, of flowers, resins, spices and so on, so if one

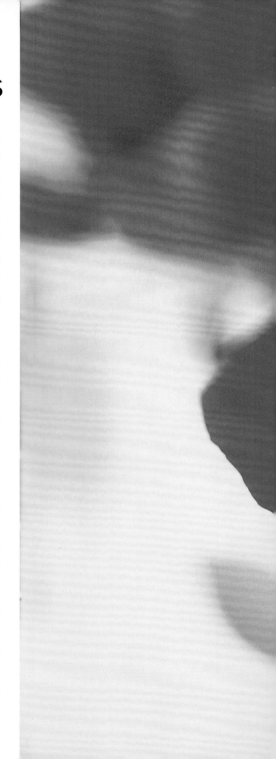

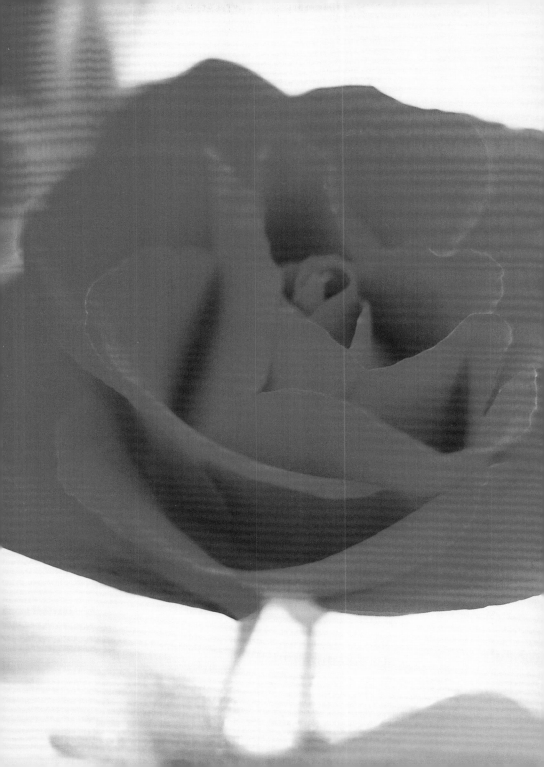

of those essential ingredients becomes impossible or difficult to obtain, then the cost can skyrocket or the scent may be discontinued – until an alternative source becomes available.

Guerlain Nahema, launched in 1979, was inspired by Catherine Deneuve. The scent contains May roses and Damask roses and the price fluctuates annually, depending on the availability of the flowers. Likewise, Jean Patou Joy is made with pure jasmine and May roses from Grasse and there is limited availability of both. Because the flowers can be harvested only once a year, Joy can be made only in limited quantities. Like both these companies, Chanel has also made long-term investments and commitments to planting, harvesting and buying the highest-quality ingredients so that the quality of their products never suffers.

Of course, not all perfume houses have such scruples when it comes to ingredients. In an effort to cut corners and costs, many downgrade their ingredients. Jasmine from Grasse becomes jasmine from Morocco, and natural flower oils become cheap, synthetic versions until the scent is a pale shadow

of its former self. Due to climate, soil acidity, strength of the sun on the petals and so on, flowers smell differently when grown in different countries, but today business decisions are often the last word. Takeovers and company restructurings often lead to a demise in quality and the end result can be a poor product. Fortunately, the flip side is that many houses that were downgraded in the 1970s and 1980s have now been bought by bigger and better consortiums, whose aims are to restore the scents to their former glory. The classic scents Lanvin Arpège and Robert Piguet Fracas are examples, and now both are glorious once again.

ROSE

'A rose is a rose is a rose is a rose,' said Gertrude Stein. Roses themselves have been worshipped and adored since ancient Roman times and rose oil, surprisingly, is antiseptic and high in vitamin C. The very best rose for perfumes is the May rose (*Rosa centifolia*) from Grasse in the South of France and from North Africa. Roses are picked by hand, very early in the morning when drenched with dew and before the sun can blanche the petals and disturb the delicate scent. A champion rose-picker will take a whole day to collect sufficient to extract just a few drops of precious rose oil. The Damask rose (*Rosa damascena*) is the one most widely used in perfumery and comes from Turkey, Bulgaria, Egypt and Russia.

JASMINE

The varieties *Jasminum officinalis* or *Jasminum grandiflorum* feature in almost all women's, and some men's, fragrances — whether you can smell them or not. Jasmine is sacred to the perfumer and known simply as '*la fleur*' to many. The best varieties come from France, but Egypt, Italy, India and China are all producers of the flowers. It is incredibly expensive, so synthetic versions are often substituted. When jasmine is combined with May roses it provides the heart of many well-known scents; for example, 10,600 jasmine blossoms (and 28 dozen roses) make one single ounce of Jean Patou Joy.

VIOLET

Much loved by the Victorians, the best violets are Parma violets from northern Italy. The fragrant oil does not come from the flowers themselves, but from the leaves of the plant. Only a tiny amount of oil is extracted, so synthetics are often substituted in perfumery today. Violets have a sweet, powdery smell, which is often reconstructed with bergamot, mimosa, sandalwood and rose, among others. A beautifully made violet scent does not need to smell old-fashioned at all. Borsari Violetta di Parma is a sensual, earthy violet fragrance, and another is Penhaligon's Violetta. Gentle notes of violet can be detected in classics like Chanel No. 19 and Givenchy L'Interdit.

NEROLI

Neroli is orange flower oil, particularly that of Seville oranges, and the flowers come from the South of France, Italy, Egypt and Tunisia. It gives an incomparable light freshness to the top notes of many high-quality scents, but it is also sweet and orangey. Neroli is irreplaceable in the classic eau de cologne. 1016 kg (1 ton) of flowers yields 907 g (2 lb) of oil and worldwide production does not exceed 2032 kg (2 tons). Neroli is traditionally linked with purity and as a result is often included in many bridal bouquets. Aromatherapists also use neroli oil as a treatment for nervous depression and anxiety, but I am sure there is no connection …

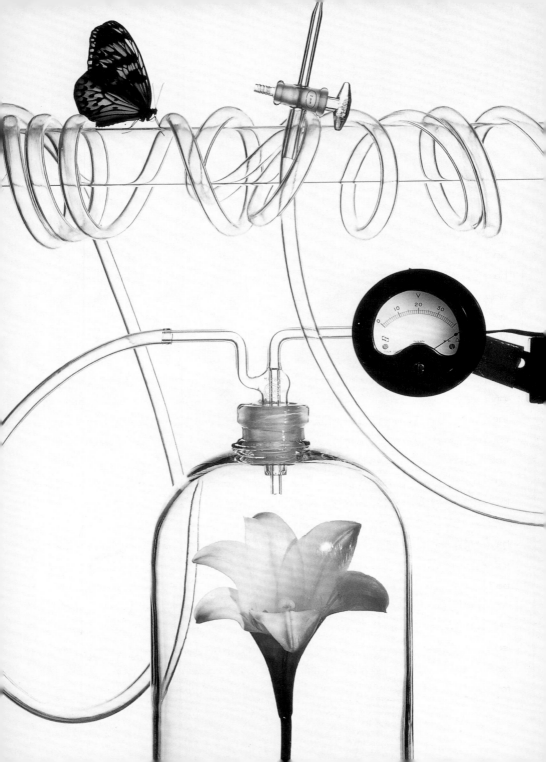

naturals & synthetics

Good-quality, natural ingredients are rare and expensive commodities, but they make the finest raw materials for perfumery. The smell is rounder, vibrant and more real than chemicals and they have more of an affinity with human skin. However, the debate between natural versus synthetic is highly complex. Many flowers, such as lily-of-the-valley, linden blossom and lilac, do not release their odour to perfumers. They yield an infinitesimal amount of oil, which makes their use impossible in perfumery, but for over 100 years perfumers have been able to make very respectable synthetic versions, many of which feature heavily in the great classics. By no means all synthetics are cheap and tacky. Some have a long heritage and provide us with extremely interesting notes that cannot be found in nature.

There are two kinds of synthetics: isolates, which mimic the molecular structure of a real smell and can be found in nature, and synthetic chemicals, which are based on unnatural smells but are a dream for the modern perfumer. As you may have noticed, many of the new scents do not actually smell like anything you have ever smelled before and that is because they do not come from nature, but from a chemist's lab. Such scents can be marketed as smelling like 'sand' or 'clouds' or 'linen', or anything else that might fit the image and concept of the new scent. Let your nose be the judge. If it does not smell completely pure, fresh and exquisite, ditch it. Likewise, if you develop a headache or it makes small children cry, then you have your answer.

AMERICAN STYLE

American women have always had their own ideas and tastes when it comes to scent. When Guerlain's Shalimar first launched stateside it was an instant success, much more so than in Europe, where it was probably too ahead of its time. American women loved Shalimar's blatant, sexual, upfront nature and the high concentration of perfume oils which gives it a warm, long-lasting scent on the skin. However, Estée Lauder was the one who gave American women purchasing power when she brought out Youth Dew in 1953. Until then women did not buy scent for themselves, but only hoped and hinted. Estée Lauder set about to change that and made the deeply oriental Youth Dew a moisturizing bath oil, which doubled up as a powerful perfume if dabbed onto the pulse points. Her strategy worked. With Youth Dew women started buying fragrance for themselves and, as a result, the perfume is often referred to as the first feminist fragrance.

While European women were happy to spritz themselves with their favourite scent several times a day, in the USA they wanted scent to last. Estée Lauder made a decision to bypass the demure eau de toilette strength when she brought out Cinnabar, Knowing, Estée, Beautiful, Private Collection and Dazzling. Only White Linen, reminiscent of crisp linen sheets drying in the sun, and Pleasures are available in the light eau de toilette.

Today, American fashion houses and their fragrances are major players. Ralph Lauren launched Polo Sport Women fragrance and body line to coincide with the active lifestyle of the 1990s. The company describes the green, fresh, herby notes as evoking 'diving into a cool pool on a hot day', 'surfing the curl' and 'parachuting for the first time'. The packaging has practical flip-top lids, easy-grip sides and is perfect for the gym. The smell? Does it really matter? This is a lifestyle scent.

Calvin Klein has charted the decades as cleverly with his fragrances as with his clothes. Obsession was truly 1980s – gutsy, ambitious and upfront – but when the mood changed and the 1990s turned the corner, Eternity was spot on yet again. One minute Klein was espousing 'obsession and sensuality' in relationships and the next it was 'intimacy'. Escape was at the forefront of the new, American ozonic note in perfumery and CK One broke ground again, using MTV advertising to capture the young crowd. In 2004 Klein had moved with the times once again, with Scarlett Johansson becoming the face of Eternity Moment.

different
moods

'What remains of a woman when she is in the dark? When she has undressed, when she has taken off her dress, when we can no longer see her make-up, her wonderful hair, her beautiful eyes, when she takes off her jewellery, what is left? Only her charming voice and her perfume.'

Jean-Paul Guerlain

No, it is not all hype and blag. There is little doubt that scent is linked to sex, or, at least, desirability. When you love someone, you love their smell and can identify them equally well in a dark room or a crowded daytime elevator. When we wear scent, we want others to love it, too. As well as our blatant, recognizable smell, each of us secretes chemical messengers known as pheromones. These are hormonal substances secreted by the skin which can alter the physiology and behaviour of others. You cannot choose or change your pheromones, just as you cannot decide or change the effect that others will have on you. Research has shown that women are attracted to men who smell least like themselves, as these men will have dissimilar immune-system genes and will, perhaps, help you produce the healthiest babies. So if you do fall madly in love, or are wildly attracted to someone, there may well be very sound biological reasons for this.

Smell is a sexual sense, but the decision-making process involved in choosing a new scent is not. All too often we buy something because it is new, we like the advertising and marketing, but not because it is really sexy. What is really beautiful and sexy about a perfume is not its image, its chemical formula or how it smells in the bottle, but how it smells when it has been on the skin for several hours and has been altered by your own body chemistry. A strong, modern scent which does not change its smell over time, or does not smell differently on different women, won't do that, which is a shame. If it is a scent with sexuality you are after, choose one with a high proportion of natural ingredients, as these are rounder, warmer and have more affinity with skin than chemical ingredients. According to Roja Dove, professeur de parfums, 'Each of us has our own, natural smell. Combine that with a high-quality perfume that is made with natural, raw materials and you will get a third scent — one that is unique to you. If you use chemical-laden perfumes, then those chemicals will either cloak your own natural scent or clash with it.'

Scent is at its most sensual when it becomes part of a woman's smell. According to Karen Hawksley, owner of London's best fragrance emporium, Les Senteurs, 'The French are wonderful at making really sexy scents. They make these beautiful, pure, floral fragrances and then add something really dirty to them, such as civet and ambergris.' When Guy Robert made Hermès Calèche in 1960, he wanted it to smell of 'the marital bed' — warm, lusty, sexy and comfortable, and funnily enough,

it does. Calèche is an easy scent to wear. It is not aggressive or too exciting; it will not tire you out, but it is definitely warm and sensual. Other classic sexy scents are Guerlain Chamade, which is supposed to be reminiscent of a heart beating wildly when a woman is in love, or Molinard Habanita, which is meant to smell like the thighs of young Cuban girls who roll cigars. So yes, there are many sexy scents out there. Really and truly.

Annick Goutal **Passion**

Aveda **Equipoise**

Caron **Fleur de Rocaille**

Chanel **Coco**

Guerlain **Mitsouko**

Guerlain **Shalimar**

Guy Laroche **Fidji**

Jo Malone **Fleur de la Forêt**

Jo Malone **Red Roses**

L'Artisan Parfumeur **Mure et Musc**

Molinard **Habanita**

Neal's Yard **Exotic Body Lotion**

Paloma Picasso **Paloma Picasso**

Robert Piquet **Fracas**

L'EAU KEY SCENTS

In the 1980s the fashion for scents with more personality than their wear-

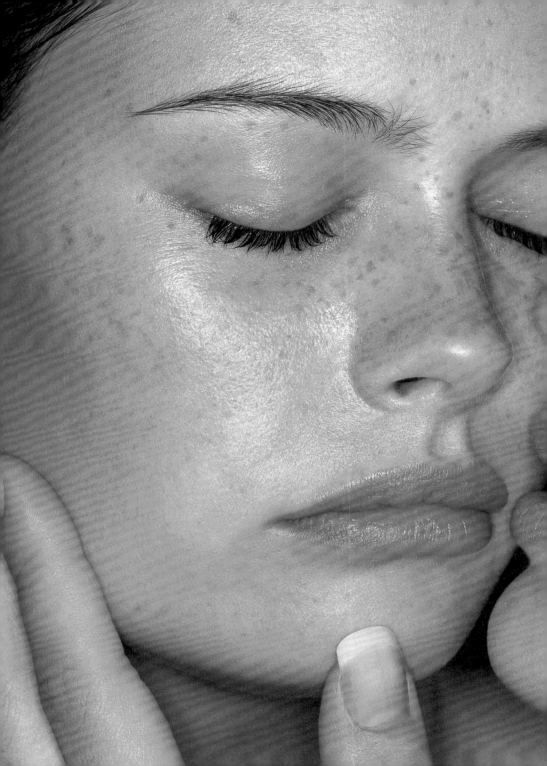

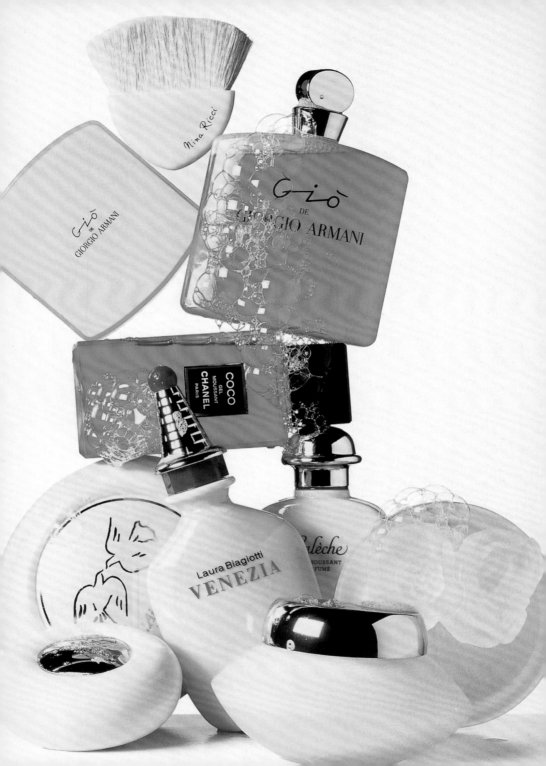

ers was, arguably, a blip on the landscape, but the correlation between overpowering scents and huge hair and shoulder pads cannot be lost on anyone. Women were breaking into the workplace during the 1980s and needed confidence and presence to spur them on. Giorgio Beverly Hills and Christian Dior Poison terrified people. But that was OK. They were outrageous, but at least they got you noticed. Fragrance ball-breakers are not in vogue now. Far from it. But some scents have been updated for the twenty-first century.

Cacharel **Eau d'Eden**
Christian Dior **Tendre Poison**
Estée Lauder **White Linen Breeze**
Giorgio **Beverly Hills Giorgio**
Guerlain **Un Air de Samsara**

NICHE SCENTS

We all know the giants – those fashion and fragrance houses that spend millions on marketing. But what about those select and secretive scent houses who make small batches for those in the know? These companies do not spend money on promotion, but rather on the 'juice' itself and the reason they have survived is their dedication to quality and exclusivity. Most of these companies make scents that are more expensive than average, but you may just find that they smell worth it.

ANNICK GOUTAL: Each scent is unique, beautiful and unmistakable. Classics are Eau de Hadrian and Grand Amour.

CARON: A great old perfume house. Royal Bain de Champagne smells like a bath filled with champagne.

CREED: Established in 1760, Creed uses only the finest natural ingredients. Grace Kelly wore Fleurissimo on her wedding day.

JO MALONE: A modern English perfumer whose scents are both innovative and classic. Lime, Basil and Mandarin is famous, but French Lime Blossom is wonderful too.

L'ARTISAN PARFUMEUR: An adventurous French house that loves breaking new barriers. Two of their irrepressible scents are Premier Figuier and Dzing (which smells of the circus).

MILLER HARRIS: Founded in 2000 by 'nose' Lyn Harris, who pioneered the bespoke market in the UK. The foundation for her fragrances are precious natural ingredients.

PENHALIGON: The epitome of English perfumery. Dedicated to quality and style, their L'Eau Sans Pareil says it all.

CLASSIC SCENTS

To define a fashion classic is very tricky; what looks cool one moment can look decidedly not right the next. Even classic fashion staples, such as jeans, need to be updated constantly to keep them modern.

Perfumes are a little bit like that. Notes that smell new, exciting and sexy one decade can begin to pall the next. Some scents transcend fashion, however, remaining as breathtaking as ever, year-in, year-out. Because they are beautifully made, with quality ingredients, these scents are more like precious jewels than fleeting fashion statements.

Cacharel **Anaïs Anaïs**

anything by Chanel and Guerlain

Christian Dior **Diorissimo**

Jean Patou **Joy**

Lancôme **Trésor**

Lanvin **Arpège**

Thierry Mugler **Angel**

LOOKING AFTER YOUR SCENT

Scents and perfumes are light- and temperature-sensitive. Leaving them open or in sunlight are probably the worst things you can do to them. 'Variations in temperature are very bad for scents, so bathrooms which fluctuate constantly are out,' says Karen Hawksley from Les Senteurs, London's perfume shop. 'Some scents now come with refills. The best thing is to buy the largest refill possible and keep the refill in its box in the fridge. The fridge is probably the only temperature-constant place in anyone's house. Decant only a small amount of scent at a time for the bottle that you keep on your dressing table.'

changing scents

For some of us, a scent is our signature. If we are the faithful type, the same scent worn over time can become a part of us, defining and enhancing our personality. But what if it is discontinued? As Julia Reed described in American *Vogue*, September 1999, 'My identity has been seriously messed with. I walked into Boyd's pharmacy, where I'd been buying my favourite – my only – perfume for 17 years, Paco Rabanne's Metal, and was told it had been discontinued. This was too much. Scent is one of those ostensibly superficial things – like a hairstyle, a look – that defines us. Also, the only man I've ever really loved told me a long time ago that Metal is the only perfume he's ever even liked ... I hadn't even seen an ad for Metal. I had simply found it. On my own. On an island. It was chemistry. Like love, like that look across a crowded room, there is no explaining the attraction.' Very occasionally, you can get a reprieve by buying up the entire worldwide stock, finding a perfume detective to trace some hard-to-source bottles or buying on the 'grey' (discount perfume shops) market. But that is not really the solution: you have to screw up your courage and find another scent. Jean Michel Duriez is the in-house perfumer for Jean Patou. He is obsessed by fragrance, and feels that the quest to find your own perfume is very important. 'Perfumes are like guys, or husbands. There is not just one out there for you. You can probably fall in love with two or three, maybe five or six, but definitely no more than ten. For men it is not the same; they usually stick to one or two, but women are more open. If you haven't found your true-love perfume yet, don't despair. It is out there — just keep sampling and be patient, it will happen.'

According to Karen Hawksley, when you need to find a new scent, do not start from scratch. Look for scents that have some correlation to your previous love. More likely than not, you are attracted to a particular fragrance family and your search should start from there. You will only find yourself overwhelmed if you walk into a store and start smelling every new scent that has just been launched. Find out your favourite fragrance family first, and then target accordingly. And do not be rushed or hassled. Like love, the perfect one often comes along when you are least expecting it.

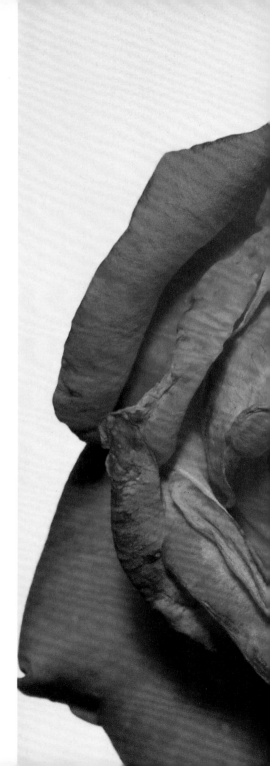

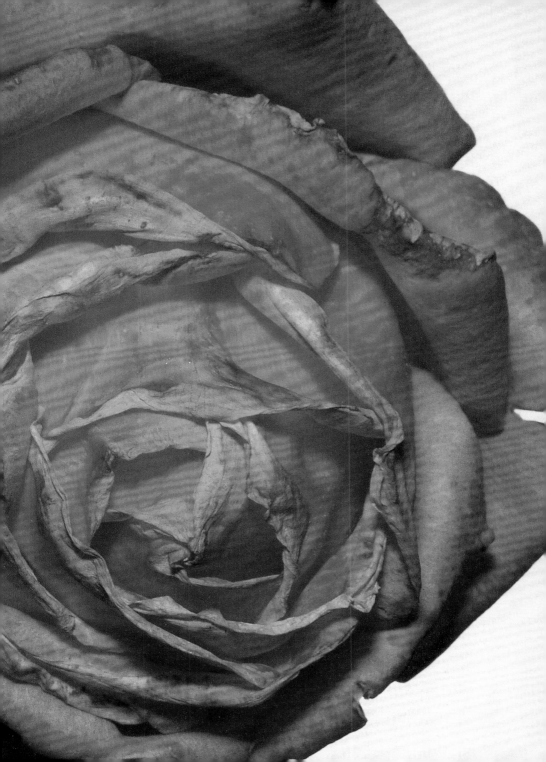

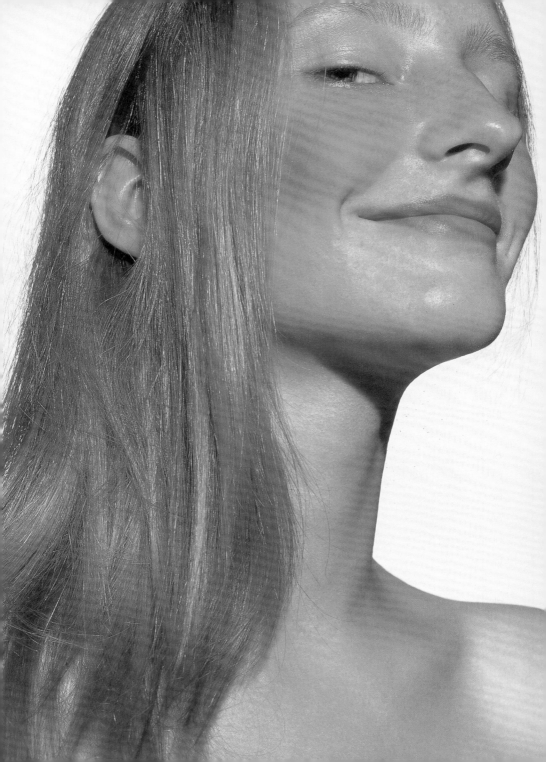

best-kept secrets

Although all quality scents have a high proportion of natural ingredients so they smell different on each woman, many of us like to have something just a little bit unique, that is not easily recognizable and that people can identify with us and us alone. So unleash the bloodhounds. The best-kept secrets of the fragrance world need to be sniffed out of each and every nook and cranny because they are not being actively advertised and promoted. Why are they not hitting the headlines and inspiring lists as long as your arm? The reasons are numerous, but nothing to do with them not being beautiful smells. Smaller scent houses do not have money to lavish on all their fragrances and the bigger houses usually splurge their budget on their latest launches. Some companies just prefer to keep their scents, well, slightly exclusive, and that's what you want, right?

Annick Goutal **Grand Amour** and
    Eau de Camille

Barneys **Route du Thé**

Borsari **Violetta di Parma**

Bulgari **Eau Parfumée**

Chanel **Cristalle**

Chanel's 'boutique' fragrances:
    Bois des Iles and **Cuir de Russie**

anything by Creed, but especially
    Fleurissimo

Clinique **Aromatics Elixir**

anything by Diptyque

D'Orsay **Tilleul**

Estée Lauder **Private Collection**
    and **Estée**

French Connection **French**
    Connection

Guerlain limited edition fragrances

anything by Jo Malone

Shiseido **Feminité du Bois**

anything by L'Artisan Parfumeur,
    but especially **L'Eau de**
    L'Artisan, **Pour un Été**,
    Dzing, **Mimosa Pour Moi**
    and **Mure et Musc**

Le No. 9 Cadolle

Parfums de Rosine

Parfums de Nicolai

making
it last

Those who like their scent to announce their arrival, stand forward. Those who like their scent to be sensed only by those close enough to smell their skin, stand back. Fragrance power is a divisive issue. For some it is the raison d'être of the fragrance, while others find it incredibly vulgar. Today, the trend for slender and more feminine, lighter fragrances has taken much of the vulgarity out of scent-wearing. The stronger, heavier and more penetrating notes of yesteryear have given way to bright, fresh, transparent notes, so you are no longer likely to offend anyone by your choice.

That aside, many of us find that scent just disappears like magic on our skin, evaporating into thin air, never to be smelled again. Other women seem to keep that lovely rosy note, fresh in the air around them, throughout the whole day. What is their secret? According to Roja Dove, it is vital to understand the various fragrance strengths available, as each strength is made for a different purpose: 'Eau de toilette is for refreshing yourself, traditionally when a woman was getting ready. Perfume is for perfuming and it is the only strength that will last.'

TYPES OF SCENT

PERFUME: Between 15 and 40 per cent of the bottle is pure fragrance oils. In 15 minutes, 20 per cent is gone; in 45 minutes, 30 per cent is gone; and 50 per cent stays all day.

EAU DE PARFUM: Between 7 and 14 per cent is pure fragrance oils. In 15 minutes, 40 per cent is gone; in 45 minutes, 30 per cent is gone; and 30 per cent stays all day.

EAU DE TOILETTE: Between 3 and 10 per cent is pure fragrance oils. In 15 minutes, 50 per cent is gone; in 45 minutes, 30 per cent is gone; and 20 per cent lasts all day.

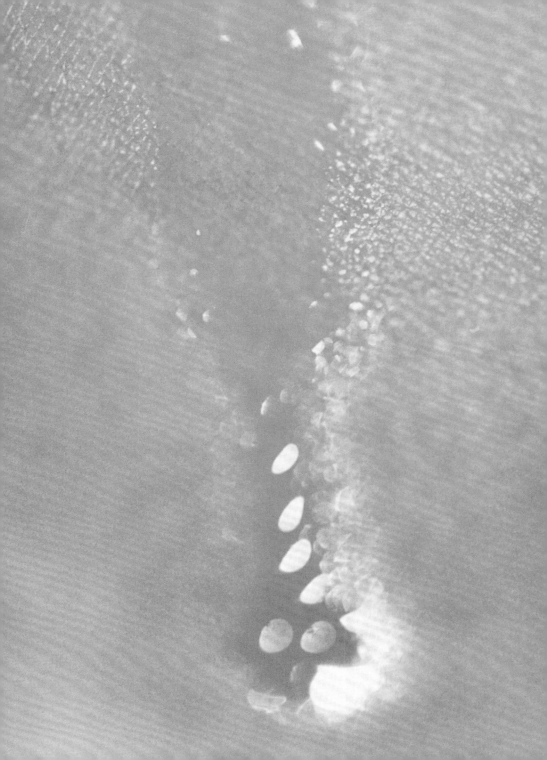

EAU FRAÎCHE: Between 3 and 7 per cent is pure fragrance oils. In 15 minutes, 60 per cent is gone and in 45 minutes 40 per cent is gone.

WEARING SCENTS

A sure way to make a scent more effective and longer-lasting is to 'layer' it with matching body products. Estée Lauder was the first to encourage the use of bath oil, body cream and deodorant to envelope you in a scent. 'Dry skin has a particular difficulty when it comes to scent,' says Roja Dove. 'Because dry skin doesn't produce enough oil, the skin's acid mantle is not intact and the skin can become too acidic. This interferes with a perfume and can make it a little unpleasant. It also means that your scent is not staying, and staying true on your skin.' And the answer to this? 'Always use bath oils and creams to moisturize your skin, and use your perfume before your creams when you get out of the bath or shower. After all, you wouldn't put moisturizer on before toner would you?'

'A common mistake that women make when applying scent is to spray it on just as they are dashing out of the house,' says Karen Hawksley. 'If you are just swooshing the scent around your clothes, then you are missing that vital X factor – the fact that perfume should react with your skin and your body chemistry. Really, scent should be the first thing you put on in the morning – well, maybe after your underwear. Then it has time to become warm and develop.'

Scent does not need to be restricted to the skin. Spray a little on a cotton-wool ball and tuck it in your bra, spray it on hems and cuffs of clothes (checking that it does not stain the fabric first) or spray it on your hair. To this day, the house of the Empress Josephine, Malmaison, still smells of the musk she lavishly used to perfume the house. Sergei Diaghilev, founder of the Ballets Russes, insisted on spraying the curtains of every place he stayed with Guerlain Mitsouko to make him feel at home. In India, blinds to keep out the midday sun are often made of vetiver grass and sprayed with water during the afternoon heat to add scent to the wafting breezes. Are you feeling inspired?

scents of time & place

Perfumers often talk about oakmoss smelling 'earthy and autumnal', a bouquet of fragrant white flowers being 'light and summery', a bunch of freesias being 'fresh and spring-like' and a bundle of cinnamon being 'spicy and wintery'. The fact is that winter, spring, summer and autumn play an integral part in perfumery. After all, ultimately perfumes are harvests of nature; they come from natural ingredients – flowers, fruit, leaves, herbs, spices, moss, wood and so on – and they are our attempt to perfect nature, making it tangible and manageable.

Christian Dior Diorissimo is a perfect example. Lily-of-the-valley are the most delicate and sweetest of flowers, but in nature they grow sparsely under the shade of large trees, appearing only during the springtime. You could never hope to gather large armfuls and bring them home to fill your living space with their precious

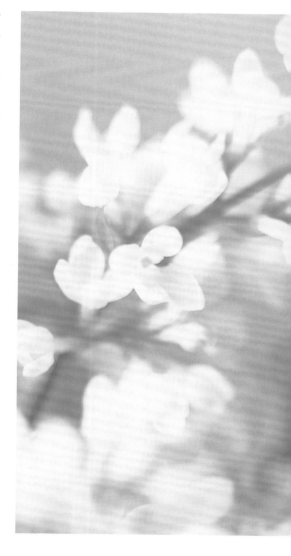

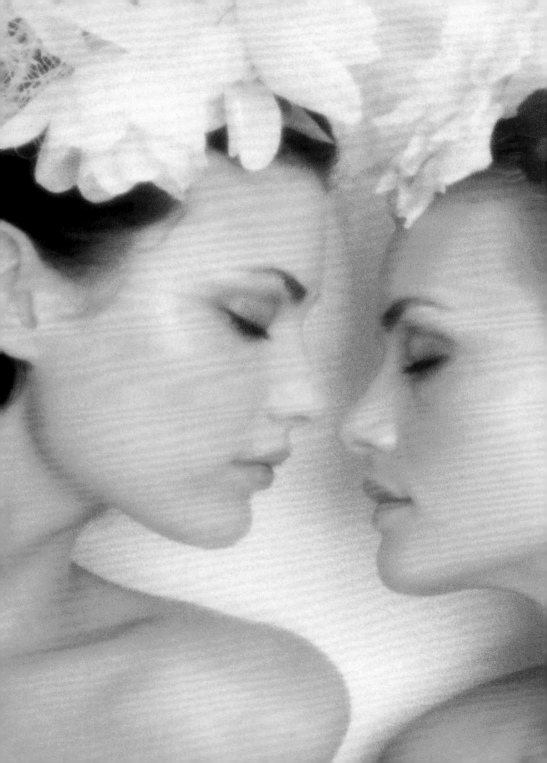

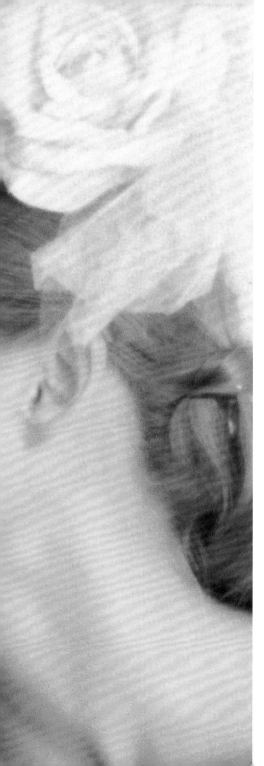

aroma, but with one squirt of Diorissimo we can dream of doing just that. The scent is pure, clean and truly smells of an abundance of the rarest wild lily-of-the-valley. That is the perfumer's art.

Ernest Beaux, the genius perfumer behind the inception of the classic scent Chanel No. 5, once described his most famous and legendary creation as 'the smell of a snowy landscape'. Apparently he was inspired by the clean, fresh smell of the rivers and lakes after sunset in the Arctic Circle, where he had spent part of his military service, and he captured this note with aldehydes, a perfume ingredient that, at the time, was new.

The snowy, midnight smell of Chanel No. 5, the springtime smell of Diorissimo, the unmistakable summer garden of Guerlain Jardins de Bagatelle ... undoubtedly, some scents are perfect for certain seasons or times of day. You would not want to smell of fresh air and coconut body oil after dark, when the air is crisp, the music loud and the atmosphere intimate, now would you?

DAY-TO-DAY SCENTS

Cacharel **Anaïs Anaïs**

Calvin Klein **CK One**

Calvin Klein **Truth**

Christian Dior **J'Adore**

Clinique **Happy**

Hermès **24 Faubourg**

Joseph **Joseph de Jour**

Lancôme **Miracle**

Nina Ricci **L'Air du Temps**

Ralph Lauren **Romance**

AFTER-DARK SCENTS

Chanel **Coco**

Chanel **No. 5**

Dolce e Gabbana **Dolce e Gabbana**

Giorgio Armani **Mania**

Givenchy **Amarige**

Guerlain **Shalimar**

Paco Rabanne **La Nuit**

Robert Piguet **Fracas**

Thierry Mugler **Angel**

Versace **Blonde**

SPRING SCENTS

Antonia's **Flowers**

Christian Dior **Diorissimo**

Diptyque **Ofresia**

Floris **Seringa** and **Stephanotis**

Sylvie Chantecaille **Wisteria**

Origins Spring **Fever**

SUMMER SCENTS

Annick Goutal **Eau de Hadrian**

Calvin Klein **Escape**

Clarins **Eau Dynamissante**

Giorgio Armani **Acqua di Gio**

Givenchy **Eau de Givenchy**

Guerlain **Eau de Fleurs et Cedrat**

Guerlain **Jardins de Bagatelle**

Guy Laroche **Fidji**

Kenzo **Parfum d'Été**

L'Artisan Parfumeur **Thé Pour un Été**

AUTUMN SCENTS

Bulgari **Black**

Cabochard **Grès**

Caron **Tabac Blond**

Clinique **Aromatics Elixir**

Donna Karan **Cashmere Mist**

Hermès **Calèche**

Jil Sander **Woman III**

Les Senteurs **Apogée**

WINTER SCENTS

Caron **Nuit de Noël**

Guerlain **Mitsouko**

Jo Malone **Nutmeg** and **Ginger**

L'Artisan Parfumeur **Mure et Musc**
    and **L'Eau d'Ambre**

Lancôme **Magie Noire**

Paloma Picasso **Paloma Picasso**

Rochas **Femme**

passionate
about scent

Jean Michel Duriez from Jean Patou: 'When I was a small boy, 10 years old, I went to the parfumerie to buy a Mothers' Day present. I smelt and smelt all the perfumes and none were right, until they gave me Calèche, by Hermès. I knew immediately that it was right for my mother ... When she opened it, she was amazed. "How did you know that this was the perfume that I was wearing when you were born?" she said. Obviously my olfactory memory had remembered the smell of my mother in those first few days, weeks and months of my life.'

Calice Becker, vice president of Quest: 'One of my favourite smells is the smell of plums cooking in red wine. I must remember it from my childhood ... it is such a powerful smell to me that it makes me feel quite dizzy with emotion. As a perfumer, I worked hard to re-create that smell and eventually I was able to put elements of it into Christian Dior

J'Adore. I also love those little incense papers that you can buy in France, Incense d'Armenia. It is a blend of vanilla, sandalwood, musk and rose and when I burn it in my apartment it makes me feel so peaceful.'

Anne Françoise Schneider of L'Artisan Parfumeur: 'A perfume is something that becomes a part of you and changes with your own body chemistry, and with some of my favourite smells I don't want that. I just want to smell them and be comforted by them ... I love the smell of old-fashioned lipsticks as it reminds me of my mother's goodnight kiss. It's a lovely, sweet blend of violets and rose. I also love oakmoss; it's beautifully earthy, mossy and woody.'

Karen Hawksley of Les Senteurs: 'My earliest scent memories come from my mother, who was half French. No matter what she was doing, or how ordinary her day, she always wore

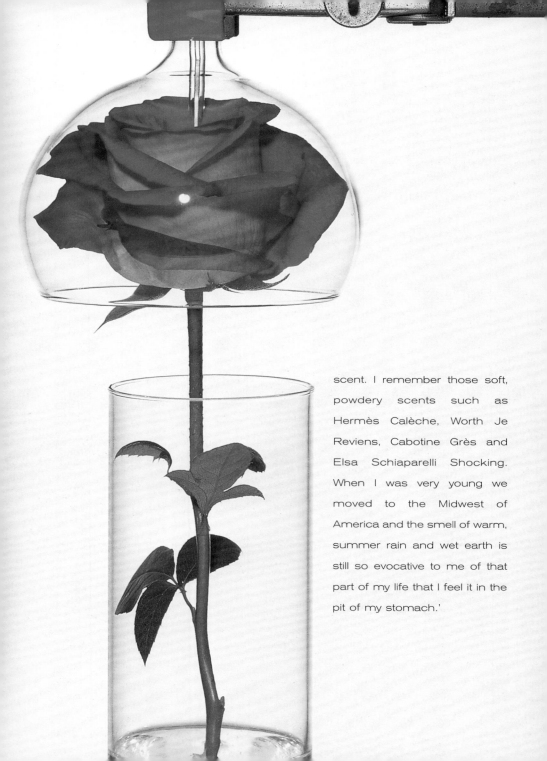

scent. I remember those soft, powdery scents such as Hermès Calèche, Worth Je Reviens, Cabotine Grès and Elsa Schiaparelli Shocking. When I was very young we moved to the Midwest of America and the smell of warm, summer rain and wet earth is still so evocative to me of that part of my life that I feel it in the pit of my stomach.'

WHAT TO WEAR & HOW TO WEAR IT

One of the golden rules of applying scent is never, ever rub it into your skin. If you do, you will be crushing the scent molecules and damaging the smell. All scents are in alcohol for a reason; alcohol is an excellent dispersant and evaporates naturally and quickly, leaving only the real scent behind. So do not be tempted to burn off your scent with friction. Dab, spray and then just be patient.

But where should you apply it? Anywhere the blood supply comes close to the surface of the skin. So that is anywhere you can see those veins pumping away: wrists, behind the ears, crooks of the arms, ankles, backs of the knees. Basically, we are into erogenous zone territory here because we're talking about those sensual places where the nerves are sensitive and blood is pumping close to the surface. Oh, and don't forget what Coco Chanel said about where to apply scent: 'Anywhere you want to be kissed.' Get the message?

According to Anne Françoise Schneider of L'Artisan Parfumeur, the best way to make sure your scent lasts is to wear the matching body lotion and bath oil. 'Wearing different products in the range adds a new dimension to your favourite scent. Also, when women say that they can no longer smell their scent on themselves any more, often after two to three years of wearing the same scent, I advise them to start wearing the body lotion, too. It's amazing how that can activate their senses again and they get newfound pleasure from their favourite scent. Personally, I love wearing scent in my hair. It's very effective, but you must be careful not to spray it on jewellery, as it will damage it. In France, the trick is to spray a cloud of scent in the air and then walk into it. That way your clothes are fragranced all over, too.'

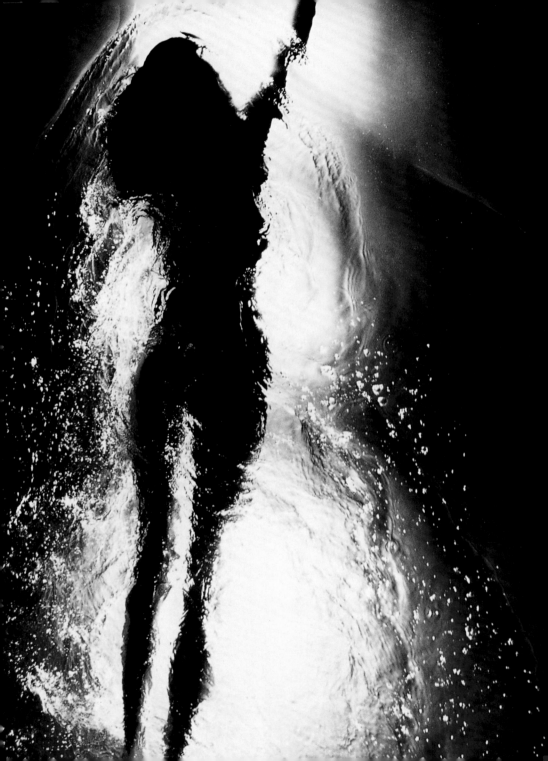

COMPLEMENTARY MEDICINE

Conventional medicine has no time for miracles, and yet there are dozens of incredible case histories which are stranger than fiction: terminal patients who recover; the paralysed who walk again; the chronic sufferer who becomes free of all symptoms. Science has proved to be less powerful than word of mouth and never more so than at the beginning of the twentieth-first century. In this time there has been not only a rising disenchantment with conventional medicine but also a widespread interest in and use of various kinds of alternative therapies. In simple terms, Western medicine focuses on scientific proof and the production of weapons (in the form of drugs) to fight disease. In the East the focus has always been entirely different: concentrating instead on building an immunity to disease by holistic means – a preventative rather than curative approach.

Orthodox medicine has proved unsuccessful for a great number of routine complaints, including allergies, headaches, insomnia, sinus trouble, skin disorders, back pain, arthritis and so on. It cannot treat viral infection, nor does it have success with depression, mental and psychosomatic illness or auto-immune diseases. Equally it has failed to educate people to be responsible for their own state of health in order to avoid disease. We now face the possibility that antibiotics, the great discovery of the previous century, may well now prove useless in the face of new and resistant organisms and viruses.

That said, it would be stupid to ignore severe and persistent symptoms without consulting a conventional doctor. The benefits of the modern hospital with its emergency care facilities in the case of, say, a serious car accident, heart attack, acute bacterial infection or appendicitis are undisputed. But scepticism of rushed treatments at the doctor's surgery and the indiscriminate handing out of dangerous drugs have sent patients on the quest for alternatives. This is where complementary medicine seems to have a lot to offer and the public is voting in favour of it with its feet and its faith. Nowadays we take vitamin C, have echinacea on stand-by if a snuffle develops, put drops of lavender oil on our pillows at night to help us sleep and take regular yoga classes. Visiting an alternative practitioner is just one step further. What was once considered quackery is now commonplace. We have embraced reiki, flower remedies, magnet therapy, shiatsu and rebirthing. Despite a lack of scientific proof as to their absolute necessity, we are stocking up on vitamin supplements, organic produce, environmentally friendly cleaning goods and 'pure' cosmetics with enthusiasm

and, it has to be said, a certain lack of discrimination. A weekend course in massage or healing does not produce a gifted therapist and many people simply do not check qualifications until it is too late. At least bad doctors have taken the Hippocratic oath and aim to do their best by their patients, whereas there are certainly charlatans of alternative health who are merely happy to take substantial amounts of money from an unsuspecting clientele.

Luckily the more open-minded doctors are taking note of empirical and anecdotal evidence about the treatments and tinctures that they might once have seen as akin to alchemy. In some surgeries you can now be offered acupuncture to treat painful musculoskeletal problems, and a few of the main teaching hospitals are researching alternative philosophies due to their apparent success with all sorts of chronic problems. As people begin to embrace alternative therapies, they are learning more about them and about themselves. Helping the body heal itself can often involve more than one therapy. Many, in fact, seem to work well in tandem. This chapter lists and clarifies many of these complementary treatments for those who want to take control of their health, and consequently their beauty, the natural way.

CAN YOU TRUST A PRACTITIONER?

Remember that anyone can set up as a homeopath, hypnotherapist or acupuncturist. Even societies that claim their members are bona fide may be too small or too ad hoc to really guarantee anything. However, osteopathy has a regulating governing body so the checks are secure, which is why asking your doctor for referrals can be a good idea.

One thing is certain. Whichever therapist you find, their concern, apart from your symptoms, will be about the way you live your life — what food you eat, how much water you drink, what exercise you take, what supplements you need and which areas of your life are causing you stress. Be prepared to look closely at your breathing, sleeping patterns, emotional and mental state, your relationships and your day-to-day choices. This is the holistic approach: the belief that all these factors add up

to the reason for illness and are the key to spontaneous healing. Holistic therapists take into account the whole person and treat you in such a way as to kick-start the body's self-healing.

INSOMNIA

Sleep deprivation undermines the immune system, and experts maintain that most people need eight hours a night. Sleep is necessary for long-term health and regeneration. Not only does it function as an antioxidant for the brain, but the growth hormone, mostly produced during sleep, stimulates tissue and liver regeneration, muscle-building, the breakdown of fat stores and other beneficial actions. Interestingly, eight times more women than men report sleep difficulties throughout their lives. If you get behind with your sleep, it is important to make up the hours when you can.

The average person over 50 years old sleeps almost two hours less than they did as a teenager. Seven million people in the UK have trouble sleeping, with 32 million suffering in the US, but there is no sense in resorting to habit-forming drugs to sort it out. The body can easily form a resistance to these so that people end up raising their normal dose to get the same effect.

HELP YOURSELF TO SLEEP

Regular daily exercise encourages deep sleep, the sleep of the physically tired. Although aerobic exercise should be done early in the day, certain yoga programmes, breathing exercises and asanas are geared toward slowing and calming the body in preparation for sleep, so these can be performed in the evening. Caffeine and alcohol are both bad news at bedtime – coffee, tea, chocolate and even cigarettes are stimulating to the system. Here are some other tips to help you get a good night's rest.

• Make sure fresh air is circulating in the bedroom.
• Try to cut out noise, even if it means resorting to earplugs.

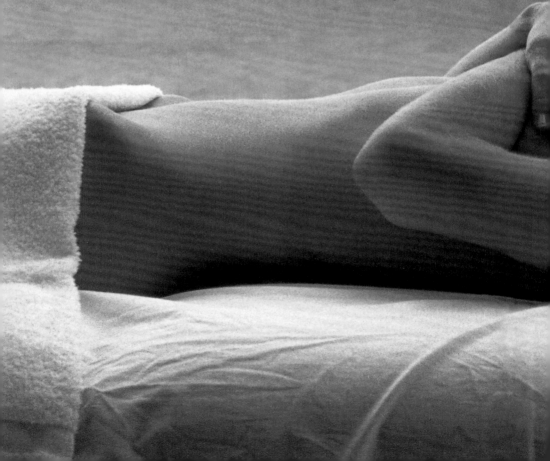

- Check your mattress for signs of deterioration. Should you change it for a better supporting one?
- Lavender essential oil sprayed onto the pillow, or added to a warm bedtime bath, can help you to relax and induce sleep.
- Acupuncture given by a qualified therapist can help insomnia.
- Consult a homeopath for a herbal sleep remedy that includes belladonna. Many herbal suppliers also sell sleep mixtures that include passiflora, hops, valerian and others.
- Drink herbal teas, especially homemade infusions using fresh organic herbs such as German camomile or lime flower.
- Drink hop tea, or take a tincture of hops before bed or if you wake during the night.
- Take 10–20 drops of valerian tincture in a little water before bedtime or in the middle of the night when you wake.

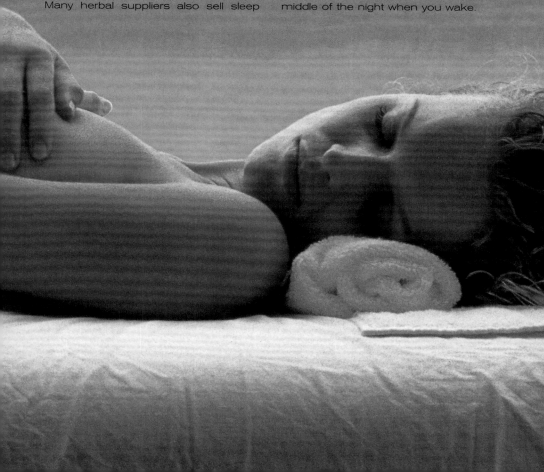

• Melatonin, a hormone from the pineal gland which regulates the biological clock, is a popular jet-lag remedy. The dose is 1–3 mg at bedtime. Use it only in synthetic form.

BREATHING

How well do you breathe? Evenly or erratically? Over the last few years books, manuals and the health industry in general have stressed the importance of breathing well. In Eastern philosophies, the breath is the hub around which the wheel of life revolves. Several thousand years ago the first yogic texts explained, with exercises and warnings, the importance of breathing. In Sanskrit, the word 'prana' means breath, wind, respiration, vitality, life, energy or strength and is similar to the Chinese word 'chi'. Pranayama is the science of the breath. A yogi's life is measured by his number of breaths rather than number of days or years. So it follows from this that the simple philosophy of breathing more slowly will inevitably help you live for longer. Proper rhythmic patterns of breathing strengthen the respiratory system, soothe the nervous system and reduce cravings. Bad breathing can be danger-

ous emotionally and physically, and can be the cause of nervous irritation, indigestion, asthma, coughs, catarrh and pain in the head, eyes and ears. 'As lions and tigers are tamed very slowly and cautiously,' says the *Hatha Yoga Pradipika* (one of the earliest yogic texts, dated between 200 BC and AD 200), 'so should prana be brought under control very slowly in gradation, measured according to one's capacity and physical limitations. Otherwise it will kill the practitioner.'

SIMPLE BREATHING

1 With practice you can use this breathing at any time, wherever you are, to steady and calm yourself. Sit up and back in a chair. Rest your hands on your knees with the palms upwards. Relax your shoulders and elongate the back of your neck, tucking your chin in.

2 Exhale. As you exhale the abdomen draws in and the hips drop. The spine straightens, the back of your neck elongates and your head finds its correct position with the pull of gravity. Inhale. As you inhale the shoulders stay down, your face relaxes, your elbows drop and your palms soften.

3 Just sitting up straight can be hard for some people. Allow the gentle, cool, calm breathing in and out to help you stay straight. If you like, close your eyes, relax your frown and unclench your jaw. Do not attempt to take or hold breaths, but just allow the breath to come naturally and evenly. This will automatically help you to sit up.

4 Believe it or not, correct breathing takes practice. As your breathing gets steadier, count the seconds so that inhalation and exhalation are equal in length. Start with a count of four exhaling and four inhaling, and then lengthen the breaths when you feel comfortable.

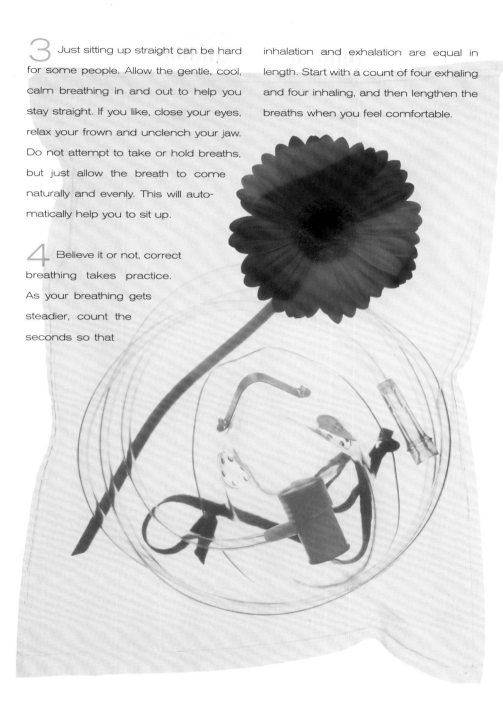

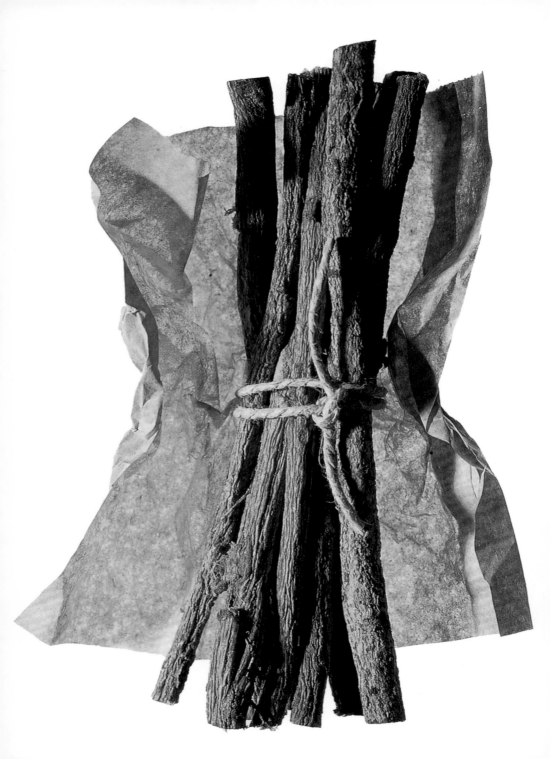

everyday maintenance medicines

NATUROPATHY

Naturopathy centres around the ancient belief that the body has the power to heal itself through lifestyle and diet. In essence, the Greek physician Hippocrates was the first naturopath when he recognized 'ponos', the way in which the body works hard to restore itself to good health. The term 'naturopathy' was coined by New York doctor John Scheel in 1895. Naturopaths work on the idea that a combination of stress, pollution, poor diet and lack of sleep and exercise result in the build-up of waste products and toxins in the body. This, in turn, can lead to disease. Naturopathy is a detoxing therapy. Practitioners stress the restorative powers of nature and use natural, non-invasive methods, such as massage, exercise, a diet rich in organic fruit and vegetables, hydrotherapy and herbal remedies to improve the overall health rather than concentrating on specific symptoms. Naturopaths aim to return the body to a state of balance and encourage its own self-healing system.

WHAT IS IT GOOD FOR?

Naturopathy tends to focus on gentle treatments. With 'do not harm' as the motto for practitioners, it is suitable and safe for the majority of people. It is most successful in treating such conditions as: asthma, arthritis, depression, fatigue, high blood pressure, skin conditions, irritable bowel syndrome, hormone imbalances, premenstrual tension (PMT) and menopausal problems.

WHAT HAPPENS?

Practitioners of naturopathy range from massage therapists to physicians. While they might have different approaches to diagnoses, they all consider the evaluation of diet and lifestyle to be crucial to treatment. During the initial consultation the naturopath will assess physical and emotional health through conventional medical tests, in addition to such naturopathic tests as analysing the hair, testing muscle strength and examining the irises of the eyes. The treatment itself then falls into two categories. The first is catabolic, or cleansing, and might include fasting to help rid the body of toxins and waste, or a fruit-only diet. The second is anabolic, or strengthening, and the practitioner may prescribe nutritional supplements, modifications to the diet, hydrotherapy and yoga. Do not be alarmed if your symptoms worsen at the initial stages of the treatment as this is often the case when detoxification takes effect.

HERBAL MEDICINE

Herbal medicine uses plants to treat illness and maintain good health and a state of balance. Plants and herbs have been used for their medicinal properties since ancient times and continue to be beneficial in treating a wide range of symptoms from arthritis, skin conditions, migraines, insomnia and PMT, to respiratory and circulatory problems. While many conventional drugs are based on plants – aspirin, for example, contains white willow which is high in salicylic acid, and foxglove is used in digoxin, a drug used to treat heart failure – herbal medicine differs from the conventional in that whole parts of the plants are used rather than extracted substances. Herbal medicines target specific organs and systems in the body due to the neurochemical reactions they trigger. The herbs can be used in various ways: some act as diuretics and laxatives to rid the body of accumulated waste and toxins; some stimulate the body's self-healing powers and target any causes of illness; and some nourish the body and its systems and help to keep it balanced.

Herbal medicines can be very potent, so it is not wise to self-prescribe. Nor does it make sense to take expensive herbal medicines while ignoring other more obvious factors in health like a good diet, sleep and exercise. In the hands of a skilled practitioner, herbal medicines can be effective for all manner of diseases.

WHAT HAPPENS?

Before prescribing, the herbalist will ask for a medical history, take your blood pressure and may examine your eyes, ears, throat and abdomen. On the basis of these checks, specific remedies will be recommended.

A FEW HERBAL REMEDIES

Horse Chestnut (*Aesculus hippocastanum*): The seeds have long been used in the treatment of varicose veins and haemorrhoids due to their ability to increase venous tone. It is often used in soothing and calming creams.

Milk Thistle (*Silybum marianum*): This herb is a wonder treatment for the liver. Many documented trials have proved that it can prevent and heal damage to the liver and that it has a significant effect on cirrhosis and chronic hepatitis. It can also be prescribed for PMT.

Feverfew (*Chrysanthemum parthenium*): In a survey of 270 migraine sufferers, 70 per cent who had eaten feverfew daily for prolonged periods claimed that it decreased the frequency and/or intensity of their attacks.

Valerian (*Valerian officinalis*): This is another herb that is well-known for treating migraine. The root was also the primary herbal sedative used on both sides of the Atlantic before the advent of barbiturate sleeping pills. Occasionally valerian can be too strong, so lower the dose if you feel a slight hangover effect in the morning.

Garlic (*Allium sativum*): Garlic can lower blood pressure, cholesterol and blood fats, and reduce the clotting tendency of the blood. It also acts as an antiseptic and antibiotic and therefore enhances the immune system.

Centella (*Centella asiatica*): Recently rediscovered by the cosmetic industry, the herb is used in products for its effects on the metabolism of connective tissue. Several experimental studies have demonstrated a positive effect in its topical and oral use for the treatment of cellulite and, to some extent, varicose veins.

Astralagus (*Astralagus membranaceous*): This herb is used widely in Chinese medicine for treating colds and flu. It is also good for bronchitis and sinusitis.

Herbs are dispensed in various guises. The most common is a tincture, which involves steeping herbs in alcohol to draw out the active ingredients of the plant material. Tinctures are similar to conventional medicines in that they are swallowed two or three times a day. If the softer parts of the plants – the leaves or flowers – are prescribed, then an infusion (very much like a cup of tea) will be sufficient. Tablets may also be used, and herbs can be added to a bath or inhaled. Creams, oils and lotions may be applied topically. Herbalists will also advise on diet and lifestyle because, like naturopaths, they aim to rid the body of toxins.

CHINESE MEDICINE

Revolution, counter-revolution and the passing of thousands of years have not diminished the importance of traditional Chinese medicine to the Chinese. The way this Eastern philosophy has become a source of inspiration to the West is fascinating. Disenchantment with modern medicine and the reliance on synthetic

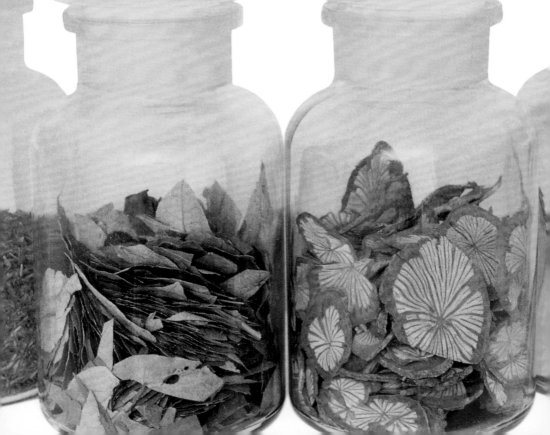

drugs have sent many patients searching for a new way. This gentler approach, with its emphasis on prevention, has proved attractive and successful, especially with nervous diseases, infertility, skin problems and chronic disorders.

Chinese diagnosis picks up surprising subtleties without the need for blood tests and complicated machinery. The secret is the tongue: each part represents a part of the body, like the foot does in reflexology (see pages 368–9). The colour of the tongue and its coating are indicators of health. The normal tongue is, of course, pink, but a paler colour might indicate a weakness such as anaemia, malnutrition or fatigue. Toxins are referred to in terms of 'heat' or 'damp' by Chinese practitioners, so a red tongue signals heat toxins in the body while purple suggests extreme heat or stagnation of the blood. The location of the colour is all-important too. Red on the tip would point to heat in the heart. If you were prone to heart attacks, this would probably manifest itself as purple at the tip. The size and texture of the tongue matters, too. Swollen or shrunken tongues can each suggest a deficiency. Cracks in specific areas or a thick or shiny coating can each point to an informed diagnosis. All conditions are treated with herbs to strengthen glands or make organs function more efficiently. This is tackling the root cause of the condition the Chinese way. By isolating parts of the body and strengthening them, the whole picture improves.

WHAT HAPPENS?

A Chinese doctor will ask questions about medical history, diet and emotional state. He will observe the bearing of the patient and look at his or her complexion. The pulse is taken at the beginning of the consultation but not in the same way as a Western doctor would take it. Pulses can indicate the state of the heart, liver and gall bladder, kidney, bladder, lungs, spleen, stomach and intestines, not only due to the speed and regularity of the pulse but also according to the depth of the pulse and its shape, size and strength. It is worth knowing that most Chinese doctors are also trained in acupuncture. In every instance the doctor aims to maintain and fine-tune the body, and so help prevent illness altogether. Note: Never buy Chinese medicines or herbs that have been stored in glass jars – the ingredients will be useless.

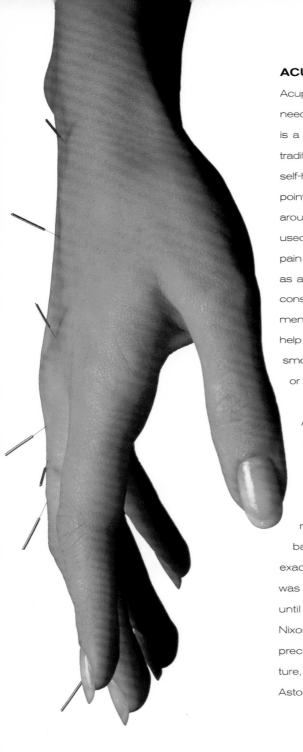

ACUPUNCTURE

Acupuncture involves the insertion of needles into specific points of the body. It is a unique therapeutic practice used in traditional Chinese medicine to stimulate self-healing powers by 'triggering' certain points and to manipulate energy flows around the body. In the West it has been used mainly to treat acute and chronic pain – for instance, some dentists use it as an anaesthetic. There has also been considerable success with it in the treatment of addictions, when it is used to help moderate addictive eating, give up smoking or even withdraw from heroin or cocaine.

Acupuncture is an ancient therapy that has been traced back to the Egyptians. But it was the Chinese who refined the practice into a system of medicine, and ancient manuscripts on the subject date back as far as 475 BC. Whatever the exact date of its origin, acupuncture was rarely used in Western medicine until about 25 years ago. Richard Nixon's state visit to China in 1972 precipitated an awareness of acupuncture, and Chinese medicine in general. Astonishingly, it is now a useful addition to the doctor's surgery since it can treat painful musculoskeletal problems.

In Chinese philosophy, there is a quest for balance of the body's natural state. Chinese medicine works on the premise that true health is both emotional and physical and comes about when the 'chi' (the life force or vital energy) flows smoothly. Acupuncture is used to rebalance the flow of chi by stimulating the relevant or blocked points of the body, which is divided into 12 meridians (pathways) and eight deeper channels. Western scientists have acknowledged that acupuncture releases neurotransmitters (key chemicals which carry messages between nerve endings), which not only block the sensation of pain, but can also have an anti-inflammatory effect, reduce blood pressure and trigger the release of hormones.

WHAT IS IT GOOD FOR?

Headaches, migraine, osteoarthritis, back pain, respiratory disorders, sinusitis, asthma, irritable bowel syndrome, gastritis and colic, allergies, painful periods, skin complaints, depression and addictions all seem to benefit from this therapeutic technique.

WHAT HAPPENS?

As in all Chinese medicine, when the acupuncturist takes down your case history, specific pulse points and your tongue will also be checked. Needles are usually inserted while you are lying down and you will be left alone for around 20 minutes for the flow of chi to correct itself. There could be around eight needles inserted but it can be less. The needles are tiny and only penetrate superficially. They should not hurt. Sometimes there can be a short, sharp pain which is related to a strong blockage. You may feel euphoric and/ or revitalized after the session and certainly you will feel relaxed. It is important to stay relaxed immediately afterwards to sustain the benefits.

HOMEOPATHY

Hippocrates was known to have used homeopathic remedies in 430 BC, but it was German physician Samuel Hahnemann who pioneered homeopathy as we know it today. Working in the late 1700s and disillusioned by such contemporary practices as leaching, purging and poisoning, he began to research and translate medical papers. His investigations involved dosing himself with quinine, which he found gave him the symptoms of malaria. By testing others in the same way he discovered that each person reacted differently, thus concluding that the patient's own healing capacity played a part in their response. These observations founded the two fundamental tenets of homeopathy: firstly, that like cures like; and secondly, that since no two people's reaction to treatment is the same, their cures must therefore be tailored individually. Some see Hahnemann as a heretic and homeopathic remedies as mere placebos. The principles certainly do not follow science, nor are they easy to assess from trials. However, there is much positive anecdotal evidence.

WHAT IS IT GOOD FOR?

An overview in the *British Medical Journal* in 1991 concluded that there was sufficient evidence from well-run homeopathic clinics to prove that it did work for the following conditions: asthma, respiratory tract infections, hay fever, irritable bowel syndrome, high blood pressure, migraines, skin conditions, depression, insomnia, and behavioural problems in children.

Distinguished health writer Andrew Weil, although in general not a fan of homeopathy, says he has seen responses from sufferers of auto-immune disease.

WHAT HAPPENS?

After exhaustive questioning on both private emotional matters and previous medical history, the patient is prescribed very small doses of highly diluted plant or mineral extracts, in the form of tinctures, which catalyze healing responses. The homeopath is not treating your symptoms, he or she is treating you. Some homeopaths insist that coffee, camphor, mint and a few other substances are antidotes to the remedies and must be avoided once you begin treatment.

TIBETAN MEDICINE

Bon was the religion of Tibet prior to the fourth century when the Buddhists first invaded from India. After a later Buddhist invasion, many Bon traditions and practices were absorbed into what became Buddhist culture. Much later, when China invaded Tibet in 1959, even more of the spiritual traditions were lost. When it comes to medicine, the West is mostly unaware of its long Chinese history. According to Christopher

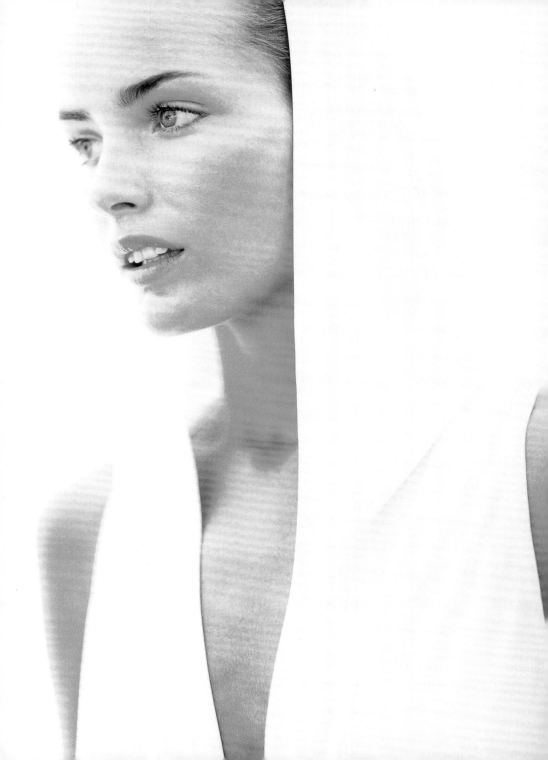

Hansard, a master physician in the Dur Bon medicine tradition who has studied the ancient culture of herbs, acupuncture and philosophy for most of his life, the history of Bon medicine goes back even further than the Chinese one and is, as such, the orthodox medicine of the East. 'Tibetan medicine is a medical and spiritual technology that enables an individual to create their own soul,' he says. 'We believe in a mind/body link, that there is a spiritual architecture on which Tibetan medicine is founded.'

As is usual with all practitioners in the preventative techniques of the East, Hansard has qualifications in many areas, including surgery, acupuncture and the preparation and prescription of herbal remedies. His training spans far more than the few years necessary to qualify in the West. Already knowledgeable and able to prepare herbal remedies at the age of 13, his training was nevertheless only considered complete at 27. He sees himself as a general practitioner and can do everything that a fully trained general practitioner can do – it is just that he does not use drugs. Hansard's mission has been to integrate East with West in a practice that offers excellence in differing medical fields. An example of an East-meets-West prescription, and one Hansard recommends, is Schweppes's tonic water (for the quinine) and angostura bitters (for the gentian) as an instant pick-me-up.

WHAT HAPPENS?

An initial consultation in Bon technique would involve a good deal of intuitive conversation, and would particularly focus on taking the pulse in the wrists and ankles. This enables the practitioner to detect evidence of any physical as well as emotional irregularities from the 'channels' of the nervous system and nerve pathways.

ANTHROPOSOPHICAL MEDICINE

The Anthroposophy Society is a worldwide spiritual movement based on the work of Rudolf Steiner, an Austrian scientist and philosopher. The basis of the thought behind it is to give a truer meaning and focus to our deeds on earth. Steiner was concerned by the one-sided materialistic view of life and looked for a more spiritual world. He extended this higher thinking in a very pragmatic and educational way into several key fields, such as farming, medicine and sociology. In order to make food more nutritious and less damaging to the body, he spawned bio-dynamic farming, which has grown in popularity since the 1920s. Bio-dynamic farming involves a new understanding of the relationships between plant, soil and animal, avoiding the use of harmful pesticides and using the cycles of the moon and the seasons to ascertain ideal planting times. It is a complicated process but can produce the optimum yield in the minimum space. Though it sounds unscientific, it has produced extraordinary results with organic food, medicine and cosmetics.

One disciple of Steiner's philosophies was Dr Rudolf Hauschka, who shared his belief that mankind should not exploit the earth. After meeting Steiner, Hauschka, who had studied not only chemistry and pharmacology but also anatomy and psychiatry, developed a method of producing remedies using the rhythmical moon, sunrise, sunset and seasonal cycles (as in bio-dynamic farming) instead of alcohol and preser-vatives. Plants are exposed to warmth

and cold, light and dark as well as still-ness and movement, and over 150 medicinal plants are grown at WALA, a manufacturer in Germany, where many of Dr Hauschka products are made. The Rose Elixir he made in 1929 is still available today.

In 1966 Dr Hauschka teamed up with a nurse, Elizabeth Sigmund, to develop a skincare range based on the same principles, which include caring for nature and a consideration for the human race. The principles applied to employment and marketing as well as to manufacturing. The company adheres to the Steiner motivations, which have advanced the methods of healing and therapeutic remedies simply by the profound study and respect for the relationship between man, animals and nature.

AROMATHERAPY

Aromatherapy has its roots in ancient Egypt where the dead were embalmed in plant essences that were believed to have antibacterial and antiseptic properties which kept the body in good condition for the next life. Plant reme-dies have also long been the medicine of ordinary peasant folk, but these age-old treatments have proved to be effective time and time again.

Aromatherapy has become a generic term for almost any smelly product with a herb or plant essence waved over it at some point during its production. Sadly, this is far removed from the medicinal and healing properties of the genuine article used by an experienced and trained practitioner. In Britain aromatherapy was practically unheard of until doyennes like French aromatherapist Micheline Arcier began to practice. Aromatherapy has become a global phenomenon, although the best oils and practitioners are still few and far between. Micheline Arcier trained with Dr Jean Valnet, whose book *The Practice of Aromatherapy* is considered to be the bible on the subject. Many respected aromatherapists, such as Robert Tisserand, acknowledge that Jean Valnet's observations and prescriptions were a seminal starting point for their own work.

Today more than 400 essential plant oils are sourced from all over the world and used for their therapeutic olfactory properties and healing powers. For instance, from almost 700 types of geranium, around seven are used to produce essential oils. Juniper can come from central and southern Europe or North America. Lavender comes not only from France but also from Italy, Corsica and Yugoslavia. Each plant has different qualities: jasmine, for example, is known for relaxation; geranium for peacefulness; rosemary to combat low vitality; and ylang ylang to relieve stress. The oils can be used in various ways, too, such as in baths, on compresses, inhaled or massaged onto the skin.

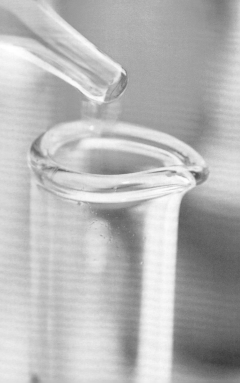

A FEW ESSENTIAL OILS

Tangerine: The best pregnancy oil, tangerine harmonizes and is good for preventing stretchmarks.

Camomile: A gentle oil that promotes relaxation, camomile can be blended in a carrier oil for massaging purposes or used to promote restful, deep sleep.

Geranium: Used in a low dosage, geranium is good for blood circulation, particularly in pregnancy. It balances the emotions and relaxes and refreshes.

Cajuput, niaouli and pine: These can be used for colds, bronchitis, influenza and sinusitis.

Lemon: A very good oil for high blood pressure and veins. Citrus oils detoxify and stimulate a sluggish system.

Eucalyptus: This oil decongests a blocked system and aids in breathing.

Neroli: A calming essential oil for the nervous system.

Rosemary: This oil can stimulate the body and mind. It can help promote clarity of thought and improve memory and concentration.

Tea tree: This is often used because of its antiseptic, healing properties.

Orange: Orange oil is fortifying and acts as a tonic for the nervous system.

Sandalwood: A helpful oil for the urinary tract and for general control of fluid retention.

Lavender: The most versatile essential oil, it relaxes and restores a sense of inner balance. It is good in cases of general fatigue, tension, aches, pains and skin irritations.

Good for the endocrine system (the glands that secrete hormones into the bloodstream): basil, cajuput, juniper, lavender, rose, sage and thyme.

Helpful for slimming: lemon, rosemary, tangerine and violet leaves.

Antifungal: lavender, patchouli, sage and thyme.

Good for eczema: camomile, geranium, juniper, lavender, neroli, peppermint, sage and sandalwood.

The quality of the oils is crucial, as is a talent for blending and prescription. Each aromatherapist uses their own prescriptions, formulas, blends and choice of oils. Aromatherapy is an art that cannot be learned in a weekend course. Micheline Arcier established her Knightsbridge, London, shop in 1981, where her products are still hand-blended on the premises. 'When it comes to oils you have to be tough,' says Arcier, now in her seventies. 'You must find the best ones, which isn't easy. Nor is the formulating. The bottles mustn't contain a speck of dust and the oils must never be cloudy. Anybody can mix oils but to make something special is different.'

Aromatherapy can be dangerous. The power of essential oils to penetrate the skin is remarkable – it takes from 20 to 70 minutes for an oil to be absorbed into the bloodstream. Some plants, if they are used in too high a dose, can be toxic. For example, sage and rosemary can induce epilepsy in a sensitive subject, while marjoram can have a narcotic effect and peppermint can cause dizziness. This is why it is essential to consult a trained aroma-therapist who can recognize the quality of oils and is knowledgeable about their functions. Micheline Arcier, is only too aware of this, particularly in the use of oils during pregnancy, which should always be supervised by a professional. Where necessary, her therapists work with obstetricians and doctors to ensure the safety of the therapy. Aromatherapy techniques during pregnancy can help circulation, lymphatic drainage, skin and muscle tone, and relax and revitalize the mother-to-be.

AYURVEDA

A complex system of healing, Ayurveda originated in India over 5,000 years ago. Based on the teachings from ancient Vedic (Hindu) scriptures, it offers a variety of healing therapies that aim to balance and heal the mind, body and spirit. It incorporates a wide range of treatments using oils, and lifestyle mea-sures such as massage, medicinal herbs, nutrition, yoga and exercise. It views the body as part of the universe, sharing in its energies, and good health is achieved via the balance of these energies. Ayurveda is derived from the Sanskrit words, 'ayus' and 'veda', mean-ing 'life' and 'knowledge/science', so in

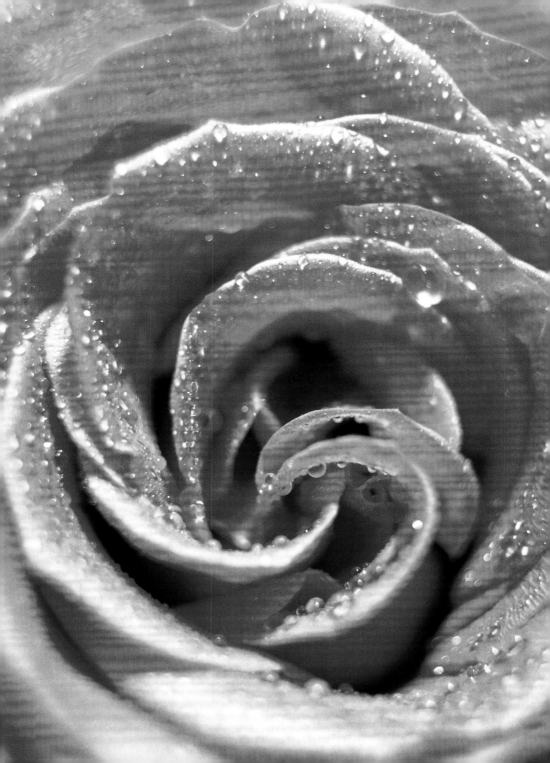

essence, this practice is based on the knowledge of life. Practitioners believe that the body is composed of the five elements of the earth – fire, water, earth, air and ether. There are also three specific constitutional types (doshas) – Pitta, Kapha and Vata – and each person has characteristics of one or more of these types. The practitioner will identify a patient's 'tridosha' – their unique combination of the three doshas – and prescribe lifestyle changes and treatments to balance it. Once the doshas are balanced, the patient should be restored to health.

The surge of interest in this system of holistic health and medicine is slightly worrying, and finding an Ayurvedic doctor with proper qualifications is all-important. Dr Andrew Weil, a renowned authority on natural and preventative medicine warns, 'Many practitioners in the West are members of the international religious organization of Mahareshi Mahesh Yogi, a Holland-based billionaire whose promotion of Ayurveda is definitely a for-profit endeavour. In India it is an inexpensive alternative to allopathic treatment.' His advice is to seek out practitioners through a registered organization or by inquiring in Indian communities.

WHAT HAPPENS?

A detailed medical and emotional history will be taken in order to determine your dosha. Your tongue may also be examined and your pulse will be checked because in Ayurvedic medicine, the pulse reveals imbalances in the doshas. The Pitta or fire type has qualities relating to heat or burning, and might be considered hot-tempered and competitive. Kapha types are calm and stable; with earth and water elements featuring strongly, they tend to be earthy, cool and pale, and are inclined to be strong, virile, slow-moving and affectionate. Vata types are dominated by the element air and tend to be thin, quick and energetic. Once your dosha has been determined, a diet and primarily herbal remedies are prescribed. Dietary advice is based on food's flavour rather than its nutritional content, and a good deal of emphasis is placed on balancing your temperamental and physical needs by adjusting your diet. You may also be told to take up exercise, and will be advised on proper breathing techniques. Therapeutic massage is also key.

Vata types: Kate Moss, Jodie Kidd, Gwyneth Paltrow.

Body type: Angular and thin – they talk a lot, and quickly.

Skin type: Tends to be dry, prone to fine, dehydrated lines.

Diet: A high metabolic rate keeps you slim. Yes to eggs, fish, rice, oats, almonds, milk. No to cold drinks, coffee, yoghurt, cabbage, cauliflower, leeks, peas, potatoes, peppers.

Exercise: Relaxing types of exercise – not too much aerobic.

Health: Joint pain, arthritis, constipation, blood pressure problems, heart disease, emotional imbalance.

Pitta types: Madonna, Christy Turlington, Cindy Crawford.

Body type: Average height and build.

Skin type: Normal but can get red and blotchy.

Diet: You need a diet high in carbohydrate and low in sour, salty, spicy foods. Yes to milk, butter, apples, avocado, watermelon, lettuce, cabbage, spinach, eggs, fish, chicken. No to sour cream, yoghurt, radishes, chillis, garlic, bananas, lemons, papayas, leeks, peppers, almonds.

Exercise: Need to exercise to burn off excess energy.

Health: Digestion, jaundice, vision problems.

Kapha types: Kate Winslet, Christina Ricci, Oprah Winfrey.

Body type: Large framed and heavy set.

Skin type: Thick, cool, pale and oily.

Diet: Lighter food. Yes to apples, apricots, peaches, broccoli, cabbage, garlic, chillis, onions, peppers, spices, tomatoes, fish, and chicken. No to milk, cheese, avocados, watermelon, bananas, dates, grapes, cashew nuts, peanuts and almonds.

Exercise: Vigorous exercise to counteract lazy tendencies.

Health: Water retention, low immunity, impotence, fatigue.

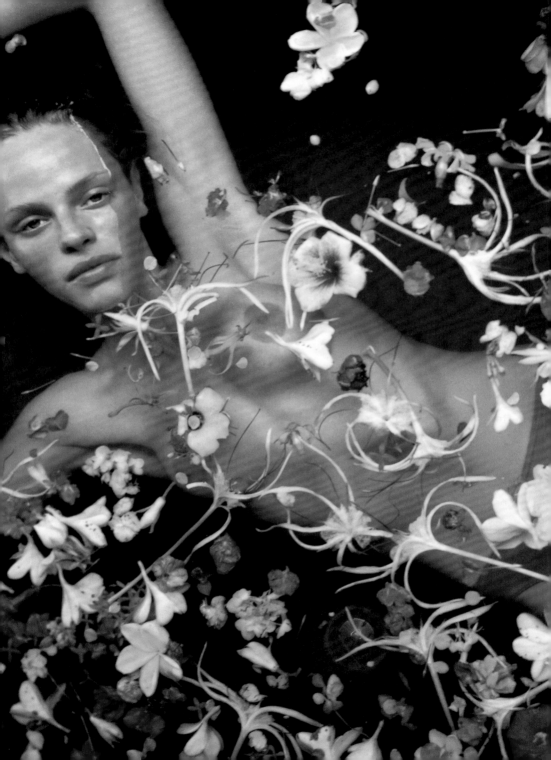

everyday maintenance therapies

FLOWER REMEDIES

The most well-known flower remedies were pioneered by Dr Edward Bach (pronounced 'Batch') who gave up his practice in 1930 to develop tinctures and perfect the method of flower healing. There are 38 different remedies in Bach's range. Although Nicholas Culpeper was working with herbal remedies in the early seventeenth century, flower remedies were prepared in a specific way and prescribed individually, according to the personality of the patient. This is another example of a complementary medicine that is tailored to both the mind and the body of the patient: emotional shock might be treated with Star of Bethlehem, for example; 'dwelling in the past' with honeysuckle; resentment with willow; depression with gentian; and so on. Sometimes several remedies are prescribed. The tinctures are taken in the form of drops added to water and you can prescribe yourself by following the instructions included.

MAGNETIC FIELD THERAPY

This treatment makes use of electromagnetic or 'energy' fields. Magnets have incredible healing properties and it is said that Cleopatra wore a magnet on her forehead to keep her looking young and beautiful. For many years it has been acknowledged that certain electric energies, radio waves and electromagnetic waves seem to increase susceptibility to cancer, but there are good magnetic fields and bad ones. Therapeutic use of the 'good' fields has only been accepted to some extent by the medical profession since the 1960s, when NASA astronauts returning to earth were suffering from nausea, loss of bone density and reduced immunity. The white corpuscles in their blood – significant in forming part of the body's immune system – were severely depleted. The astronauts proved to be afflicted by withdrawal symptoms from the earth's magnetosphere. After this, magnetic fields were placed in the astronauts' capsule, thus stimulating blood flow and attracting oxygen.

Electromagnetic applications induce changes in the tissue voltage, improve the activities of the body's enzymes and enhance ion transport at a cellular level. This means that magnetic therapy is good for healing wounds, reducing bruising and swelling, as well as increasing oxygenation of the blood.

One of the most knowledgeable people in the field is London-based naturopath and homeopath Bob Jacobs, who has spent more than 30 years developing cutting-edge equipment. His crystal magnetic bed is designed to re-establish order and relieve stress on a molecular level. Magnetic field therapy is very popular in Japan, where many homes have a magnetic therapy couch.

WHAT IS IT GOOD FOR?

This therapy is especially beneficial in speeding up the healing of injuries, torn muscles, ligaments and tendons. It also helps alleviate headaches and migraines, eases insomnia, improves circulation and also helps to provide increased energy.

WHAT HAPPENS?

Lying on Jacobs's crystal magnetic bed, wearing earphones that add therapeutic sound waves, induces deep relaxation, stimulates circulation, improves the elimination of wastes and enhances the use of oxygen and the assimilation of nutrients. The quartz crystals act rather like a tuning fork, opening up areas of blocked energy – some people experience tingling sensations. In the case of sports injury, some orthopaedic specialists use pulsed magnetic field treatment to heal soft tissue and bone. Magnetic soles for the shoes, pads to place under pillows and mattresses, as well as wraps and discs containing magnets are recommended for circulatory problems and low-energy levels. Unfortunately, there are some ineffective magnetic products where the manufacturers have wrongly mixed positive and negative fields. Only the negative fields can bring long-term benefit to the body.

massage

Massage is a healing art. It can be stimulating or soothing depending on the speed and depth of the strokes. Despite some scepticism from the scientists, it is more and more regularly used to counteract stress of all kinds. Hippocrates wrote about the power of 'rubbing' as far back as the fifth century and there is historical and pictorial evidence of reflexology massage and shiatsu from ancient Egypt and Japan, as well as from Greece and Rome. Many different types of massage can help bring about relaxation, relieve

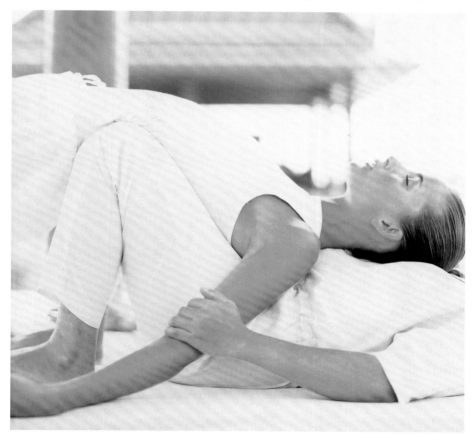

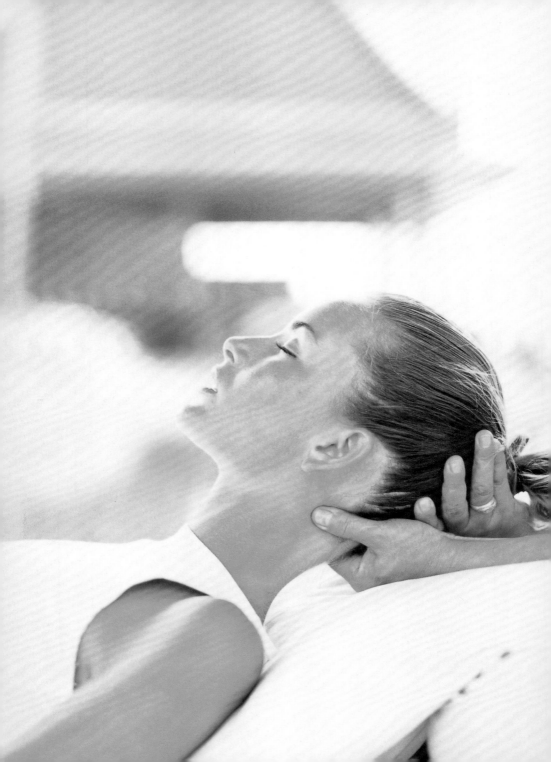

aches and pains, soften tension in muscles, assist lymphatic flow and encourage blood circulation. At the beginning of the nineteenth century a Swede called Per Henrik Ling developed what is now known as Swedish massage, and the first college offering massage on the curriculum opened in 1813 in Stockholm. The fascination of the West with all things Eastern has seen a recent interest in and integration of many Eastern techniques and theories. From Thailand, Japan, China and India come massage procedures that can be done through clothing or on a naked body using oil to lubricate the skin. Massage can be given with hands, feet, thumbs, fingers, elbows or knees. Depending on the system, it works on muscles, ligaments and tendons or, as in shiatsu, concentrates on pressure points in order to affect vital energy flow. These days therapists train and observe methods from a mix of cultures and develop them into their own personal system. The skill of

MASSAGE STROKES INCLUDE:

Kneading: Using the whole hand to knead flesh like dough.

Gliding: The hand floats rhythmically over the skin in a soothing, light action.

Effleurage: A sliding, soothing movement.

Feathering: Using the fingertips of alternate hands in a light, fast action.

Deep tissue: Using the thumbs, fingertips or heels of the hands to reach right down into hidden tension points.

Percussion: This term encompasses various stimulating movements, which are all quite noisy. These improve tone and circulation on soft tissue areas such as the thighs and buttocks. These include:

> **Cupping:** The cupped hand claps against the skin.

> **Hacking:** The hands are bounced up and down alternately and rapidly with the palms facing each other.

> **Plucking:** Pinching or plucking small bunches of flesh.

> **Pummelling:** The fists are clenched to bounce up and down.

massage is all in the hands of the practitioner, a touch therapist who can relax and heal, and there is no doubt that the best masseurs and masseuses are both gifted and truly dedicated.

SHIATSU

This is a traditional healing art from Japan developed in the early twentieth century by a Japanese practitioner Tamai Tempaka. The word means 'finger pressure' and the technique involves using hand pressure and manipulative procedures to adjust the body's physical structure and its natural inner energies. As with other Oriental healing techniques, the goal is to balance the chi, or ki, the life force which creates a harmonious, healthy, breathing and functioning body. Very simple pressure techniques work on a subtle level to find balance and increase energy flow. Most shiatsu sessions take place on the floor. The recipient should breathe evenly and consciously 'let go', while the practitioner applies pressure with their hand, knee, elbow, foot and sometimes their whole body, gently alleviating tension, pain and discomfort. As with acupuncture, the pressure points are related to the 12 primary 'channels' or meridians associated with the main organs. Pain, when pressure is applied, suggests a blockage in the flow of chi. The correct pressures can realign and heal.

London-based practitioner Max Forsyth, who has over 30 years of experience in shiatsu, kiatsu and setai (Japanese chiropractic), says, 'Shiatsu is much more than just focusing pressure on the body's meridians. It is about finely tuned intuition combined with a thorough knowledge of the human structure.'

SPORTS MASSAGE

This is fairly obvious, in that sports massage has been developed for those involved very actively in sport or dance of all kinds. It tends to be 'deeper' than ordinary massage, working on muscle groups that may be overexercised. It is very anatomically based, allied to a knowledge of the working of muscle groups and of physiotherapy – using touch techniques that go deeply into the joints and muscles. The sports masseur may use Swedish strokes of massage but will also know how and where to stretch and rehabilitate the body after

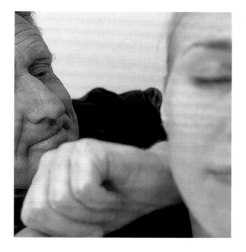

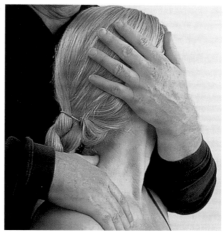

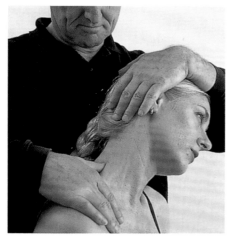

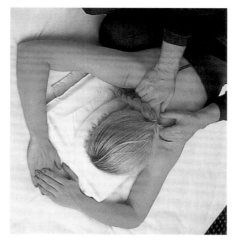

sport and extreme athletics, as well as how to deal with torn and sprained muscles, ligaments or tendons.

TUI NA

Tui na is Chinese medical massage and works alongside its sister therapies, acupuncture, Chinese herbal medicine and qi gong (page 375). It has a long history. Research from archaelogical digs suggests that it was first practised over 3,000 years ago. A famous ancient text completed between the first century BC and the first century AD refers to 12 massage techniques and how they should be used in the treatment of certain diseases. In the Tang dynasty (AD 618–906) a further text was written listing the range of diseases that could be treated with massage. From this point the idea began to spread to other countries – Japan, Korea, Vietnam and Islamic countries. Later, in the Ming dynasty, texts were written on paediatric tui na, and up until the early part of the twentieth century Chinese massage therapy flourished. Then the influence of Western medicine took hold and Chinese doctors were forced to train in Western ways. Not until 1948, under the People's Republic of China, was traditional Chinese medicine once more encouraged and tui na training courses became available in the big teaching hospitals. Tui na massage is inseparable from the theory of Chinese medicine and from the quest for balance of Yin (negative, dark and feminine) and Yang (positive, bright and masculine) in the body.

WHAT HAPPENS?

The flow of vital energy or qi stagnates (gets blocked) and this must be rectified by looking at the whole picture of the person and the ailment. So, as with Chinese medicine there is a lengthy diagnostic process where the overall manner of the patient, his or her skin colour, texture, pulse, tongue, emotional state and symptoms are considered. The technique of tui na is physical and demanding. The patient usually remains clothed and the practitioner uses hands, fingers and sometimes elbows to apply pressure. Legs and arms are pulled and stretched. The patients may have to sit, stand or lie, and a session can last for two or three hours if necessary.

ROLFING

A more invasive form of body work than some other treatments, rolfing was developed by Ida Rolf. She called her system Structural Integration, and Rolfing aims to restructure the musculoskeletal system by working on patterns of tension held in deep tissue. This connective tissue (fascia) holds the body together both directly under the skin and on deeper levels such as around the internal organs. Subtle changes to the body over the years, through injury and emotional stress, add up to pain and discomfort. Ida Rolf developed the system using her PhD in biological chemistry, a knowledge of osteopathy and the theories of yoga.

WHAT HAPPENS?

Rolfing involves ten sessions, which each focus on a separate part of the body. The therapist applies firm pressure to different areas, which can be painful, and during the session the body is encouraged to work with, rather than against, gravity. As in yogic positions, the body twists and elongates in order to achieve alignment, as the therapist manipulates the bodily structures, aided by the pull of gravity. In this way, repressed emotions are released at the same time as muscular tension is dissipated. In fact, one helps to release the other and vice versa.

WHAT IS IT GOOD FOR?

Rolfing relieves long-standing pain and fatigue brought about by poor postural habits. It helps to regain a feeling of lightness and flexibility and hence can enhance the performance of athletes, dancers and actors. This treatment also helps children's growing bodies develop in a balanced way.

AROMATHERAPY MASSAGE

As a trained aromatherapist it is not enough just to blend oils (see also pages 344–5). The massage given with the oils is a therapeutic and holistic experience, with the prescription of oils used in the therapy and the pressure points where those oils are applied being all-important. A straightforward massage with aromatherapy oils is not the true therapeutic procedure.

WHAT HAPPENS?

Part of the process involves the therapist spending a considerable time on consultation with the client before the hands-on process in order to diagnose the general state of health and the toxicity of the body. The essential oils then work in three ways. The first is by absorption. When you inhale, molecules drift to the top of your nose where they stimulate nerve endings that report to the brain. At the same time the molecules can pass through the lining of the nose and breathing passages into your blood. The second mechanism behind aromatherapy is the absorption of the oils through the skin. The third way is through massage. The massage technique works on the nervous system and the whole body, from the feet to the head and neck are treated using pressure points along the spine. Massage movements are based on reflexology and some help lymphatic drainage and blood circulation. The whole effect produces a release of tension and an ability to relax. All treatments should last at least one hour. A well-trained aromatherapist will take great care when dealing with clients who have suffered or still are suffering from anything approaching a serious medical condition. They should not work without a doctor's consent.

WHAT IS IT GOOD FOR?

Aromatherapy can be a real help with morning sickness, backache and general wellbeing throughout pregnancy, as well as helping to prevent stretchmarks. At this time, however, it is essential to make sure that the therapist is fully qualified before they use and prescribe oils. Aromatherapy massage can also be an effective treatment for skin disorders, dehydrated skin, menstrual problems, digestive problems and general aches.

TRAGER WORK

Like many subtle forms of body work, Trager work, the discovery of Milton Trager in the 1930s, works on the nervous system as well as the muscles, helping one to 'communicate' with the other and function better. Trager, who at the time was a young boxer and acrobat, decided that rather than pushing himself to his physical limits, he would see if he could jump and land in the softest possible way. He changed his whole thinking because of this and later trained as a doctor in order to give his form of body work a scientific basis.

WHAT HAPPENS?

The technique involves a gentle rocking and bouncing motion to induce deep relaxation. There are also movements which involve stretching, rolling and shimmering, during which the practitioner moves their hands very swiftly backwards and forwards over a muscle or group of muscles to soothe the central nervous system. The Trager method's gentleness means that it is particularly helpful as rehabilitation, especially for people suffering from traumatic injuries, disabilities and chronic neuromuscular diseases. 'This feels unusual if you are used to pressure point massage – but wonderful after heavy exercise as the whole body loosens up,' says therapist Jananda Bird, who suggests three sessions for full benefit.

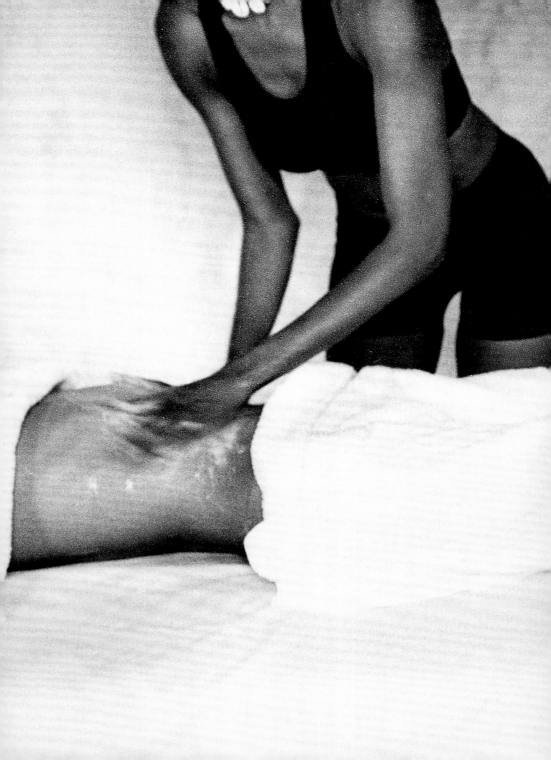

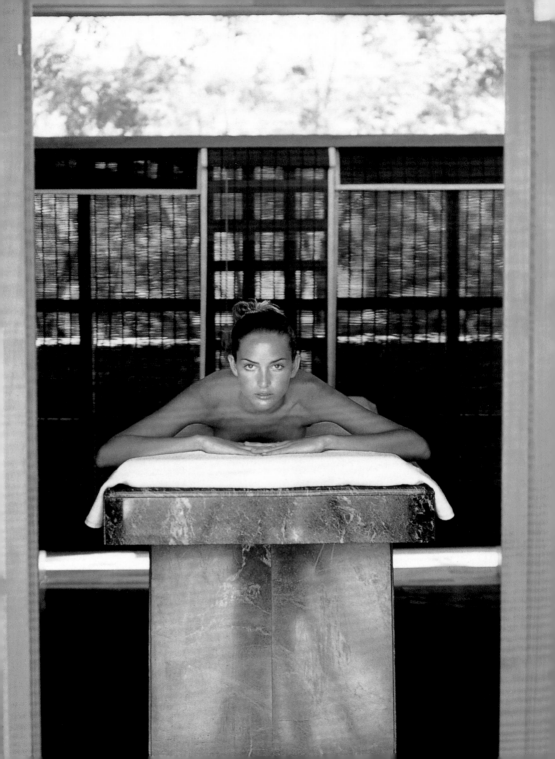

body manipulation

In 1990 and 1995 the British Medical Journal published results of trials showing patients receiving chiropractic for lower back pain improved more than those receiving standard hospital out-patient care. It was concluded that chiropractic would be a useful addition to the National Health Service. As with osteopathy, the medical profession have come round to the beneficial healing powers of several techniques of body manipulation. Practices that were once thought alternative are now considered mainstream.

OSTEOPATHY

Developed in the 1870s by American physician, Dr Andrew Taylor Still, osteopathy is today one of the most commonly sought after complementary therapies. So much so that people have forgotten that it was once treated with scorn. In the UK it was given the seal of approval in the 1993 Osteopathy Act and can be considered mainstream. Dr Still recognized that the musculoskeletal system (the bones, joints, muscles, ligaments and connective tissue) plays a major role in maintaining health. If a person is particularly stressed, encounters an injury or has bad posture, this system will not work sufficiently and ill health will ensue, as the nerve supply from the spinal cord will be disrupted and the organs it supplies will in turn be affected. The osteopath aims to rebalance the system using various manipulative techniques which allow blood to flow freely and the nerves to continue their proper functioning. The idea behind this therapy is that if the anatomy and physiology are functioning properly then you will be healthy.

WHAT IS IT GOOD FOR?

Osteopathy is predominantly used for back and neck pain, but also provides relief from the following: sciatica, joint pain, sports and strain injuries, headaches and migraines, high blood pressure, irritable bowel syndrome, insomnia, depression and asthma.

WHAT HAPPENS?

The practitioner will inquire about your medical history details before assessing posture, spine, joints and balance. You may be asked to strip to your underwear, so that the osteopath can see your body structure. This examination may be followed by a number of techniques that can vary from light pressure on the tissues to gentle massage, depending on the severity and type of problem. For example, light massage and stretching may be used for lower back pain to relax the muscles and increase the blood flow to that area. Often the osteopath will administer a high velocity thrust, which although not painful, causes the joint to 'click' loudly. It is quite normal to experience some stiffness for a couple of days after your session. In addition to the treatment, the osteopath will also offer advice on exercise, posture and diet.

CHIROPRACTIC

Derived from the Greek words 'cheir' (hands) and 'praktikos' (done by), this treatment is based on 'hands-on' joint manipulation. Discovered in the late nineteenth century by Canadian, Daniel David Palmer, chiropractic is now the most widely practised complementary therapy in the West. Legislation in Britain in 1994 enabled chiropractors to become state-registered health professionals. Chiropractors always stress the importance of the spine in the body structure, and realize that as it protects the nervous system, disruptions to either will affect the functioning of the entire body. The chiropractor focuses on an area of pain and manipulates the joints to rebalance and realign the entire structure. Pain will also be eased and movement restored as the muscles are relaxed. There are many similarities between chiropractic and osteopathy, and indeed differences are becoming less and less pronounced. However, the major distinction between both therapies is that while osteopaths work on the whole body, chiropractors concentrate more on the spine.

WHAT IS IT GOOD FOR?

Chiropractic is administered to patients with back pain, sciatica, joint stiffness, headaches and migraines, postural problems, gastrointestinal problems, asthma and vertigo.

WHAT HAPPENS?

Chiropractors take a medical history before examining the muscles and bones in your body, paying particular attention to the spine. They then use manipulation, mobilizations (moving a joint within its normal range) and palpation (feeling) to locate stiff or 'locked' joints. 'Unlocking' a joint involves creating tension around it and then applying pressure in order to return it to its proper position. This is a painless procedure, and although an unnerving popping sound might be heard and even felt, it offers immediate pain relief. The chiropractor may also give you advice on bending and lifting objects, and may recommend exercises to prevent further problems.

CRANIOSACRAL OSTEOPATHY

Craniosacral osteopathy is a specialized area of osteopathy which makes use of very gentle and specific techniques of manipulation of the skull and minute joints (sutures) within it, and the skeletal system. This manipulation releases stress patterns. The touch is so light that you may not feel it at all – however, the results are impressive. It is this gentle touch that forms the basis of the difference between conventional osteopathy and craniosacral osteopathy, and that's why the latter is so appealing to many people – because it appears to be a lot less traumatic and abrupt. In addition, while they both work on the same principal, conventional osteopathy uses a much larger range of movements.

WHAT IS IT GOOD FOR?

Physical traumas, stress, headaches, migraines and posture. Craniosacral osteopathy can be treated from birth onwards (conventional osteopathy cannot) and it is especially beneficial for babies born with distortions in the cranial bones.

KINESIOLOGY

Structural kinesiology is the study of muscles as they are involved in the science of movement and the muscular system as a whole. The term comes from the Greek word kinesis meaning 'motion'. Applied kinesiology was the name given to the system of muscle testing diagnostically by an American Doctor of Chiropractic, Dr George Goodheart, in the 1960s.

From this starting point more than half a dozen different branches have evolved, including health kinesiology which was developed in 1978 by a Canadian, Jimmy Scott. His initial concern was to find how a combination of physical, psychological and environmental stresses affected a health issue. In general, kinesiology can be described as a system of healthcare that combines muscle-testing with the principles of Chinese medicine. It is based on the belief that the body, at some unconscious level, knows precisely what it needs to cure itself, and the muscles and the subtle energy of the body can indicate this by weakening in answer to pertinent questioning.

Although this is a holistic treatment and not acknowledged by the medical profession, it has scientific roots, and the International College of Applied Kinesiology (ICAK) only accepts students with medical or scientific qualifications. Some doctors of medicine like Dr Rodney Adeniyi-Jones now integrate it with their medical diagnoses, and some dentists are finding they can use it alongside their dental work.

WHAT HAPPENS IN
APPLIED KINESIOLOGY

A lengthy case history will be taken, including questions about work, relationships, stresses, diet, home and lifestyle. The first muscle tests will assess the energy balance of muscles, meridians, related organs and glands. The patient is usually lying down fully clothed, although a few movements involve having to stand. The kinesiologist moves your arm into a particular position and then asks you to 'hold' while they apply light pressure in a particular direction for a few seconds. Surprisingly, sometimes the arm or leg gives way unexpectedly. This process is not to test strength but the response of the muscle and the energy immediately available to it. When a weakness shows up it can be corrected, sometimes immediately, by adjustments made with fingers and hands. When an allergy appears, the offending substance can be eliminated from the diet and so on. The number of sessions needed depends on the problem.

WHAT IS IT GOOD FOR?

The list is very long and varied and includes accident trauma, myalgic encephalomyelitis (ME), allergies, food intolerance, addictions, nausea, eczema, digestive problems, eating disorders, neck ache, bed-wetting, insomnia, phobias, sciatica, sports injuries, tennis elbow and hyperactivity.

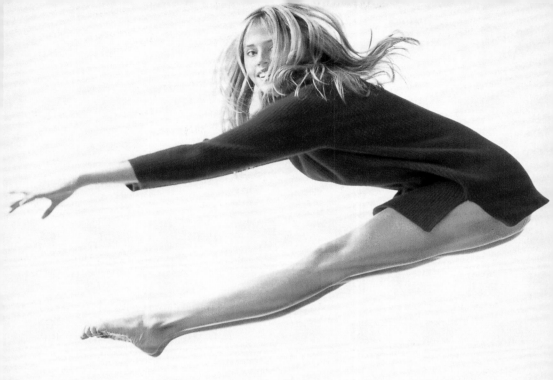

HEALTH KINESIOLOGY

The patient usually lies down and, as is the case with all holistic therapies, the practitioner will note their demeanour, their bearing and the answers to many questions. The main focus of health kinesiology involves the patient stretching out an arm and the practitioner applying light pressure to it while asking relevant questions. The body will answer the questions by its automatic response to the applied pressure. The muscles weaken and the arm drops if there is a negative response. It is difficult to describe this procedure, which seems hardly scientific. The practitioner asks the body a stream of questions, pausing to gauge response from the outstretched arm. They can even ask the body what they should prescribe and receive a positive or negative answer. The treatment seems bizarre, but the results can be truly extraordinary and it has become quite widely used in Germany and Switzerland, even by vets. Patients are prescribed homeopathic treatments, tissue salts, flower remedies and sometimes essential oils.

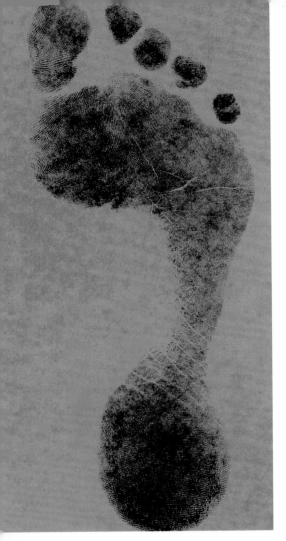

as well as a raft of psychological problems like panic attacks, anxiety, phobias, stammering, shyness, lack of confidence and grief.

REFLEXOLOGY

An ancient technique which has been practised for thousands of years, reflexology is the therapeutic massage of pressure points on the feet to relieve symptoms elsewhere in the body. Reflexologists suggest that energy flows through our bodies in ten zones that run from the head down to the toes and fingers; the flow of energy ends in the reflex points in the hands and feet. Different parts of the toes and feet relate to different organs or systems of the body. For example, the big toe corresponds to the head and brain; the heel relates to the lower back; and the ball of the foot to the lungs. If there is an imbalance in the body, the energy will become blocked at the reflex points and toxins (uric crystals) will form. The reflexologist will be able to feel these blockages and will massage them to break down the crystals and restore the flow of energy. The massage will also stimulate the circulatory and lymphatic systems, and help to flush away toxins.

WHAT IT'S GOOD FOR?

Practitioners report success with chronic problems that have not been successfully treated elsewhere. Eczema, migraine, arthritis, bronchitis, acne, Chronic Fatigue Syndrome, Candida Albicans, menopausal problems, irritable bowel syndrome and food allergies,

WHAT IS IT GOOD FOR?

Reflexology can help to alleviate stress and anxiety, headaches, migraines, insomnia, asthma, eczema, PMT, digestive disorders, back pain and high blood pressure.

WHAT HAPPENS?

An initial reflexology session is likely to last for 90 minutes, with a detailed consultation taking place before the actual therapy is commenced. Subsequent sessions usually last for between 30 minutes and 60 minutes, and these will generally take place on a weekly basis. There are reflex points on the hands as well as on the feet, so reflexologists can work on those, too; the majority, however, prefer working on the feet because there are far more reflex points there. 'People with the best feet don't wear shoes at all,' says London-based reflexologist Michael Keet.

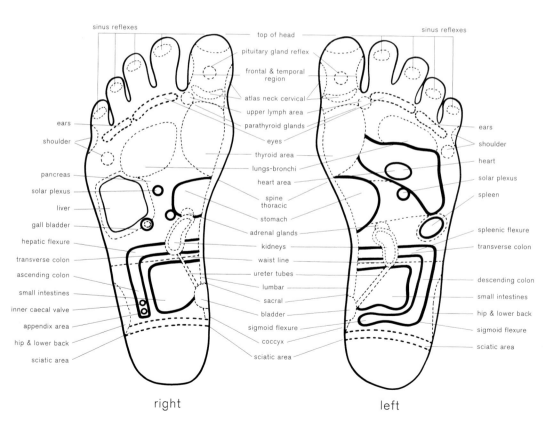

right   left

body & soul

It is now acknowledged that the mind can have an extraordinarily potent effect on the body. Mind/body therapies aim to relax, but often gentle movements can have powerful long-term results, re-establishing equilibrium, energy and optimism, and ultimately becoming impressive preventative health measures.

YOGA

The theosophists discovered yoga at the beginning of the twentieth century, although it originated in the subcontinent of India thousands of years ago as a physical and ethical discipline and meditation, focused, ultimately, on union with God. Part of the teaching of yoga is an emphasis on posture and breathing, and this is the aspect that is best known outside India today.

B K S Lyengar, whose seminal book *Light on Yoga* details hundreds of postures and breathing exercises, was one of the first Indian teachers brought to

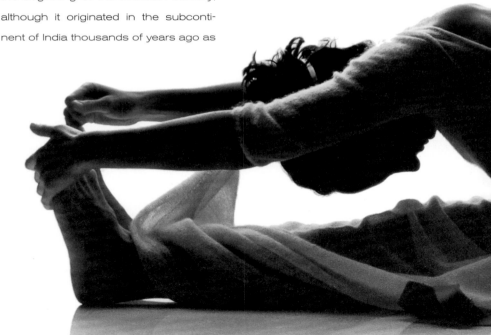

London in the 1960s by eager would-be pupils. There was a trend for all things Oriental at the time — the Beatles were off to visit their Maharishi — and it may also have become popular as a reaction to the fact that organized religion and the practice of it was breaking down. Yoga, at that time, seemed totally different and magical, an Eastern package with a new vocabulary that included words such as 'guru', 'inner peace' and 'freedom', and books with pictures of esoteric Indian experts wrapping their bodies into exotic positions.

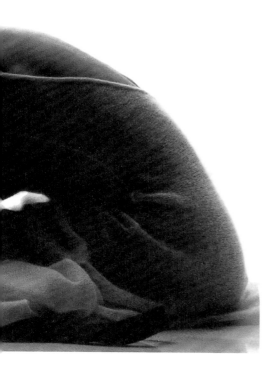

American movie star and fitness queen Jane Fonda's insistence on 'going for the burn' was the passion killer for the yoga craze of the 1960s and for the following two decades we were persuaded that jumping, sweating and aerobic exercise were the only route to a beautiful body. The new century, however, has brought with it a desire for more than just muscle tone. Today we want wellbeing as well as aesthetics, balance as well as fitness, a quiet mind as well as an energetic body. The renewed interest in yoga may well have sailed in from America again, with Hollywood's invention of power yoga, classes based on astanga yoga, which involve both jumping and complicated postures. It is a yogic system which was originally only for young Indian boys, chosen for training especially by the Brahmins, and it is indeed suitable for young and flexible bodies. Mary Stewart, who has taught a simpler, more traditional yoga with the emphasis on breathing for more than 30 years, believes that 'power yoga is fine but it could be just a keep-fit trip, and the worst that can happen is that devotees end up with a bad back. Some of the yoga postures like back bends are quite extreme and you need to be mindful.'

Taught well, yoga is the combination of an exercise system that works the body safely and thoughtfully, coupled with a philosophy that teaches calm, mindfulness and moderation. The postures, each being a therapy in themselves, stimulate the internal systems of the body and stretch and elongate the spine, giving better posture, improved circulation and no aches and pains, not to mention strength and stamina. Yoga requires no special clothing or props, no appropriate location, and has no age limit — and I enjoy the prospect of being mobile in my old age. 'If you quieten your mind a bit,' says Mary Stewart, 'it can make you more powerful because you can give more attention to things that will increase your potential. So just as you can clear clutter from your physical body by detoxing, so you do the same with your mind.' Mary Stewart, now in her sixties, says that she stayed with yoga all these years 'because it worked, physically and emotionally together. It helped me through some pretty bad times in my life and I'd hate to be getting old without it.' People often start yoga because they are tense, unhappy or they have a bad back. Men, historically, have only turned up at yoga classes when they've been injured in sport and told by doctors to try it. Yoga can certainly be very powerful, but without a good teacher, it can be dangerous. Some modern instructors distort the principles of yoga by trying to bring it in line with present-day fitness crazes. Yoga practice is not about working out. It should not make you feel tired, nor should you experience a 'high' followed by exhaustion later. You should feel grounded and calm, and your energy and potential for life should increase day by day. *The Bhagavad Gita*, a philosophical book written in around 600 BC and widely read all over India, explains, 'Yoga is a harmony. Not for him who eats too much, or for him who eats too little; not for him who sleeps too little, or for him who sleeps too much.' You can change the chemistry of the body with yoga breathing if it's taught badly. Reading *The Yoga Sutras* (the earliest writings about the systems of Yoga by Patanjali, who is thought to have lived between 200 BC and AD 200) helps to explain the simplicity of yoga breathing. The texts explain that yoga is not a way of having weird out-of-body experiences, nor has it evolved to lift people onto a higher plane. 'Yoga plus meditation (or sitting in prayer/silence/contemplation,

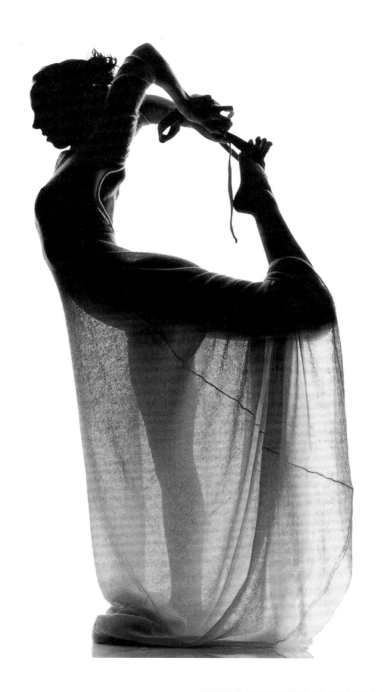

whatever you like to call it) helps you meet life a bit better,' says Mary Stewart, 'It should teach you humility, in union with the physical and the mental.'

FELDENKRAIS

Feldenkrais is a system of simple movements, floor exercises and body work designed to retrain the central nervous system. It is very gentle and was conceived to help in the rehabilitation of trauma, cerebral palsy and stroke victims. Moshe Feldenkrais, who died in 1984, applied his background in physics and engineering to the study of human movements because of his own chronic knee problems. It is a physical therapy that really unlocks stiffness for those unused to and unable to contemplate complicated or strenuous exercise. The key aim is body and sensory awareness and it can be very surprising how a small, slow movement can unlock tension and allow flexibility. Often the physical action happens without the intellect interfering.

WHAT IS IT GOOD FOR?

Improving posture and voice projection; easing pain in the back, neck and shoulders; learning how to avoid repetitive strain injury, developing greater awareness and flexibility.

ALEXANDER TECHNIQUE

The Alexander Technique is not a set of exercises to help posture, as is often thought. It is a programme for releasing unnecessary tension and bad postural habits by consciously controlling the way our bodies work in unison with how we feel. It was developed by Australian, Frederick Matthias Alexander, at the beginning of the twentieth century. In trying to solve his own throat problems, he discovered by watching his posture in the mirror, that he was standing and moving his body in ways he was unaware of. He found that if he was standing better, he could also breathe better — if the neck was free, the head could go forward and up, and the back could lengthen. By working his body harmoniously, he found that his throat problems disappeared and his general health improved. It sounds simplistic, but doctors agreed with Alexander that constant bad habits over time can alter us both physically and mentally. The technique, now taught all over the world and particularly used by art, drama and music schools and colleges, aims to re-educate the senses, teaching new ways to sit, stand, lie down, bend, breathe and walk, all designed to enable the body to choose correct and efficient postures, which in turn allow ease of movement.

QI GONG

Like yoga in India, there are several branches or systems of qi gong (chi gung) in China, where it is apparently practised regularly by around 60 million people. It is a form of exercise that develops more than just physical strength; it also promotes balance and wellbeing. 'Qi gong' means 'energy cultivation' and, along with acupuncture and herbalism, forms one of the bases of traditional Chinese medicine. Though the movements may be small, they can be powerful and dynamic. They strengthen muscles and bones, and develop the qi, or internal force, of the individual, helping to keep the mind focused. It has been described as 'meditation in motion' and has similar health benefits to meditation. Qi gong would be considered essential training for anyone practising massage; the theory being that you must be in balance and harmony yourself before you can give a treatment to another person.

T'AI CHI

Various different branches, styles or systems of t'ai chi are practised all over China and the West today. In China people practise in parks and offices at the most beneficial time of day, sunrise — according to Chinese philosophy, nature's chi flows at its strongest at sunrise. The more martial-arts-orientated styles of t'ai chi are called t'ai chi ch'uan. Ch'uan means 'the supreme ultimate fist'. T'ai chi, which offers health, meditation, self-defence and physical exercise in one package, is not competitive. It involves a series of movements, each called a form. They are performed in slow, fluid, continuous movements, one leading into another. The weight is very solidly grounded in the feet and the flow, or chi, of the person can then move freely from this centred starting point. Again, like yoga, the postures reflect nature: the tree with its roots, the mountain large and strong, the bird flying rhythmically. But due to the control, whichever position, there is great strength. In China it is done by young and old, weak and strong, and it benefits the body and mind, as well as the circulation of blood and lymph systems, movement of joints, strengthening of the lower back, massaging of the internal organs, and improves breathing, which results in more oxygen to heart and brain. It also promotes concentration, confidence, self-control and awareness.

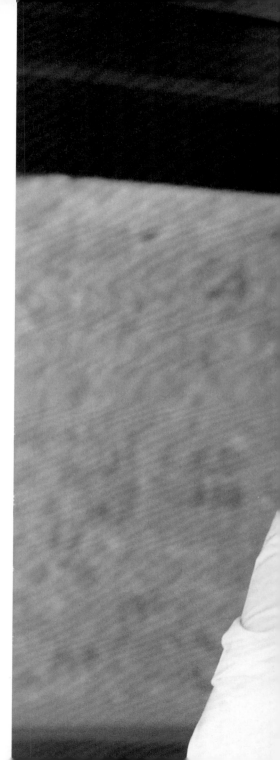

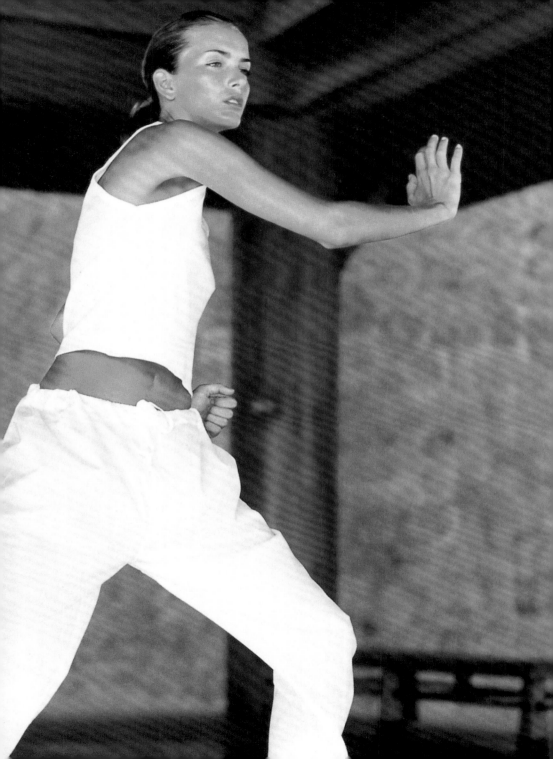

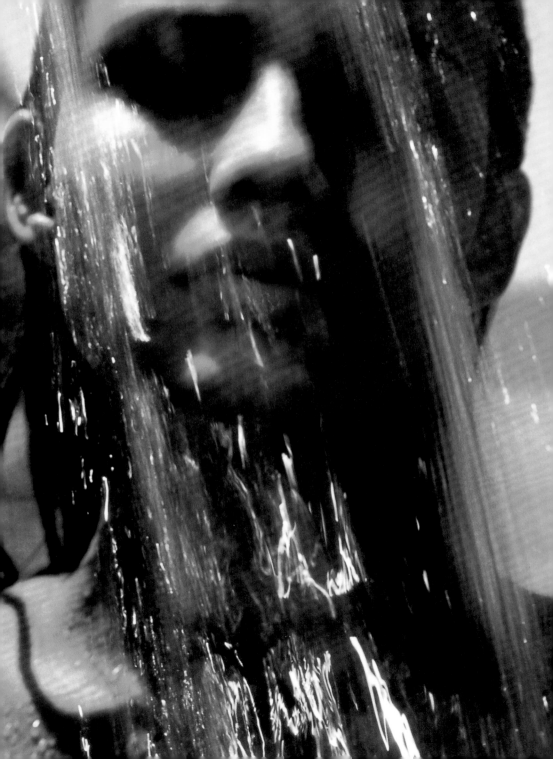

mind

New ways of healing in the twenty-first century suggest that the mind as a healing tool is underdeveloped in our conventional culture. Our belief systems in the past have relied on going to a doctor when we get sick and expecting them to come up with a cure. Alternative practitioners suggest that the innate intelligence of the body should be used to enable people to heal themselves. They believe that medicine should be preventative and that the mind can play the largest part in the healing process. But the 'new age speak' of some of these practitioners has been controversial and difficult to understand. Only because so many people have tried and been impressed with the results have the alternative ways gained momentum. Certain practices and therapies help us to clear the mind of preconceived ideas. Others hope to bypass the intellectual to get to the body's innate intelligence directly by 'clearing clutter'.

treat both mental and physical problems. Contrary to popular belief, you are not unconscious during hypnosis; your state is similar to when you daydream or when you become so enthralled in a book that your mental attention is fully focused. You are in a trance-like state — neither fully awake nor fully asleep. This is the unconscious level of the mind, which people have no control over. During hypnosis you are aware of other people and are in control, however, you are unable to detach from your surroundings. Hypnotherapy has been administered since ancient times to cure hysteria and anxiety. In the eighteenth century, Austrian physician, Anton Mesmer, used a technique called mesmerism to put people into a trance and subsequently cure their ills. Later, English surgeon Dr James Braid coined the term 'hypnotism' after observing a demonstration and he thus developed his own theories and techniques.

HYPNOTHERAPY

Hypnotherapy relies on the induction of an altered state of consciousness to

WHAT IS IT GOOD FOR?

This treatment does not work for everybody — it has been estimated that one in ten people cannot be hypnotized. However, it is successful in helping people overcome addictions (alcohol, smoking, drugs), weight loss, stress-related conditions, anxiety, pain relief, bedwetting and phobias.

WHAT HAPPENS?

A session will last no longer than an hour. Initially, you will be made to feel comfortable and at ease by the hypnotist, who will ask you to relax on a reclining chair. The first task will be to determine whether or not you are a suitable candidate, and whether hypnosis will work for you. There are several tests that the therapist can use, including asking you to imagine that your hand is too heavy for you to lift, or to close your eyes and fall forwards or backwards. The hypnotist can then use various techniques to put you into a hypnotic trance; the most common being to ask you to watch a moving object as it swings back and forth and then to suggest in a soothing voice that your eyes are so heavy you cannot keep them open, or being told to concentrate on the hypnotist's voice as they give you instructions; or counting slowly backwards from 30 to 0.

REIKI

Pronounced Raykee, this Japanese hands-on healing system was developed in the late 1880s by theologian Dr Mikao Usui. He discovered ancient Buddhist texts describing a formula for healing and worked through them to revive the reiki process. Reiki means universal life energy — 'rei' is the Japanese word for 'universal' and 'ki' for 'life energy'. Healing is derived from and based on channelling spiritual energy through one's hands. The Reiki healer channels this energy, which flows through all living things, into the patient through placing a hand in contact with them. Practitioners believe that this healing dissolves any energy blockages in the body, increases the circulation and rebalances body, mind and spirit, ridding the body of toxic waste. It is a democratic system which is difficult for most people to grasp since all Reiki masters insist that anyone can do it. It is not about being told what's wrong, more about laying on the hands and letting them do the healing for you.

WHAT IS IT GOOD FOR?

Reiki aims to relieve acute emotional and physical conditions and helps overcome stress, anxiety, migraines, irritable bowel syndrome, and menstrual pain. It is also used for general wellbeing and relaxation, leaving the patient feeling revitalized and refreshed. It is often used in tandem with other complementary therapies.

WHAT HAPPENS?

Treatment typically lasts for 90 minutes and you remain clothed. The practitioner will place their hands on your body in a unique sequence of positions to assist the flow of energy, and you should feel a pleasant warmth and tingling sensation, and might even see bright colours. You may feel very emotional and even fall asleep. It is not uncommon to cry or laugh during the therapy as deep-rooted problems and emotions surface.

SPIRITUAL HEALING

For centuries, healing has played an important role in the religious and magical practices of most cultures. Spiritual healers consider themselves the conductors of supernatural healing forces and they aim to repair damaged auras (the energy that supposedly surrounds all humans). There are strong connections between the mind and the immune system, and between the immune system and the nervous system. Spiritual healers suggest that they tap into this connection and unlock the healing potential of the immune system. Most healers claim that they themselves do not heal – they simply help patients unlock their body's own healing powers.

WHAT IS IT GOOD FOR?

Healing is generally used to ease pain and relieve stress, although it is often administered to terminally ill patients to offer them peace and a sense of acceptance.

WHAT HAPPENS?

Spiritual healing is often performed in group sessions, but it can also be done on a one-to-one basis; it will typically last 30 to 60 minutes. The healer will talk to you to help you relax, and will then use a hands-on approach as the two of you work together. Either their hands will be placed very lightly on you, or will hover above you. This light touch will allow the healing energies to flow through you and subsequently heal your aura. You may experience warm, tingling sensations, and should be left with a pronounced feeling of wellbeing.

LIGHT THERAPY

Light has been used in medicine for centuries and today full-spectrum lighting is mainly used to treat physiological and psychological problems. The therapy was introduced in the 1980s as doctors recognized that when deprived of light, people suffer from lethargy, depression, insomnia and an inability to concentrate. Research has suggested that such problems arise from a disruption to the body's 'circadian rhythm' – our internal 24-hour 'dark-light cycle clock'. This rhythm governs the timing of such functions as sleep, hormone production and body temperature, and it is regulated by the pineal gland, which is controlled by the presence or absence of light. When it is dark, the pineal gland produces melatonin to promote sleep. If you disturb the circadian rhythm by sleeping during daylight hours, travelling across time zones or not getting enough exposure to light, your health may suffer. Two striking examples of this are jet lag and SAD (Seasonal Affective Disorder). Light therapy is probably the best and most common treatment for SAD.

WHAT ELSE CAN IT TREAT?

There are few disorders that would not benefit from light therapy. Other than SAD, it is especially recommended for low energy levels, depression, high blood pressure, infertility, PMT, joint problems and sleep disorders.

WHAT HAPPENS?

Most people take this treatment at home, although you can visit a therapist. If you choose to do the latter, the therapist will take a medical history and then ask you to lie on a couch, removing as much clothing as you like, as well as glasses or contact lenses, which restrict the light reaching the pineal gland. A lamp about 1 m (3 ft) above your body emits light, which is roughly half the intensity of sunlight, and you are advised to keep your eyes open during the treatment for maximum benefits. A session might last an hour and you should come away feeling brighter and more cheerful, with increased energy levels. Should you decide to do the treatment at home, you will be advised

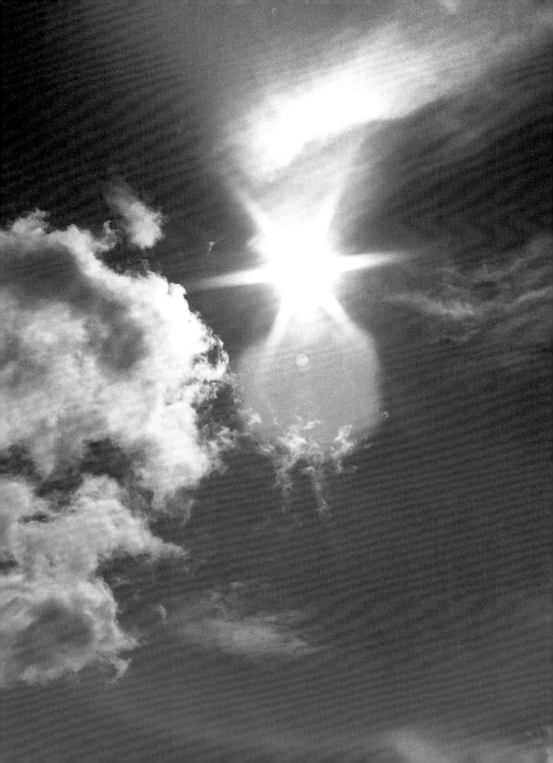

to buy a lightbox, which you place on a table at eye level. Sit about 45 cm (18 in) from the box, facing the light source but never looking directly at the bulb. As long as you are constantly facing the light, you can perform other activities during the treatment. Depending on the brightness of the light source, the treatment time can range from 15 minutes to three hours.

COLOUR THERAPY

Healing with light and colour has been used for thousands of years. In ancient Egypt special diagnostic rooms were constructed in such a way that sunlight was refracted into the colours of the spectrum. The patient was then placed in a room flooded with the appropriate colour for their problem. Closer to the present day, it is no coincidence that hospital walls are painted pale green, which is known to induce calm, or that seeing the world through rose-tinted glasses makes it a more beautiful place. The recent global trend for coloured gemstone bracelets (pink for love, orange for joy, and so on) harks back to ancient customs and cultures who believed that the correct choice would produce results. Today even cosmetics are being conceived with colour therapy in mind: nail colours to calm or energize; lipsticks in tones to attract, give courage or comfort.

Painting colours on walls or wearing colours is only one way the therapy works. There are scientific studies, too. One written up in *The American Journal of Psychology* found that using red and green light to treat depression reduced symptoms by 20 per cent after two hours. Some therapists work by directing coloured lights, in the form of lamps or torches, onto specific areas to promote healing. The theory is that our bodies are sensitive to colour, and therapists use one of the seven energy centres of the body – chakras – which are each associated with a particular colour, as a focus. For example, the heart chakra, which when imbalanced leads to heart disease and high blood pressure, is green. So a colour therapist will use green to treat such conditions. The spleen chakra, which is related to circulation, creates problems with the lungs and kidneys when it is out of balance. Its colour is orange, so such conditions should be treated with orange. Research suggests that orange has been used to successfully treat asthma, bronchitis and emphysema.

Colour Puncture, a more concentrated form of light and colour therapy, uses coloured light at acupuncture points, so directing the necessary light at the body's meridians. It was invented by a German naturopath, Peter Mandel, in the 1970s.

WHAT IS IT GOOD FOR?

Colour therapy is a beneficial treatment for psychological problems, infertility, high and low blood pressure, coughs, colds, constipation, digestive disorders, insomnia and amnesia.

WHAT HAPPENS?

There are lots of methods for treating with colour and each therapist will choose a different one. Using a 'Kirlian' photograph is a popular technique. This shows the electromagnetic field, or aura, around the body and is an indication of health and wellbeing. If it displays problems in your aura, colour will be used on the relevant areas to treat the problem. Other therapists may show you colours and ask you to choose the ones that most appeal to you. Some suggest that our bodies know exactly what healing we need and so we are likely to pick out the right colours. The Luscher colour test is frequently used. This involves putting colours in order of preference, and in doing so you reveal areas of imbalance and any potential illnesses. An unusual method is adhering to a colour diet — eating food that is carefully balanced in colours, or predominantly eating one colour to rebalance the body.

BEST (BIO-ENERGETIC SYNCHRONIZATION)

Most chiropractors limit themselves to spinal column — the crunch and crack technique. Fix the bone, manipulate the neck and send the patient away feeling relieved until next time. Some chiropractors, like Douglas Diehl, have taken the whole thing further. He believes that there are emotional, physical and neurological factors in any one trauma. 'You cannot cure someone by treating the symptom, you must treat the cause,' he says, and now uses a technique, called BEST in the USA, which combines his chiropractic and scientific background with both applied kinesiology, reiki and toxicity analysis. The BEST technique, coupled with chiropractic practice in the way Diehl practises it, aims to clear out the clutter, both physical and emotional. This is on the cutting edge of what is known as mind/body medicine.

WHAT HAPPENS

Sessions take 30 minutes and the patient is clothed and often lying down. Quick, light muscle-testing movements of the legs and arms, and application of pressure to specific points, plus simple breathing and visualizing techniques are used. Results are uncanny – the patient becomes a computer and by pressing the salient 'buttons', the therapist can delete emotional memory blocks as you would an obsolete file. As the emotional pains are deleted, the physical problems disappear.

Diehl's analogy is as follows: imagine that you have a car crash, where you break your arm. The bone breaks, the body responds and reacts. That response and reaction is stored in the memory as what we do and what happens when we're hit by a car. As well as the physical damage, if the car was brand new, you're probably angry. That's the emotion associated with the trauma. Six months later, bones mended, incident over, you don't remember anything. Two years on, a friend asks after your fabulous silver Jaguar. This first triggers off the anger. The anger then triggers off the neuro, or body's response stored in the memory. Suddenly your body/arm starts to hurt again. You go to a chiropractor perhaps and he asks you what you've done. You say, 'nothing'. They treat the arm pain.

The reverse analogy is when someone unwittingly thumps you on the arm. The body remembers the bad arm pain and suddenly from being fairly mellow, you're angry. You yourself don't understand why you're angry. The therapist can treat the pain or even the mood swings, but they'll keep on coming back unless you delete the memory from the nervous system, which is what this technique claims to do. Ultimately the conflict in the mind of how you would like life to be and the reality of how it is, is a major cause of stress. Once you take responsibility for your own reality, the choice to be well or sick becomes yours.

MEDITATION

Meditation has been practised in all major world religions for centuries, either in prayer and contemplation, or as a way to achieve a state of bliss. Today many people use it to induce a state of relaxation and harmony. It has almost become fashionable since it is heralded in the media as a way of helping with stress. It can be very powerful and should be practised with care. Altered awareness during meditation is associated with the pattern of electrical impulses in the brain. Research has shown that brain waves associated with quiet, receptive states – alpha waves – are of a higher intensity during meditation than during sleep. Transcendental meditation (TM), which was introduced to the West in the 1960s, is still a common form of meditation and is used to treat stress. Various techniques are practised, however all involve focusing the mind on an object, activity or phrase (mantra), to which it can always return if distracted. A quiet setting and a comfortable position (usually sitting in a straight-backed chair) are necessary.

WHAT IS IT GOOD FOR?

Studies suggest that meditation may help to reverse or reduce heart disease and improve circulation. Other common ailments it can improve are stress, anxiety, high blood pressure, fatigue, headaches, migraines, depression, insomnia and addictions.

WHAT HAPPENS?

Books and videos are available to teach you to meditate, but it is always better to be guided by a teacher with experience. A beneficial session will probably last 15 to 20 minutes, and it is recommended that sessions take place at the same time each day. However, be aware that it takes some time to learn to get the hang of it. It is not something that necessarily comes easily. The number of sessions required will depend on how difficult you find it. You may prefer to keep your eyes closed to avoid any distractions and to enhance concentration, and you must breathe slowly and rhythmically, all the time concentrating on your focus object, activity or phrase. Stay as still as possible during this time, and should your mind wander, always return to your point of focus. Meditation should not be a trend that you pick up and put down because the more you practise it, the easier it will be.

directory

The following listing is a compilation of the finest experts in their fields – beauticians, therapists, health practitioners, fitness trainers, hair stylists and colourists, spas and salons. Also included are organizations, who can supply general advice and information, as well as lists of recommended practitioners.

UK

BODY

BEAUTY THERAPISTS & SALONS

Amanda Griggs at Balance
250 King's Road
London SW3 5UE
Tel: 020 7565 0333
www.balancetheclinic.com
Nutrition assessment, colon hydrotherapy, food intolerance.

Bharti Vyas Holistic Therapy & Beauty Centre
5 & 24 Chiltern Street
London W1U 7QE
Tel: 020 7935 5312
www.bharti-vyas.com
Holistic skincare, beauty treatments and hair removal, including threading.

Bliss Spa
60 Sloane Ave
London SW3 3DD
Tel: 020 7590 6146
www.blissworld.com
Skincare and facials.

Eve Lom
2 Spanish Place
London W1U 3HU
Tel: 020 7935 9988
www.evelom.co.uk
Facialist with product range and spa treatments.

Fay Wancke
Tel: 07973 325 645
Private aromatherapy and Swedish-style massage in your own home.

The French Cosmetic Medical Company Ltd
25 Wimpole Street
London W1M 7AD
Tel: 020 7637 0548
Soft peeling, mesotherapy, facials, light therapy for cellulite and lymphatic drainage.

Martyn Maxey
18 Grosvenor Street
London W1K 4QQ
www.martynmaxey.co.uk
Tel: 020 7629 6161

Norma Newman
154 New King's Road
London SW6 4LZ
Tel: 020 7731 2323
Facials, manicures, pedicures, eyelash perming, San Tropez, waxing and massage.

The Spa at The Aveda Institute
174 High Holborn
London WC1V 7AA
Tel: 020 7759 7355
www.aveda.co.uk

Urban Retreat at Harrods
Fifth Floor, Harrods
Knightsbridge
London SW1X 7XL
Tel: 020 7893 8333
www.urbanretreat.co.uk

AROMATHERAPY

Aromatherapy Associates
Unit 6, Great West Trading Estate
Great West Road
Brentford
Middlesex TW8 9DN
Tel: 020 8569 7030
www.aromatherapyassociates.com

Eve Taylor
No 1 Mallard Business Centre
Mallard Road
Brettan
Peterborough
Cambridgeshire PE3 8YR
Tel: 01733 260 161
www.evetaylor.com
Private aromatherapy treatments, own product range.

Micheline Arcier
Tel: 020 7235 3545
www.michelinearcier.com
Aromatherapy products and treatments and online shopping.

Tisserand Aromatherapy Products Ltd
Newtown Road
Hove
East Sussex BN3 7BA
Tel: 01273 224 084
www.tisserand.com
E-mail sales@tisserand.com for stockists and salons.

SPECIALIST TREATMENTS

Dr Andrew Markey
at St John's Institute of Dermatology, St Thomas's Hospital, and privately at **The Lister Hospital**
Chelsea Bridge Road
London SW1W 8RH
Tel: 020 7928 9292
Laser hair removal and Botox.

Anne Rivlin
Vascular & Vein Unit
25 Wimpole Street
London W1G 8GL
Tel: 020 7436 1931
www.vascularandveinunit.com
Varicose veins and thread veins.

Gemma Ireland Bodyflow
For private sessions, call
Tel: 020 7376 5278
www.bodyflow.co.uk
Reflexology, yoga, Pilates, fertility, pre- and post-pregnancy massage, shiatsu, nutrition.

Jane Clarke
53 Upper Montagu Street
London W1H 1SE
Tel: 020 7467 5470
www.janeclarke.com
Dietitian and nutritionist.

Dr Jean-Louis Sebagh
9 Wimpole Street
London W1G 9SG
Tel: 020 7580 3343
www.drsebagh.com
Botox and fillers.

The Life Centre
15 Edge Street
London W8 7PN
Tel: 020 7221 4602
www.thelifecentre.com
Energy healing, shiatsu,
acupressure and yoga.

Michael Keet
Reflexology Limited
Marlborough House
14–16 Betterton Street
Covent Garden
London WC2H 9AB
Tel: 020 7240 1438
www.www.reflexologypages.co.uk
Reflexologist.

Michael Skipwith
1 Oldbury Place
London W1U 5PA
Tel: 020 7486 2875
Cranial osteopath.

Nicholas Lowe at
The Cranley Clinic
3 Harcourt House
Cavendish Square
London W1G OPN
Tel: 020 7499 3223
www.drnicklowe.com
Botox, dermatology and
anti-ageing.

Smile Beautiful
22 Wimpole Street
London W1G 8GQ
Tel: 020 7436 8989
www.smilebeautiful.co.uk
Orthodontics, teeth whitening and
other cosmetic treatments.

Wendy Lewis
Tel: 001 212 861 6148
www.wlbeauty.com
Contact ilana@wlbeauty.com
for dates in London and New York.
Cosmetic surgery consultant.

MANICURES & PEDICURES

Iris Chapple
3 Spanish Place
London W1U 3XH
Tel: 020 7486 6001

Midge Killen at
Amazing Nails
22 Weighhouse Street
London W1K 5LZ
Tel: 07775 780 744
www.amazingnails.co.uk

Nails Inc
For branches nationwide visit
www.nailsinc.com

HAIR

SALONS

Adam Reed at Percy & Reed
157c Great Portland Street
London W1W 6QS
Tel: 020 7637 4634
www.percyandreed.com

Charles Worthington
7 Percy Street
London W1T 1DH
Tel: 020 7631 1370
www.cwlondon.com

Daniel Galvin
58–60 George Street
London W1U 7ET
Tel: 020 7486 9661
www.danielgalvin.co.uk

Derek Thompson at Michaeljohn
25 Albemarle Street
London W1S 4HU
Tel: 020 7629 6969
info@michaeljohn.co.uk

Errol Douglas
18 Motcomb Street
London SW1X 8LB
Tel: 020 7235 0110
www.erroldouglas.co.uk

Luke Hersheson at
Daniel Hersheson
45 Conduit Street
London W1S 2YN
Tel: 020 7434 1747
www.danielhersheson.co.uk

Michael van Clarke
1 Beaumont Street
London W1G 6DF
Tel: 020 7224 3123
www.vanclarke.com

Nicky Clarke
130 Mount Street
London W1K 3NY
Tel: 020 7491 4700
www.nickyclarke.co.uk

Richard Sorrell at
Hugh & Stephen
161 Ebury Street
London SW1W 9QN
Tel: 020 7730 2196

Toni and Guy
For branches nationwide
call 0800 731 2396
www.toniandguy.com

Trevor Sorbie
27 Floral Street
London WC2E 9DP
Tel: 020 7379 6901
www.trevorsorbie.com

The Aveda Institute
174 High Holborn
London WC1V 7AA
Tel: 020 7759 7355
www.aveda.co.uk

Windle
41 Shorts Gardens
London WC2H 9AP
Tel: 020 7497 2393
www.windlehair.com

COLOURISTS

The Aveda Institute
28–9 Marylebone High Street
London W1U 4PL
Tel: 020 7224 3157
www.aveda.co.uk

Jo Hansford
19 Mount Street
London W1K 2RN
Tel: 020 7495 7774
www.johansford.com

John Frieda
6–8 Kingly Court
London W1B 5PW
Tel: 020 7851 9800
www.johnfrieda.co.uk
Susan Baldwin and David Adams.

Real
8 Cale Street
Chelsea Green
London SW3 3QU
Tel: 020 7589 0877
www.realhair.co.uk
Josh Wood and Belle Cannon.

TRICHOLOGY

Philip Kingsley Trichology
54 Green Street
London W1K 6RU
Tel: 020 7629 4004
www.philipkingsley.com

SKINCARE

Allergenics
For stockists call
02920 388 422

Clarins
For stockists and salons
see uk.clarins.com

Clinique
For stockists and salons
see www.clinique.co.uk

Darphin
For stockists, spas and salons
see www.darphin.co.uk

Decleor
For salons, stockists and mail
see www.decleor.co.uk
Essential oil-based skincare.

Elemis
The Lodge, 92 Uxbridge Road
Harrow Weald, Middlesex
HA3 6BZ
Tel: 020 8954 8033
www.elemis.com
Noella Gabrielle for aromatherapy.

Gatineau
For stockists and mail order call
0800 731 5805

Guinot
For stockists and salons
call 01344 873 123

Jurlique
Holly House
300–303 Chiswick High Raod
London W4 1NP
Tel: 020 8995 2293
Australian skincare and spa.
www.apotheke20-20.co.uk

La Prairie
For stockists and salons
see www.laprairie.com

SCENT

Annick Goutal
For stockists and online shopping
ssee www.annickgoutal.com

Caron
For stockists and online shopping
see www.parfumscaran.com

Creed
For stockists and online shopping
see www.creedfragrances.co.uk

Estée Lauder
For stockists and online shopping
www.esteelauder.co.uk

Guerlain
For stockists and mail order
see ww2.guerlain.com

Jo Malone
150 Sloane Street
London SW1X 9BX
Tel: 08701 925 121
www.jomalone.co.uk

Les Senteurs
71 Elizabeth Street
London SW1W 9PJ
Tel: 020 7730 2322
www.lessenteurs.com

Miller Harris
21 Bruton Street
London W1J 6QD
Tel: 020 7629 7750
www.millerharris.com

Scent Direct
International gift delivery service
for perfume and aftershave.
Tel: 08454 502 450
www.scentdirect.com

MAKE-UP

Chanel
For stockists and information
call 020 7493 3836
www.chanel.com

Cosmetics à la Carte Ltd
19b Motcomb Street
London SW1X 8LB
Tel: 020 7235 0596
cosmeticsalacarte.com

Farmacia Urban Healing
169 Drury Lane
Covent Garden
London WC2B 5QA
Tel: 020 7394 7995

Molton Brown Cosmetics
58 South Molton Street
London W1K 5SL
Tel: 020 7499 6474
www.moltonbrown.co.uk

Pixi
22a Fouberts Place
London W1F 7PA
Tel: 020 7287 7211
www.pixibeauty.com

Screen Face
48 Monmouth Street
London WC2 9EP
Tel: 020 7836 3955
www.screenface.com

Shiseido
For stockists and product finder
see www.shiseido.co.uk

Space NK
For stockists and online shopping
see www.spacenk.co.uk

HEALTH CLUBS & SPAS

Grosvenor House Health Club
86–90 Park Lane
London W1K 7AW
Tel: 020 7499 6363

The Harbour Club
Watermeadow Lane
London SW6 2RR
Tel: 020 7371 7700
www.harbourclubchelsea.com

Lambton Place Health Club
11 Lambton Place
Westbourne Grove
London W11 2SH
Tel: 020 7229 2291

DAY SPAS

The Berkeley Health Club and Spa
Wilton Place
Knightsbridge
London SW1X 7RL
Tel: 020 7235 6000
www.the-berkeley.co.uk

Bliss London
60 Sloane Ave
London SW3 3DD
Tel: 020 7590 6146
www.blissworld.com

Champneys Piccadilly
21a Piccadilly
London W1V 0BH
Tel: 020 7255 8000
www.champneys.com

Chewton Glen Hotel, Health
and Country Club
New Milton
Hampshire BH25 6QS
Tel: 01425 275 341
www.chewtonglen.com

The Cowshed
Babington House
Babington
Near Frome
Somerset BA11 3RW
Tel: 01373 812 266
www.babingtonhouse.co.uk
For spas in London, Cornwall and
New York, and for online shopping
see www.cowshedonline.com

The Dorchester Spa
Park Lane
London W1K 1QA
Tel: 020 7629 8888
www.thedorchester.com/
dorchester-spa

The Grove Health Centre
182–4 Kensington Church Street
London W8 4DP
Tel: 020 7221 2266

The Lygon Arms
Broadway
Worcestershire WR12 7DU
Tel: 01386 852 255
www.broadway-cotswolds.co.uk/
lygon.html

The Phillimore Club
45 Phillimore Walk
Kensington
London W8 7RZ
Tel: 020 7937 2882

The Royal Crescent Hotel
and Bath House Spa
16 Royal Crescent
Bath BA1 2LS
Tel: 01225 823 333
www.royalcrescent.co.uk

The St David's Hotel & Spa
Havannah Street
Cardiff CF10 5SD
Tel: 08715 088 768
www.thestdavidshotel.info

The Sanctuary Day Spa
12 Floral Street
Covent Garden
London WC2E 9DH
Tel: 01442 430 330
www.thesanctuary.co.uk

Spa NK
127–131 Westbourne Grove
Notting Hill
London W2 4UP
Tel: 020 7727 8002
www.spacenk.co.uk

The Westin Turnberry Resort
Maidens Road
Ayrshire
Scotland KA26 9LT
Tel: 01655 331 000
www.turnberryresort.co.uk

PERSONAL TRAINERS

Josh Salzmann
at the Wentworth Club
Wentworth Drive
Virginia Water
Surrey GU25 4LS
Tel: 01344 842 201
www.wentworthclub.com

Matt Roberts
16 Berkeley Street
London W1J 8DZ
Tel: 020 7491 9989
www.mattroberts.co.uk
For park boot camps call
0207 491 9989

COMPLEMENTARY MEDICINE

Asanté Academy of
Chinese Medicine
Clerkenwell Building
Archway Campus
2–10 Highgate Hill
London N19 5LW
Tel: 020 7272 6888
www.asante-academy.com
Call for a list of practitioners
in your area.

The Association for
Therapeutic Healers
Acorn Centre
57a Railway Approach
East Grinstead
West Sussex RH19 1BT
Tel: 07074 222 284
www.ath.org.uk

The Association of
Holistic Biodynamic
Massage Therapists
87 Huntingdon Road
Thrapston, Kettering
Northamptonshire NN14 4NF
Tel: 07889 356 745
info@ahbmt.org
www.ahbmt.org

The Association of Reflexologists
5 Fare Street
Tauton
Somerset T1A 1HX
Tel: 01823 351 010
www.aor.org.uk

The Ayurvedic Company
of Great Britain Ltd
81 Wimpole Street
London W1G 9RF
Tel: 020 7224 6070

The Bowen Technique
European College of
Bowen Studies
The Corsley Centre
Old School, Deep Lane
Corsley, Wiltshire BA12 7QF
Tel: 01373 832 340
www.thebowentechnique.com

The British Acupuncture Council
63 Jeddo Road
London W12 9HQ
Tel: 020 8735 0400
www.acupuncture.org.uk

The British Association of
Aesthetic Plastic Surgeons
The Royal College of
Surgeons of England
35–43 Lincoln's Inn Fields
London WC2A 3PE
Tel: 020 7430 1840
www.baaps.org.uk

The British Chiropractic
Association
Blagrave House
59 Castle Street
Reading
Berkshire RG1 7SN
Tel: 01189 505 950
www.chiropractic-uk.co.uk

The British Complementary
Medicine Association
PO Box 5122
Bournemouth
Dorset BH8 OWG
Tel: 08453 455 977
www.bcma.co.uk
Covers most major therapies,
except acupuncture, homeopathy
and herbalism.

The British Federation of
Massage Practitioners
78 Meadow Street
Preston
Lancashire PR1 1TS
Tel: 01772 881 063

The British Herbal
Medicine Association
PO Box 583
Exeter
EX1 9GX
Tel: 08456 801 134
www.bhma.info

The British Homeopathic
Association
Hahnemann House
29 Park Street West
Luton
Bedfordshire LU1 3BE
Tel: 01582 408 675
www.trusthomeopathy.org
Practitioners plus research
and training.

The British Medical
Acupuncture Society
BMAS House
3 Winnington Court
Northwich
Cheshire CW8 1AQ
Tel: 01606 786 782
www.medical-acupuncture.co.uk
The society runs acupuncture

courses for doctors and dentists
and can supply names of those
who have completed training.

The British Osteopathic
Association
3 Park Terrace
Manor Road
Luton
Bedfordshire LU1 3HN
Tel: 01582 488 455
www.osteopathy.org

The British School of Shiatsu
Unit 3
Thane Works
Thane Villas
London N7 7NU
Tel: 020 7700 3355
www.shiatsu-do.co.uk

The Hale Clinic
7 Park Crescent
London W1B 1PF
Tel: 020 7631 0156
www.haleclinic.com

Jessica Loeb and Douglas Diehl
at Danceworks
16 Balderton Street
London W1K 6TN
Tel: 020 7629 2927
www.natureworks.co.uk
Holistic health clinic

Robert Jacobs
Tel: 020 7487 4334; in Los
Angeles 001 310 822 6077
www.drrobertjacobs.com
Homeopath and naturopath.

YOGA

There is a traditional belief in
yoga that you will find a teacher
when you are truly in need of
one. Learning yoga is like being
a member of a family and what
you learn depends on the style of
your teacher. Be prepared to try
different classes until you find a
teacher you feel comfortable with.
Some teachers organize yoga
holidays abroad and intensives,

which are an extension of their regular classes and a safer way of extending your practice than setting off for an unknown ashram.

Amy Redler at Metta
The College of Traditional Thai Yoga Massage
17 Cranworth Street
Glasgow, Scotland
G12 8BZ
Tel: 07956 911 159
www.yogamassage.co.uk

Anne-Marie Zulkahari
Quex Road Methodist Church
Quex Road
London NW6 4PR
Tel: 020 7624 3948
Private tuition and classes.

Catherine James
27 Portland Road
London W11 4LH
Tel: 020 7727 9998
Private tuition and classes.

Dominique Morrsom
37 Sterndale Road
London W14 0HT
Tel: 020 7602 9437
Private tuition and classes.

Jeanne Davies
Tel: 01255 436 781
www.yogainclacton.co.uk
Private tuition (one-to-one and groups); also therapeutic yoga for pregnancy and back problems.

Jiwan Brar at the Integrated Medical Centre
43 New Cavendish Street
London W1G 9TH
Tel: 020 7224 5111
Therapeutic yoga for joint or back problems.

Sophy Hoare
21 Gateway House
2a Balham Hill
London SW12 9EE
Tel: 020 8675 5721
www.sophyhoare.co.uk
Private tuition and classes.

YOGA CENTRES

The Innergy Yoga Centre
Acorn Hall, East Row
Kensal Road
London W10 5AW
Tel: 020 8968 1178
www.innergy-yoga.com

The Iyengar Yoga Institute
223a Randolph Avenue
Maida Vale
London W9 1NL
Tel: 020 7624 3080
www.iyi.org.uk

The Life Centre
15 Edge Street
London W8 7PN
Tel: 020 7221 4602
www.thelifecentre.com

The Light Centre
9 Eccleston Street
Belgravia
London SW1W 9LX
Tel: 020 7881 0728
www.lightcentrebelgravia.co.uk

Sivananda Yoga Vedanta Centre
51 Felsham Road
London SW15 1AZ
Tel: 020 8780 0160
www.sivanda.co.uk

Triyoga
6 Erskine Road
Primrose Hill
London NW3 3AJ
Tel: 020 7483 3344
www.triyoga.co.uk

BOOKS ON YOGA

Desikachar T K V, *The Heart of Yoga: Developing a Personal Practice*, Inner Traditions, 1999
Mascaro, Juan (translator), *The Bhagavad-Gita*, Penguin Classics, 2003
Mascaro, Juan (translator), *The Upanishads,* Penguin Classics, 2004
Stewart, Mary, *Teach Yourself Yoga*, Hodder & Stoughton, 2003

FURTHER INFORMATION ABOUT YOGA

The British Wheel of Yoga helps people find local yoga classes, runs a teacher training course and gives general information about yoga.

The British Wheel of Yoga
25 Jermyn Street
Sleaford
Lincolnshire NG34 7RU
Tel: 01529 306 851
www.bwy.org.uk

SHOPS

The Food Doctor
76–78 Holland Park Avenue
London W11 3RB
Tel: 020 7792 670
www.thefooddoctor.com
Nutrition, weight loss and online food shopping.

Neal's Yard Natural Remedies
15 Neal's Yard
Covent Garden
London WC2H 9DH
Tel: 020 7379 7222
www.nealsyardremedies.com

L'Occitane
For store locations and online shopping see www.loccitane.com Aromatherapy products from Provence.

Planet Organic
42 Westbourne Grove
London W2 5SH
Tel: 0207 727 2227
www.planetorganic.com
Organic supermarket.

Whole Foods
The Barker's Building
63–97 Kensington High Street
London W8 5SE
Tel: 020 7368 4500
www.wholefoodsmarket.com
Organic supermarket.

ASSOCIATIONS

The British Association
of Dermatologists
Willan House, 4 Fitzroy Square
London W1T 5HQ
Tel: 020 7383 0266
www.bad.org.uk

The British Association of Plastic
Surgeons (BAPRAS)
The Royal College of Surgeons
35–43 Lincoln's Inn Fields
London WC2A 3PE
Tel: 020 7831 5161
www.bapras.org.uk

The British Institute & Association
of Electrolysis
40 Parkfield Road
Ickenham UB10 8LW
Tel: 0870 128 0477
www.electrolysis.co.uk

The Institute of Optimum Nutrition
Avalon House
72 Lower Mortlake Road
Richmond
Surrey TW9 2JY
Tel: 08709 791 122
www.ion.ac.uk

The National Register of
Personal Fitness Trainers
PO Box 870
Sywell
Northhamptonshire NN6 0ZB
Tel: 08448 484 644
www.nrpt.co.uk

The Society of Chiropodists
and Podiatrists
1 Fellmonger's Path
Tower Bridge Road
London SE1 3LY
Tel: 0207 234 8620
www.feetforlife.org

USA

BODY

BEAUTY THERAPISTS & SALONS

Aveda Salon and Spa
456 West Broadway
New York NY 10012
Tel: 212 473 0280
www.aveda.com
Professional facials, skincare
and make-up products.

Frédéric Fekkai Beauté
de Provence
712 Fifth Avenue
New York NY 10019
Tel: 212 753 9500
www.fredericfekkai.com

Bliss Spa
2nd Floor
568 Broadway
New York NY 10012
Tel: 212 219 8970
www.blissworld.com
Facial treatments and
skincare to suit.

Elizabeth Arden Red Door Salon
691 Fifth Avenue
New York NY 10020
Tel: 212 546 0200
www.reddoorspas.com

SPECIALIST TREATMENTS

Eastside Massage
Therapy Centre
351 East 78th Street
New York NY 10021
Tel: 212 249 2927
www.eastsidemassage.com

MANICURES & PEDICURES

Arsi Skincare Clinic
162 West 56th Street
New York NY 10019
Tel: 212 582 5720

Celina Nail and Skincare Salon
156 West 72nd Street
New York NY 10023
Tel: 212 595 4100

HAIR SALONS

Art Luna
8930 Keith Avenue
West Hollywood CA 90069
Tel: 310 247 1383

John Barrett at Bergdorf Goodman
754 Fifth Avenue
New York NY 10019
Tel: 212 872 2700
www.johnbarrett.com

John Frieda Salon Inc
30 East 76th Street
New York NY 10021
Tel: 212 675 0001

Kris Sorbie
Global Artistic Director for Colour
Redken
575 Fifth Avenue
New York NY 10017
Tel: 212 818 1500
www.redken.com

Louis Licari Salon
343 North Camden Drive
Beverly Hills CA 90210
Tel: 310 247 0855
www.louislicari.com

Michaeljohn
414 North Camden Drive
Beverly Hills CA 90210
Tel: 310 278 8333

Salon Ishi
70 East 55th Street
New York NY 10022
Tel: 212 888 4744

SCENT

Anitra Earle Perfume Detective
615 Warburton, Suite 7J
Yonkers NY 10701
Send a SAE to track down any
fragrance within 48 hours.

MAKE-UP

Aveda
Tel: 1 800 644 4831
www.aveda.com

Avon
1 800 265 AVON
www.avon.com

Benefit
Tel: 1 800 781 2336
www.benefitcosmetics.com

Bobbi Brown Essentials
Tel: 1 877 310 9222
www.bobbibrowncosmetics.com

Chanel
Tel: 1 800 550 0005
www.chanel.com

Clinique
Tel: 1 800 419 4041
www.clinique.com
Skincare products and make-up.

Elizabeth Arden
Tel: 1 800 326 7337
www.elizabetharden.com
Skincare products and make-up.

Lancôme
Tel: 1 800/LANCOME
www.lancome-usa.com

L'Oréal
Tel: 1 800 322 2036
www.loreal.com

M A C
Tel: 1 800 588 0070
www.maccosmetics.com

Revlon
Tel: 1 800 473 8566
www.revlon.com

Shiseido
www.us.shiseido.com
Skincare and cosmetics.

Shu Uemura Boutiques Worldwide
Tel: 1 888 SHU 5678
www.shuuemura-usa.com

HEALTH CLUBS & SPAS

The *Day Spa Association Directory*, produced by Club Spa USA, lists top spas across the USA.
Tel: 201 865 2065
www.dayspaassociation.com

Origins Feel-Good Spa
The Sports Center (Pier 60)
Chelsea Piers
New York NY 10011
Tel: 212 336 6780

Penninsula Spa
700 Fifth Avenue, 21st Floor
New York NY 10019
Tel: 212 956 2888
www.peninsulaspa.com

Sanivan Holistic Retreat and Spa
12 Columbia Drive
Hurleyville, NY 12747
Tel: 845 434 1849
www.sanivan.com
Retreat and spa getaways

Susan Cimenelli Day Spa
754 Fifth Avenue
Penthouse Suite
New York NY 10019
Tel: 212 872 2650
www.susanciminelli.com

ASSOCIATIONS

Academy of Facial, Plastic and Reconstructive Surgery
Tel: 1 800 332 3223
www.aafprs.org

The American Board of Dermatologists
Tel: 313 874 1088
www.abderm.org

The American Society of Plastic Surgeons
www.plasticsurgery.org

Bioelements Alpha-Hydroxy Acid Hotline
Tel: 1 800 533 3064

AUSTRALIA

BODY

BEAUTY THERAPISTS & SALONS

Aesop
153 Toorak Road
South Yarra
Victoria
Tel: 03 9866 5250
www.aesop.net.au

Aveda Institute
465 Elgar Road Box Hill
Victoria 3128
Tel: 03 9286 9486

The Beauty Room
220 Goulburn Street
Darlinghurst 2010
Sydney
Tel: 02 9212 4844
www.thebeautyroom.com.au
Dermalogica appointed skincare centre and beauty salon.

Guinot
marketing@guinot.com.au
Salons across Australia.

SPECIALIST TREATMENTS

Ayurvé Beauty, Health and Skin Care
99 York Street
Sydney City
Tel: 02 9262 3466
www.ayurve.com.au
Holistic treatments.

MANICURES & PEDICURES

Park Hyatt Melbourne
1 Parliament Square
Off Parliament Place
Melbourne VIC 3002
Tel: 03 9224 1234
www.melbourne.park.hyatt.com
Manicures and pedicures using
Aveda and La Prairie products.

HAIR SALONS

Adam Noble at Next Hair
34 Mort Street
Braddon ACT 2612
Tel: 02 6247 2062
www.nexthair.com.au

Cataldo's
The Melbourne Building
55 Northbourne Ave
Canberra City ACT 2601
Tel: 02 6249 6666
www.cataldos.com.au

Dare & Dare
272 Unley Road
Hyde Park SA 5061
Tel: 08 8271 2516

Toni & Guy
Tel: 1300 131 412 (for salons)
www.toniandguy.com.au

Wildlife Hairdressing
12a Ennis Road
Milsons Point NSW
Tel: 02 9955 4990

SCENT

Jo Malone
Tel: 02 9266 5544

The Perfume Connection
Tel: 1300 306 459
perfumeconnection.com.au

MAKE-UP

Becca
Myer Sydney
436 George Street
Sydney NSW 2000
Tel: 02 9238 9111
www.beccacosmetics.com

Bethany Cosmetics
56 Fifth Avenue
Eden Hill
Western Australia 6054
Tel: 08 6278 1854
www.bethanycosmetics.com.au

Bloom
www.bloomcosmetics.com

Bobbi Brown
Tel: 07 3243 9189

Brandmakers
Tel: 02 9267 3611
www.brandmakers.com.au
International beauty brands.

Elizabeth Arden
Tel: 02 8877 5000
www.elizabetharden.com/au

Estée Lauder
Tel: 1800 061 326
www.esteelauder.com.au

L'Oréal
Tel: 1300 659 359
www.beautyclub.loreal.com.au

Mecca Cosmetica
Tel: 1800 007 844
www.meccacosmetica.com.au
Plus skincare and hair products.

HEALTH CLUBS & SPAS

The Azabu Spa
Byron Bay
New South Wales
Tel: 011 61 26680 9102
www.azabu.com.au
Full range of Aveda treatments.

Blaze Rock Retreat
3757 Arat
Halls Gap Road
Pomonal VIC 3381
Tel: 03 5356 6171
www.blazerock.com.au
Spa featuring desert salt
exfoliations and therapeutic
ochre wraps.

The Sensory Spa
LivingWell Corporate Office
3/255 Pitt Street
Sydney NSW 2000
Tel: 2 92738800
www.livingwell.com.au
Manicures, pedicures and more.

DAY SPAS

Blush Urban Spa
253–5 Oxford Street
Leederville
Western Australia 6007
Tel: 08 9201 1088
www.blushbody.com.au
Packages and treatments
using Sothys products.

For recommendations across
Australia, visit SpaFinger at
www.static.spafinder.com/locations/
australia

WEBSITES

www.adorebeauty.com.au
www.beautysupplies.com.au
www.cbeauty.com.au
www.cosmeticdentistryin
australia.com
www.efragrance.com.au
www.getfit.com.au
www.jurlique.com.au
www.revlon.com.au
www.superiorskincare.com.au
www.wella.com.au

ASSOCIATIONS

**Australasian College
of Dermatologists**
PO Box B65
Boronia Park NSW 2111
Tel: 02 9879 6177
www.dermcoll.asn.au

**Australian Society
of Plastic Surgeons**
33 Atchison Street
St Leonards NSW 2065
Tel: 02 9437 9200
www.plasticsurgery.org.au

**International Association
of Trichologists**
185 Elizabeth Street
Suite 919
Sydney NSW 2000
Tel: 02 9267
www.virtualhaircare.com

SUGGESTED FURTHER READING

Aston, Sherrell J (MD), Beasley, Robert W (MD) and Thorne, Charles H M (MD), *Grabb & Smith's Plastic Surgery* (5th ed.), Lippincott, Williams & Wilkins, 1997

Baran, Robert (MD) and Maibach, Howard I (MD) (eds), *Textbook of Cosmetic Dermatology*, Martin Dunitz Ltd, 1998

Iyengar, Yogacharya B K S, *Light On Yoga, Schoken Books, 1995*

Draelos, Zoe Diana, *Cosmetics in Dermatology* (2nd ed.), Churchill Livingstone, 1995

Foreyt, John P, *Living Without Dieting*, Harrison Publications, 1992

Gordon, Marsha (MD) and Fugate, Alice E, *The Complete Idiot's Guide to Beautiful Skin,* Alpha Books, 1998

Harvey, Clare, *Hatha Yoga Pradipika: The Healing Spirit of Plants*, Godsfield Press, 1999

Harvey, Clare and Cochrane, Amanda, *The Encyclopaedia of Flower Remedies*, Thorsons, 1995

Hayes, Kate, *Working It Out: Using Exercise in Psychotherapy,* American Psychological Association, 1999

Macdonald, Glynn, *The Complete Illustrated Guide to Alexander Technique,* **Harper Collins, *1998***

Roth, Geneen, *Feeding the Hungry Heart,* Signet Books, 1983

'Sunscreen Gives You Cancer', *The Journal of Chemical Research in Toxicology*, January 1999

Valnet, Jean, *The Practice of Aromatherapy: Holistic Health and the Essential Oils of Flowers and Herbs*, Inner Traditions

Willett, Michael J, *Facial Surgery*, McGraw-Hill, 1997

SOURCES

Alexander, Jane, *Supertherapies*, Bantam Books, 1996

Jessel-Kenyon, Julian and Shealy, Norman C, *The Illustrated Encyclopaedia of Well Being*, Sterling Publishing, 2000

Kenton, Leslie, *Passage to Power: Natural Menopause Revolution*, Vermillion, 1998

Peters, David and Woodham, Anne *The Encyclopaedia of Complementary Medicine*, Dorling Kindersley, 1997

Weil, Andrew, *Spontaneous Healing*, Warner, 1996

Wilson, Elizabeth and Lewith, George, *Natural Born Healers*, Collins and Brown, 1997

index

A

acne 95, 98–101, 107
acupuncture 338–9
ageing 102, 104, 115
Alaïa, Azzedine 29
Alexander technique 67, 374–5
Almeras, Henri 287
alpha-hydroxy acid (AHA) 108, 114–15, 122–3, 137
alpha-lipoic acid 114, 122–3
Annick Goutal 290, 304, 307, 313, 320
anthroposophical medicine 342–3
antiageing 11, 30
antioxidants 15, 96, 97, 115–16, 127
Antonia's Flowers 292, 320
Aramis 292
Arden, Elizabeth 292
Armani, Giorgio 34, 292, 320
aromatherapy 80, 343–6
aromatherapy massage 359–60
Ashley, Laura 26
astringents 108
Aveda 304
ayurveda 346, 348–9

B

B vitamins 49–50
Bardot, Brigitte 24
Barneys 313
Beaton, Cecil 16
beauty defined 8–15
Beaux, Ernest 287, 319
Becker, Calice 289, 321
BEST (Bio-Energetic Synchronization) 385–6
beta-hydroxy acid (BHA) 115, 122–3, 137–8
Biba 16
bleaching 73–4
blood pressure 56
body art 269–71
body brushing 77, 78
body work 66–8
bones 75, 77
Borsari 299, 313
breasts 77
breathing 330–31, 375
British National Register of Personal Trainers 61
Bronnley 292
browlift 158
Brown, Bobbi 34
Bulgari 313, 320

C

Cabochard 320
Cabotine 322
Cacharel 307, 308, 320
capoeira 63
Caron 290, 304, 307, 320
carotenes 127
Cartier 291
cellulite 77–8
Centre Nationale de Recherche (CNRS) 12
ceramides 116, 118
Chanel, Gabrielle 'Coco' 12, 29, 249, 252, 284, 287, 288, 291, 298, 299, 304, 308, 313, 319, 320, 323
Chantecaille, Sylvie 219, 320
Chinese medicine 336–7
chiropractic 364–5
Chloé 34, 290
cholesterol levels 56
chypre 291–2
Clarins Eau 320
cleansing 73, 106–8
Clinique 26, 290, 292, 313, 320
Clinique La Prairie 45
co-enzyme Q-10 116, 122–3
Colby, Anita 20
collagen 118, 148
colonic hydrotherapy 69–70
colour therapy 384–5
complementary medicine 324–87
body manipulation 362–9
body and soul 370–77
breathing 330–31
everyday maintenance medicines 333–49
everyday maintenance therapies 351–2
insomnia 327–30
massage 353–61
mind 378–87
practitioners 327
cosmeceuticals 118
cosmetic dermatology fillers 147–51
hair removal 146
peels 134–42, 144–5
resurfacing 143, 145, 147
cosmetic surgery
the consultation 154
procedures 155–62
Coty, François 283, 292
craniosacral osteopathy 365
craniosacral therapy 67
Creed 292, 307, 313
Crown 292

D

dandruff 207
de Gunzberg, Terry 34, 35, 36
depilation 74
dermabrasion 144–5
detoxifying 69–71
diet 43–8, 56, 96–7, 179–80
dietary supplements 49–54
Dior, Christian 12, 20, 30, 34, 241, 249, 289, 290, 292, 307, 308, 317, 320, 321
Diptyque 292, 313, 320
Dolce e Gabbana 320
D'Orsay 313

E

echinacea 50
eczema 207
elastin 78, 91, 102
electrolysis 74
Elson, Karen 14
emulsions 110
Etro 292
exercise 55–9, 78
exfoliation 73, 78, 108
eyelashes 236–8
eyelid surgery 156, 158
eyeshadow 227–35

F

Fabergé 292
face shape 176–7
facelift 161
facials 120–21
Factor, Max 24
fashion 16–37
   the 1950s 20–21
   the 1960s 22–4
   the 1970s 25–7
   the 1980s 28–30
   the 1990s 31–4
   post-millennium 35–7
Fawcett, Farrah 26
feet 84–7
Feldenkrais 374
fish oils 50
fitness options 60–65
Fitouri, Susie 272–3
floral scents 290
flower remedies 351
folic acid 50
food 43–8, 49, 56
forehead lift 158
Foreyt, John P 43
fougère 292
free radicals 96, 102, 116
French Connection 313
Frieda, John 23–4, 30, 171, 173, 183, 195

G

Galliano, John 18, 34
ginkgo biloba 50, 53

ginseng 53
Giorgio 30, 307
Givaudan-Roure 288
Givenchy 34, 292, 299, 320
Guerlain, Jean-Paul 15, 252, 278, 281, 283, 291, 292, 298, 301, 303, 304, 307, 308, 313, 314, 316, 319, 320

H

hair 166–211
   colour 188–93
   fashion 170
haircare 179–86
haircut 175–6
hairdresser 171–4
health 207, 209
   styling 194–206
   types 177–8, 185–6
hair removal 73, 146
Hale, Teresa 39, 43, 45, 49
Hall, Jerry 55
hands 80–83
hangover 57
Hansford, Jo 171, 173, 183, 189, 193
Hawksley, Karen 304, 308, 310, 316, 321–2
health kinesiology 367–8
Hellerwork massage 67
Hepburn, Audrey 21
herbal medicine 334–6
Hermès 292, 304, 320, 321, 322
home gyms 61
homeopathy 339–40
hormones 87
Houbigant 290
humectants 110
Hunt, Maggie 220, 222, 265
Hurley, Elizabeth 241, 268, 271
hypnotherapy 379–80

I

IFF Firmenich 288
insomnia 327–30
Isaacs, Greg 63

J

jet-lag 57
Joseph 320

K

Karan, Donna 320
Kenzo 320
keratin 118
kinerase (kinetin) 116, 122–3
kinesiology 365–8
Kingsley, Philip 179–80, 184, 207, 209
Klein, Calvin 26, 34, 291, 292, 302, 320

L

Lacroix, Christian 30
Lancôme 241, 290, 308, 320
Lanvin, Jeanne 287, 298, 308
Laroche, Guy 304, 308, 320
L'Artisan Parfumeur 290, 291, 292, 304, 307–8, 313, 320, 321, 323
laser technology 143, 145–7
Lauder, Estée 15, 26, 219, 241, 252, 290, 291, 292, 302, 307, 313, 316
Lauren, Ralph 26, 290, 292, 302, 320
light therapy 382, 384
liposomes 111
liposuction 155–6
lipstick 239–47
Lobell, Janine 34
Longo, Vincent 11–12, 34
L'Oréal 12, 183, 190
Lotte Berk method 62
Luscher colour test 385
Lutyens, Serge 291

M

MAC 34, 249
McCartney, Stella 34
Macdonald, Julien 269
McEvoy, Trish 34
McQueen, Alexander 34, 269, 272
magnetic field therapy 351–2
make-up 212–75
  body art 269–71
  cheeks 248–55
  concealer 222–3
  Elizabeth Hurley's five-minute make-up 268
  eyebrows 224–6
  eyelashes 236–8
  eyeshadow 227–35
  foundation 214–19
  get the look 256–65
  lips 239–47
  manicure and pedicure 272–5
  powder 220–21
  tools of the trade 266–8
Malone, Jo 290, 292, 304, 307, 313, 320
manicure 6, 80, 83, 272–3, 275
manicure kit 82
Marsden, Kathryn 69
martial arts 62–3
masks 110
massage 42, 67–8, 77, 353–61
meditation 387
menopause 207, 209
menstrual cramps 78, 80

Mercier, Laura 34
Method Putkisto 63
minerals 49, 53, 54
Mitchell, Paul 183
Miyake, Issey 292
moisturization 73, 108, 110
Molinard 304
Moss, Kate 14
Mugler, Thierry 308, 320
multigym 61

N

nails 80, 82–3
Nars, François 30, 34, 241, 242, 249, 252
naturopathy 333–4
Neal's Yard 304
Neil, Kate 49
night creams 118
Nike 34

O

oriental scents 291
Origins Spring 320
osteopathy 363–4
osteoporosis 75
oxygen 118
ozonics 292

P

Palau, Guido 14
Parfums de Nicolai 313
Parfums de Rosine 313
Patou, Jean 287, 290, 298, 299, 308, 310, 321
pedicure 273–5
Penhaligon 292, 299, 308
Penn, Irving 16
personal trainers 61–2
Phillips, Stuart 177, 178
Picasso, Paloma 292, 304, 320
Piguet, Robert 292, 298, 304, 320
Pilates 15, 56, 63–4, 78
Pilates, Joseph 64
placenta 118
Poiret, Paul 284
polyphenols 119
pregnancy 209
Prescriptives 290
psoriasis 207
Putkisto, Marja 63

Q

qi gong 63, 375
Quest International 288, 289, 321

R

Rabanne, Paco 320
reflexology 68, 368–9
reiki 68, 380–81
retinoids 113–14, 137
retinol 122–3
Revlon 26, 30, 241

Revson, Charles 30
Ricci, Nina 320
Rochas 320
rolfing 358–9
Roth, Geneen 47
Ruby and Millie 34

S

St John's wort 53
Saint Laurent, Yves 35, 223, 241, 249, 291, 320
Sander, Jil 320
Sassoon, Vidal 23, 24
scent 276–323
  Best-kept secrets 313
  changing scents 309–310
  choosing 278, 280
  different moods 303–8
  the emergence of fashion 284–9
  fragrance families 290–92
  ingredients 296–9
  making it last 314, 316
  naturals and synthetics 300–302
  passionate about scent 321–3
  perfume pyramids 293–4
  scents of time and place 317–20
  the world of perfumery 281–3
Schiaparelli, Elsa 288, 322
selenium 53
Senteurs, Les 304, 308, 320, 321
shaving 74
shiatsu 356
Shiseido 291, 313
skin cancer 126
skincare 88–165
  cleansing 73, 106–8
  cosmetic dermatology 134–51
  cosmetic surgery 152–62
  the environment 95–6
  the facts 90–91
  the future of 163–4
  hair removal 73, 146
  miracles in a jar 113–23
  nutrition 96–7
skin complaints 100–101
skin damage 124, 126, 131
skin types 92–3
sun and skin cancer 124, 126
sleep 42, 97, 327–30
soaps 106–7
Sorbie, Trevor 23, 183, 185, 198, 199
spiritual healing 381–2
spirulina 53, 77–8
sports massage 356–7
Stila 34, 249

stress 6, 12, 14, 41–2, 57, 67, 77, 97
stretching 59
submental lipectomy 156
sunbeds 130–31
sunscreens 127–8, 130
Szabo, Dominic 15

T

t'ai chi 15, 62–3, 375–7
tanning 11, 15, 35, 128, 130–32
teeth 6, 11
Tibetan medicine 340, 342
toners 108
Toskin, Frank 34
Trager work 360
treadmill 61, 78
tui na 357–8
tumescent liposuction 155–6
tweezing 74
Twiggy 24

U

Uemura, Shu 220, 249

V

varicose veins 80
Versace 34, 320
vitamin C (L-ascorbic acid) 115–16, 122–3, 137
vitamins 49–50, 53, 96–7
Voyage 34

W

waxing 74
weight 39, 43, 55, 56
Wella 190
Westwood, Vivienne 34
wheatgrass 53–4
wing chun 63
Wood, Josh 173, 174, 193
Worth 322
Worthington, Charles 173, 175, 176, 183, 184, 186, 204–5
wrinkles 104

Y

yoga 15, 56, 57, 64, 78, 370–74

Z

zinc 54

acknowledgements

PICTURE CREDITS

The publishers would like to thank the following sources for their kind permission to reproduce the pictures in this book:

All images are copyright © Vogue, The Condé Nast Publications Ltd. except where indicated.

t: top, b: bottom, l: left, r: right, tl: top left, tr: top right, bl: bottom left, br: bottom right, bc: bottom centre, bcl: bottom centre left, bcr: bottom centre right.

Miles Aldridge 215
Enrique Badulescu 1, 4–5, 210, 324, 376–7
David Bailey 22, 24,25, 27
Andrea Blanch 76
Paul Bowden 163, 178, 239, 332
Regan Cameron 94–5, 129, 132–3, 166, 178
Elinor Carucci 102, 276, 294–5, 315
Clifford Coffin 18–19
Paddy Cook 250–1
Sean Cunningham 187, 197, 202, 204tr, 206tl, 207tl, 207br, 230tl, 230c, 230b, 233, 237, 244, 246tl, 246c, 246bl, 247, 250bl, 253, 259
Corinne Day 31
Robin Derrick 42, 109, 188, 216, 234, 269, 305, 368, 369
Matthew Donaldson 43, 160, 161, 267
Arthur Elgort 10–11, 65, 362
Simon Emmett 6, 176, 260
Robert Erdmann 28, 44, 66, 88, 106, 125, 181, 191, 274–5, 336, 350, 353, 361, 373
Fototheme 245
Nathaniel Goldberg 72
Pamela Hanson 71, 120–1, 328–9, 357, 383
Hugh Johnson 306
Neil Kirk 32–3, 58–9, 200–1, 285
Nelly Klein 55, 168–9, 228–9

Nick Knight 13, 17, 35, 37, 38, 87, 153, 212, 231, 240, 248, 264, 318–19
Craig McDean 9
Tony McGee 172
Raymond Meier 40–1, 138–9, 140–1, 156–7, 159, 164–5, 182, 243, 256, 347, 367
Barbara Metz 112
Guido Mocafico 99, 309
Dudley Mountney 107
Tom Munro 93
Cindy Palmano 332
David Parfitt 75, ???
Sudhir Pithwa 48, 52, 84, 85, 117, 171, 198, 199, 206r, 221, 238, 272
Prigent 21
Demetrios Psillos 46–7
Rapid Eye 214, 219, 225
Terry Richardson 262–3
Ian Skelton 114, 300
David Slijper 81, 138–9, 211
Mario Testino 2, 194, 253
Donna Trope 270–1, 282, 310–11, 312, 322
Jenny van Sommers 214, 218br, 242
Tim Walker 79, 119, 378
Quintin Wright 353
Paul Zak 51, 208, 222–3, 286, 332, 387

The following images are copyright © Carlton Books Ltd.

Graham Atkins Hughes © Carlton Books 341, 344
Nadav © Carlton Books 90, 367
Polly Wreford © Carlton Books 278–9, 290, 291, 293, 296–7, 317, 383

Every effort has been made to acknowledge correctly and contact the source/copyright holder of each picture, and Carlton Books Limited apologizes for any omissions or unintentional errors which will be corrected in future editions.

AUTHOR ACKNOWLEDGEMENTS

Juliet Cohen
I would like to thank my husband Stuart and daughter Anouska for their patience, their honest opinions, and for being there, and to thank my parents for their years of encouragement. I would also like to thank Venetia Penfold for commissioning me.

Bronwyn Cosgrave
I would like to thank Venetia Penfold.

Rachel Marlowe
I would like to thank Marcia Kilgore, Eve Lom, Ole Henrikson, Dr Laurie Polis, Dr Bryan Mayou and Peter Thomas Roth skincare.

Lizzie Radford
I would like to thank Calice Becker, Barbara Daly, Terry de Gunzburg, Roja Dove, Fiona Dowal, Jean Michel Duriez, John Frieda, Sarah Griffiths, Jo Hansford, Karen Hawksley, Michael Keet, Philip Kingsley, Vincent Longo, Guido Palau, Stuart Philips, Anne Françoise Schneider, Trevor Sorbie, Dominic Szabo, Josh Wood and Charles Worthington.

PUBLISHER ACKNOWLEDGEMENTS

The Publishers would like to thank Elizabeth Barnett and Jane Donovan for compiling the directory